THE HORMESIS EFFECT

Books by Jane G. Goldberg, Ph.D.

The Psychotherapeutic Treatment of Cancer Patients
The Dark Side of Love: The Positive Role of Negative Feelings
Deceits of the Mind (and their effects on the body)
InSPArations: If You Can Do It at a Spa, You Can Do it at Home
The Inner Lives of Mothers (and every daughter's search for a separate self)

AVAILABLE FROM SEA RAVEN PRESS
Princess Diana, Modern Day Moon-Goddess: A Psychoanalytical and Mythological Look at Diana Spencer's Life, Marriage, and Death (with Lochlainn Seabrook)
The Hormesis Effect: The Miraculous Healing Power of Radioactive Stones (with Jay Gutierrez)

Books by Jay Gutierrez

AVAILABLE FROM SEA RAVEN PRESS
The Hormesis Effect: The Miraculous Healing Power of Radioactive Stones (with Jane G. Goldberg, Ph.D.)
The Divine Three: Healing Yourself With Frequencies, Water, and Microbiology (by Jay Gutierrez and Faye Cox-Gutierrez)

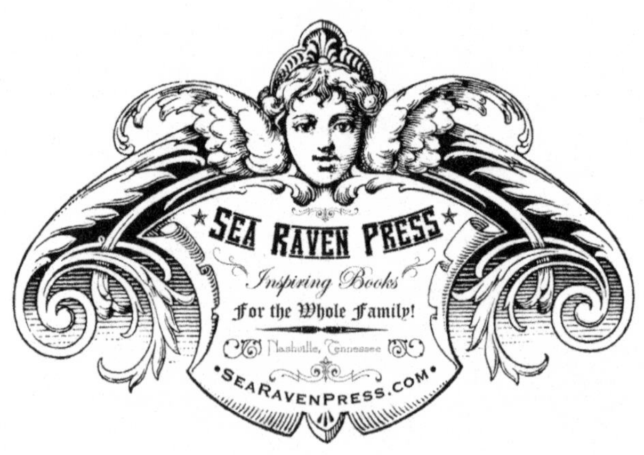

The HORMESIS EFFECT

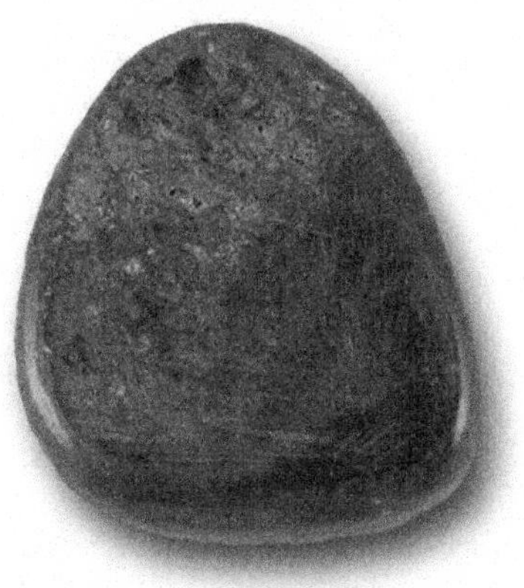

The Miraculous Healing Power of Radioactive Stones

JANE G. GOLDBERG, PH.D.

with Jay Gutierrez

Foreword by Dr. Raphael d'Angelo

Lochlainn Seabrook, Editor

SEA RAVEN PRESS, NASHVILLE, TENNESSEE, USA

THE HORMESIS EFFECT

Published by
Sea Raven Press, PO Box 1484, Spring Hill, Tennessee 37174-1484 USA
SeaRavenPress.com • searavenpress@nii.net

First Sea Raven Press Edition: June 2014
ISBN: 978-0-9913779-2-3
Library of Congress Catalog Number: 2014940743

The Hormesis Effect: The Miraculous Healing Power of Radioactive Stones, by Jane G. Goldberg and Jay Gutierrez. Foreword by Dr. Raphael d'Angelo. Edited by Lochlainn Seabrook. Includes bibliographic references, an index, and an annotated bibliography. This newly revised and updated book was previously published by Sea Raven Press in March 2009 under the title *Because People Are Dying: The Story of a Rock, an Apple, and Cancer*, ISBN: 978-098-218-9924.

Front and back cover design and art, book design, layout, and interior art by Lochlainn Seabrook
Typography: Sea Raven Press Book Design
All images, graphic design, graphic art, and illustrations © Lochlainn Seabrook
Cover image: © Lochlainn Seabrook

The paper used in this book is acid-free and lignin-free. It has been certified by the Sustainable Forestry Initiative and the Forest Stewardship Council and meets all ANSI standards for archival quality paper.

PRINTED & MANUFACTURED IN OCCUPIED TENNESSEE, FORMER CONFEDERATE STATES OF AMERICA

CONTENTS

Publisher's Note - 7
Prologue: What is a Cure?, by Paula Gloria Tsakona - 9
Foreword: A Journey Outside the Box, by Dr. Raphael d'Angelo - 13
Acknowledgments - 17
Update to the New Edition: An Introduction to the Culture of Hormesis, by Jane G. Goldberg, Ph.D. - 19

Introduction: Karma's Pit-Stop in Desolate Nature - 39
1 Serendipity or Divine Guidance - 43
2 What You Think You Know - 55
3 Saving the Penguins but Killing the Cars - 71
4 The Up-side of Radioactivity - 89
5 The Healthy Cell is a Suicidal Communist - 97
6 Who's Hungry? (and the Cancer Connection) - 107
7 Lethally Exposed or Living Longer - 119
8 Because People Are Dying - 133
9 Who's Dying? And Who's Not? - 147
10 Therapeutic Soul Sisters - 151
11 If You Can Do it in Jachymov, You Can Do it at Home - 161

Appendix A: Testimonials from Jay's Patients Using Radiation Hormesis - 183
Appendix B: What's So and What's Not on Radiation and Nuclear Power, by Theodore Rockwell, Sc.D. - 223
Appendix C: Excerpt from the Unpublished Memoir of Stafford Warren, M.D. - 229
Appendix D: On the Life-span of Nuclear Physicists, Researchers and Engineers - 231
Appendix E: Places to Go for Radon Therapy - 233
Meet Jane G. Goldberg - 235
About La Casa Day Spa - 237
Meet Jay Gutierrez - 239
About Night Hawk Minerals - 241
Meet Raphael d'Angelo - 244
The Wisdom - 245
Bibliographic References - 247
Annotated Bibliography - 257
Index - 286

Publisher's Note

In our first publication of this book in 2009 under the title *Because People Are Dying*, the "Mineral Palace" is mentioned numerous times. Today, however, the Mineral Palace is no longer in operation.

However, in this our newly revised, retitled edition, *The Hormesis Effect*, we have left in all references to the Mineral Palace in order to preserve the integrity of the original text.

The facility's hot tub and frequency room at Pritchett, Colorado, are still available to the public. To make an appointment please contact the staff at Night Hawk Minerals.

Sea Raven Press

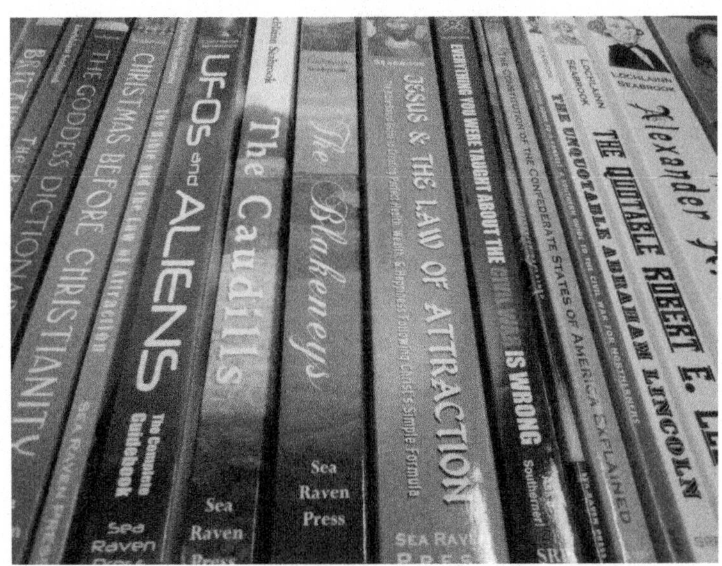

DISCLAIMER

This book is for educational and informational purposes only and may not be construed as medical advice. It is not intended to replace the services of a physician, nor does it constitute a doctor-patient relationship. You should not use the information in this book for diagnosing or treating a medical or health condition. Always consult a physician in all matters relating to your health, and particularly in respect to any symptoms that may require diagnosis or medical attention. Any action on your part in response to the information provided in this book is at your own discretion.

The Authors

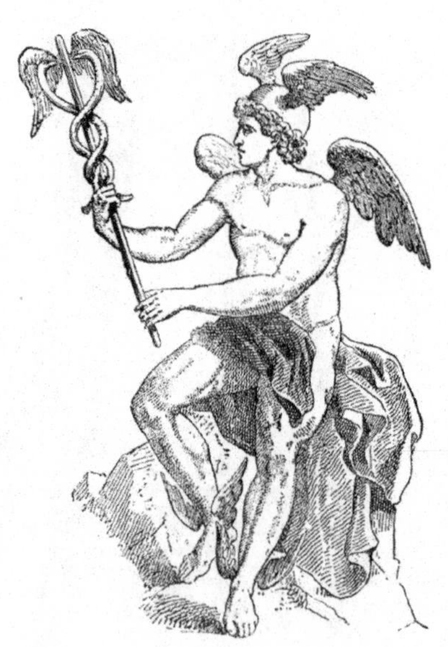

PROLOGUE

What Is A Cure?

What is a cure . . . for anything? Is it something that is accomplished on a personal level, or is it something wider? As surely as knowledge and well-being of our body is influenced by the society in which we find ourselves, does it not also make sense that any cure on a personal level will, similarly, involve that very wider society?

Today, when alternative health care is challenging old methods of treatment of diseases—methods that have been institutionally and officially embraced—there seems to be a lack of careful attention to something beyond traditional therapies and theories. Between the lines of the hard work done to bring this book together, Jane G. Goldberg, Ph.D. points with skill what the critical eye of the concerned reader will appreciate. She addresses the vulnerability of medical systems, both here and abroad—systems that have been based on scientific dead-ends. These conceptual dead-ends are, perhaps, the root cause of the failure of today's official oncology.

To rectify such a dismal state of affairs takes an ability to look deeply into the bad, and still see the good. It demands an attitude of maintaining a scientific bent of mind in the midst of great emotion. And, it means overcoming the horror of reaction as commonly held beliefs dissolve before new ones are finally understood. The lack of steady obvious cures is, as much as anything else, a function of old beliefs that are too tightly held onto. And while old systems may be comforting for both allopathic and alternative practitioners, ultimately they must be seen as mere suppositions without foundation, or worse, premises put forward based on lies and falsehoods.

It is within this environment—of revelation of past errors, at best, or outright deception, at worse—that Jane Goldberg presents her work. The diligence with which she proceeds is an example of the critical need to forge ahead in order to shape a new and more effective paradigm. Her concern here has been dual: to make therapies available cheaply, as well as proposing concrete remedies based in hard science.

Despite Jane's pointing out to me, in a friendly sort of way, my irrationally positive attitude, I realize there is a great distance to be traveled between these two places: the place of ineffective yet familiar medical approaches, and the one yet to be embraced.

How does one proceed in the face of such heartbreak and disappointment in the casting away of old belief structures? In the case of Jay Gutierrez, it happened because he noticed that people are dying. He saw, first hand, how pretty stones, originally made as jewelry, were first admired for their beauty, and then valued for their healing powers. He moved forward with this knowledge, sharing what he learned in his healing journey. And then a fortuitous thing happened along the way of Jay's journey. We encountered each other: me, Jay and Jane. We met at a small lecture that Jay was giving, sponsored by Alan Steinfeld and New Realities. Jane and I quickly discovered that we were a stone's throw-away neighbors—with only half a block between our respective homes.

But, if Jay proceeds in working so hard against our bereft medical paradigm because people are dying in their bodies, Jane works equally hard because people are dying in their minds. Jane, from childhood on, wanted to grow up to become a parapsychologist to study phenomena like ESP, because she had a strong belief and affinity for that which is not seen. She distinguished herself in college, majoring in Religious Studies, and in graduate school, working under the country's leading parapsychology researcher, Dr. Gertrude Schmeidler. Upon completing her Ph.D., Jane moved her interest in the "unseen" from religion and paranormal events to the events of the unconscious, and acquired training as a psychoanalyst. Today, this is where she puts her total joyful absorption—into her private practice.

As well, in 1993, she founded New York City's first holistic day spa, La Casa Day Spa, managed today by Gregg Lalley. Since committing to these two endeavors—health of the mind and health of the body (and the interface between the two)—Jane has never looked back. She doesn't have the time! Waking up at 4:30 am every morning for the past 5 months to write this book (she gave herself a deadline of six months), she poured over the data by the light of many dawns, attempting to reconcile contradictions and to understand scientific language about

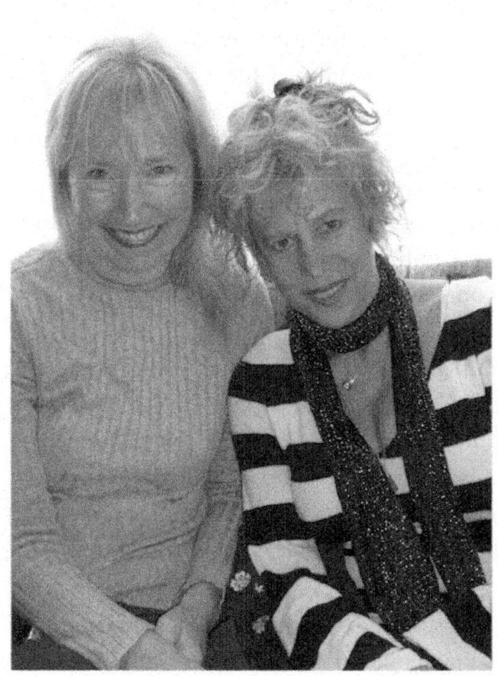

Paula Gloria (left) and Jane.

concepts that were entirely new to her. By 8 am, after worlds and universes of scientific data were processed first one way, and then another, she was armed with her knowledge from her early morning's work, and usually felt ready to discuss her latest understanding and questions with me.

True to the friendly spirit of this Gramercy Park area that we both live in, one of the oldest and nicest neighborhoods in Manhattan, I contributed as much as I could, meeting some mornings on the corner, as we sun-gazed together. But, truthfully, I more often benefitted from her than she did from me. She held my hand through my own professional frustrations and impediments. She always had sage advice to lend to me. One particularly upsetting event was when YouTube removed one of my postings. I had worked on this posting for months, but YouTube apparently didn't like the title I gave the piece.

Jane, as a psychoanalyst, understands well the seriousness of this YouTube censorship. Jane understands as well as anyone the importance of freedom of speech—both for a free democracy, and for a free psyche.

So, we two girls, originally from altogether different worlds—she, raised in New Orleans, I, in Berkeley—now call home an area rich in historical contribution—from the planning of the first transatlantic telephone cable, to the many great writers who frequented these stomping grounds. Even the legacy of the great actor of his day, Edwin Booth, lives on in the Player's Club, situated about half way between Jane's house and mine. What better physical location to surrender to and roll up your sleeves, fortified by the great esoteric principle that "what you focus on grows in your life"?

Read between the lines and see if you don't agree that as a pure scientist, Jane addresses the crying need for an overarching principle of cure and wellness . . . but if I haven't told you enough, she is also a really sparkling writer bringing to dense topics a really nice flair. And, in her writing, there is a breath of a chance for a novice to penetrate (perhaps not totally) critical understandings needed for a more balanced society.

One of her many published books, *The Dark Side of Love*, was received with critical acclaim. Three more books are finished, and were waiting to be polished and published when she undertook the task of writing *The Hormesis Effect*. When she took the carefully allocated six month break to research and write about radiation hormesis, she had been working on her most ambitious project yet: "The Collected Works of Jane G. Goldberg, Ph.D., Volumes I-IV." Her love for her work with cancer patients, and for the patients themselves, is evident in her writings, as well as in any dialogue one is fortunate enough to have with her about her work. Now, with the evidence of radiation hormesis, she has added yet another tool to her forty years of experience as an analyst, as a holistic health healer, and as an adult human woman.

Jane decided to write this book on radiation hormesis for the same reason that Jay does his work: because people are dying. The book whispers the long awaited hope that we can better help medical malfeasance by collaborating and cooperating with each other rather than competing with each other. Jane's spirited and passionate writing reminds us that no matter what the odds, we should never forget that "the greatest of things are done with a light heart."

Paula Gloria Tsakona
President, The Concordia Foundation
Gramercy Park, New York, NY
ConcordiaFoundation.org

FOREWORD

A Journey Outside The Box

Many years ago *Reader's Digest* ran a monthly series called "The Most Unforgettable Person I Ever Met." Unequivocally for me it would be Jay Gutierrez, whom you will come to know and even more appreciate as you investigate his healing work. Dr. Jane G. Goldberg eloquently examines the fundamental principles of Jay's special kind of healing scientifically described in *The Hormesis Effect: The Miraculous Healing Power of Radioactive Stones*. I have never met Dr. Goldberg, but through the writing of this book I have come to know her as one who has dedicated her life and career to the pursuit of health and wholeness.

I am an integrative holistic family physician. In 2006 Jay Gutierrez walked into my office with a briefcase of stones he had mined and cut, along with a stack of emails from grateful people he had helped. I was a bit skeptical but nevertheless curious to hear what he had to say. As he started laying out some beautiful stones on my desk I quickly went through some of the emails noting that many of them were giving Jay credit for saving their lives. He asked me what I knew about radiation hormesis. I had never heard the term. I told him that the best radiation was no radiation. Jay said I had a lot to learn, and I must say that since that day I have come to appreciate and value his point of view.

At that time I was suffering from a partially torn rotator cuff of the right shoulder and was unable to sleep on my right side. I asked Jay if one of his stones would help with the pain, so he gave me one to try. I slept with the stone against the skin of my right shoulder using a pillow to hold it in place. A week later I found myself waking up on my right shoulder without any pain. This really got my attention and I was determined to learn more about radiation hormesis.

In this book you will read many of the things that I learned from my own research. I am happy to say that three months after placing that stone on my shoulder it was completely healed without any other modality of treatment. I then turned my attention to Dupuyytren's contracture, a benign fibrotic tumor-like process of the palm of my right hand which can lead to fingers that look like a claw. Jay had me sleep with the stone in the palm of my hand and again, three months later this fibrotic process had completely melted away.

During this time I had Jay come back to the office periodically to bring stones that I could give out to my patients. I'll never forget the first patient to receive a stone from me. He was a vigorous, intellectually bright 88-year-old gentleman with biopsy proven prostate cancer and a PSA blood test of 11.5. Normal is around 1. His wife figured out a way to attach the stone to a spot in his underwear so that it would rest up against the skin over the prostate area. Eight weeks later he returned and his PSA test was 6.5. I was elated! He was satisfied that he was on the right track.

At that point he left my practice promising to use the stone, even though I wanted to have him stay with me until the prostate problem was resolved. Two years later we crossed paths. He was happy to report his PSA had been normal for quite some time. It was obvious that he was not going to die of prostate cancer.

In *The Hormesis Effect* you are going to read stories of people determined to get well from chronic, disabling and dangerous diseases. Many of them have been to their medical doctors, who were unable or unwilling to help them. Never giving up in their search, somehow they found Jay Gutierrez and his Night Hawk Minerals program. From that point they started on the road to true healing and I have been fortunate to be a witness to many of the healings reported.

Now I want to share with you why I find Jay Gutierrez unforgettable. The first day I met Jay in my office I was somewhat argumentative and disbelieving of his radiation stones, but this did not deter him in the least. His buoyant personality, gleam in his eyes, and broad smile spoke of a man undeterred by criticism. Jay often says that he has found answers. The hard part is figuring out what the questions are. He would be the first to admit that he works hand-in-hand with God's purposes in bringing healing to the individual and to the planet.

Jay is humble about this. There have been times when he questioned what he was doing and started to walk away. But being the visionary that he is, he always comes back to question what "they say" about problems and solutions.

Consequently, his own research has gone beyond the common thinking about the process of radiation hormesis—and what's more, he can validate it. I have found him to be highly perceptive and very analytical. This is no surprise as he was a highly respected and valued helicopter diagnostician in both military and civilian settings. Given any problem he just never gives up, but keeps penetrating the depths of the issue from many different angles. In time he sees a way to fix something that nobody else has thought of.

The concept of radiation hormesis may be an unfamiliar one to most people, as it was to me at first. But it is just a door to a whole world of the power of frequencies and wave phenomena that seems to be the undergirding principle of how these stones "do what is right and avoid doing what is wrong," as Jay would put it.

Together we have done a number of different experiments with water and the stones. Learning from these simple experiments Jay has gone out of his way to make sure that there are applications that can be applied to the solving of everyday problems such as keeping the water troughs of cattle clean, helping bees overcome colony collapse disorder, and using the stones and water to invigorate soils for luxuriant growth of crops. What Jay has learned from helping people he has applied to these other areas. And what he has learned from his applications in agriculture he is applying to people.

In 2011 I was retiring from my integrative family medicine practice, wondering what the next step for me would be. At that time Jay had come to the conclusion that parasitic infection of the human body was a major player in chronic inflammation especially in cancer and degenerative diseases. Little did he know that I had been active in the direct diagnosis of parasitic diseases and the natural treatment of them.

For me it started in the United States Air Force, being trained in this modality and really set into motion with an unforgettable year of parasite diagnosis in Vietnam. Following medical school I always kept the laboratory going and relied on my own microbiology training to supplement laboratory testing. When Jay found this out he asked me to consider performing parasite tests for his people, and I was happy to provide this type of help.

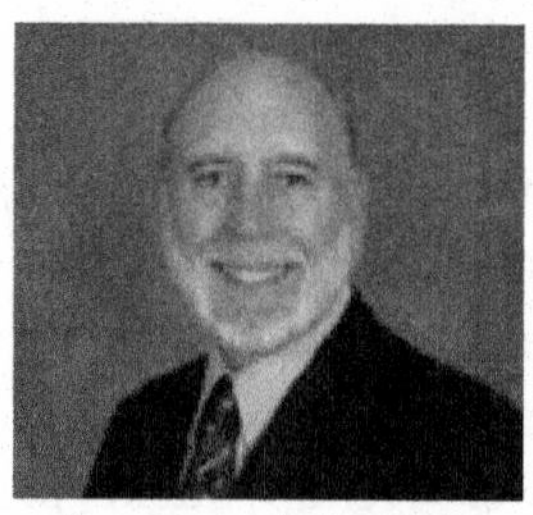
Dr. Raphael d'Angelo

My program is called the ParaWellness Research Program, which is a private research laboratory setting providing comprehensive parasite testing. I work with individuals who want to be tested as well as physicians and other practitioners who need this type of examination for their patients or clients. I started this simply because Jay had a need, and it is my privilege to corroborate with such a dedicated man.

The Hormesis Effect: The Miraculous Healing Power of Radioactive Stones, by Dr. Goldberg and Jay, brings to light the details and particular insights that I have only alluded to. Some people will say that this is way outside the box. But keep in mind the box itself is just a means of limiting one's vision. Jay started out inside the box and then stood up and viewed an entirely different picture, which he was brave enough to seek out, thoroughly examine, and bring to fruition. This book will introduce you to Jay's alternative, cutting edge tools for attaining vibrant health—for our planet and ourselves.

Raphael d'Angelo, MD
ParaWellness Research Program
Aurora, Colorado

ACKNOWLEDGMENTS

I would like to thank God for listening to people's prayers and sending an answer. I have had many that have helped and believed in what we are doing. Some have given up everything they were doing in life to help with this project. Thank you, Faye, for giving all of yourself to see us through the journey. Thank you, Jane, for having the patience and still driving through to make this book a reality. Thanks, Paula, for your support. A special thanks to Carol, Adam, Jim Biggs, Cisco, Don, My Brother Jeff, Amy, Teresia, Tana, Chris, Dr. d'Angelo and Nancy, Tom, Vic, and the numerous people who have always helped with the vision. Also, a big thanks to the people in and around Pritchett, Colorado. — **JAY GUTIERREZ**

The *sine qua non*—Lochlainn Seabrook: more than my editor, more than my formatter, more than my book cover designer, more than my publisher, above all, a man who I have high regard for and count as a friend. Also, special thanks to Paula Gloria, who was the enthusiastic engine that kept me company in so many places, both physical locations as well as in emotional and cognitive spaces. Also, a deep gratitude to Ted Rockwell, who has been so very generous in his imparting of valuable information and knowledge as well as a sense of the history of our country in terms of its struggle with the complex moral, political and scientific issues surrounding nuclear energy. And, of course, ultimate thanks to Jay, whose commitment to his work has saved so many lives, and whose trust in me to write his story enabled this book to happen. — **JANE G. GOLDBERG**

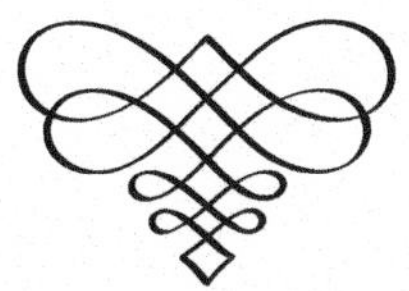

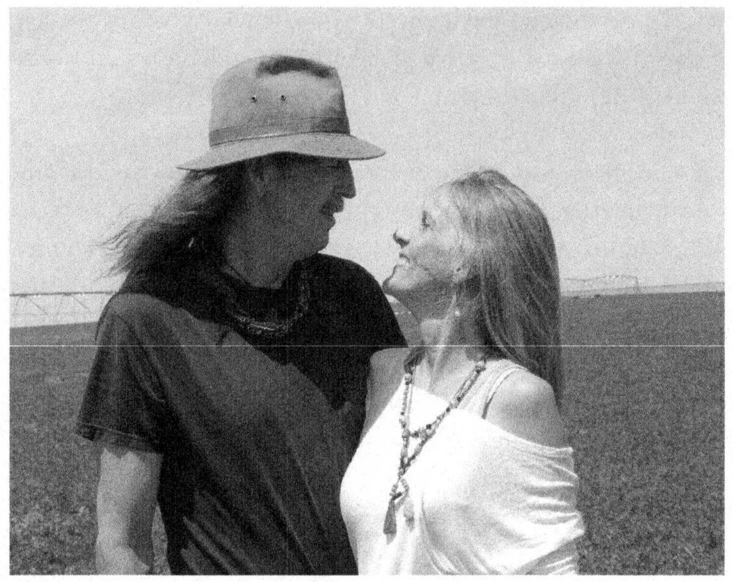

Jay Gutierrez and Faye Cox-Gutierrez

UPDATE TO THE NEW EDITION

An Introduction to the Culture of Hormesis

Much has happened in the last 30 years in the world of hormesis that makes any work on the concept, and underlining theories, much more important, even essential, not only for the on-going health of our bodies but, indeed, for our very culture. It may well be that our future depends on our thorough understanding of how hormesis works in the natural world, and how we can tap its ability to improve our health as well as the functioning of all biological systems.

The first conference specifically on hormesis was held in Oakland California in1985, with such titles for papers as: *What is Hormesis and Why Haven't We Heard About It Before*, presented by Leonard Sagan. In 1990, a group of scientists from federal agencies, the private sector, and academia convened to begin thinking about how to research the biological effects of low-level exposures to chemical agents and radioactivity. They felt it was necessary to explore this issue because of their understanding that most human exposures to chemical and physical agents are at relatively low levels, yet most toxicological studies assessing health effects look at high levels of exposure. These researchers grasped that with this contradiction between research protocols and real-life phenomena, we are destined to have little real understanding of how agents, both those artificially created as well as those from the natural world, are impacting on us.

The year 2001 marked the first annual conference on *Adaptive Responses in Biology and Medicine Translational Biology*. In

August, 2008, an entire issue of the *American Journal of Pharmacology and Toxicology* was dedicated to the subject of hormesis. *Dose-Response*, the online journal of the *International Dose-Response Society* has now published its 12th volume. And most recently, hormesis meets holistic health in the newsletter *Belle* (*Biological Effects of Low Level Exposures*), as the entire journal is devoted to the hormesis properties of resveratrol.[1]

After writing this book, I began to understand that the hormesis effect is widespread, and not just applicable to drugs, potions or radiation. I realized that I had been using it (unwittingly) in a myriad of ways. Hormesis is a fundamental part of being alive, and it is ubiquitous. Over 5600 dose-response relationships for hormesis have been identified.[2]

As we discuss in this new updated edition of our book, *The Hormesis Effect*, hormesis describes beneficial stimulation that is induced by low doses of an agent which, when applied in a higher dose, would be harmful, even lethal. Although the concept is not limited to humans and health, it has been most widely understood within the applications of medicine and pharmacology. It is the theory behind the effectiveness of immunizations, vaccinations and homeopathy. It is an effect that is used in everyday life to create better heath and robustness. Exposure to a potentially offending agent causes a reaction—even an over-reaction—within the exposed organism. It is precisely the reaction that has the effect of strengthening the organism. Within the human body, the hormesis effect is evident in exercise, smoking, alcohol, eating, not eating, and many other activities on all levels of our biological systems.

The differences between the effects of high dose and low dose are seen easily. While not eating for one day a week on a regular basis, for example, can improve lean mass retention, and boost fat burning, on the other hand, starvation will cause major

---

1. Belle, vol 16, no 2.
2. Calabrese EJ1, Blain R. "The occurrence of hormetic dose responses in the toxicological literature, hormesis database: an overview." *Toxicol Appl Pharmacol.* 2005 Feb 1;202(3):289-301.

weight loss, and the shutting down of bodily systems and eventual death. Similarly, an hour of moderately strong sun leads to a mild tan, and a healthy infusion of vitamin D; on the other hand, five hours of strong sun leads to a skin coloration that we call sunburn which can alter DNA, prematurely aging skin, and over time, this DNA damage can contribute to skin cancers, including deadly melanoma. As a final illustration: a single stressful life event leads to the stimulation of adrenaline and cortisol, which has the effect of positively increasing vigilance and alertness; yet, a year of chronic stress will lead to adrenal fatigue.

We don't yet know all of the mechanisms that create the hormesis effect within the body, but there is one candidate that seems to be intimately involved in the process: Nrf2. Nrf2 is a protein that is latent within each cell in the body. It is considered to be a gatekeeper of longevity.[3] It is involved in antioxidant defense, detoxification, and cellular protection. Stressors that stimulate the hormesis effect trigger Nrf2, including exercise, calorie restriction, and most importantly for our purposes, radiation.[4] Although Nrf2 is expressed in all tissues, and levels vary among organs, the key detoxification organs of kidney and liver exhibit the highest levels. It is not mere coincidence that Night Hawk Minerals (Jay's center in Pritchett, Colorado) and La Casa Day Spa (my holistic spa in New York City) both emphasize detoxification, as our detox procedures activate the release of Nrf2.

BEATING UP BONE TO LIVE LONGER

I first learned about how I had been experiencing the hormesis effect from a piece of equipment we purchased for my holistic spa (though I hadn't yet heard the term). The therapy is called Whole Body Vibration, and it involves standing on a platform that gives you a good shake, rattle and roll. In other words, the platform

3. Lewis KN1, Mele J, Hayes JD, Buffenstein R; "Nrf2, a guardian of healthspan and gatekeeper of species longevity". *Integr Comp Biol.* 2010 Nov;50(5):829-43. doi: 10.1093/icb/icq034. Epub 2010 May 6.
4. Pubmed.gov: www.ncbi.nlm.nih.gov/pubmed?term=nrf2.

vibrates, and thus your body, from feet to head, vibrates accordingly. You can actually feel your teeth vibrating when you stand on the platform.

The vibration platform is especially useful for people who can't get exercise in any normal way. It's the non-exercise exercise solution, and it is frequently used in rehabilitative centers. But exercise is a funny thing. Although numerous studies show that exercise promotes health, understanding *why* exercise promotes health is not as clear-cut as one might surmise. The truth is: in a literal sense, exercise per se has no intrinsic health benefit to the body. Exercise doesn't make the body live either longer or healthier any more than using a computer for ten years makes it more efficient. It is, rather, the wear and tear that happens over time and use (to bodies, but not to computers) that confers the healing effect. The biological response to the damage caused by the stress of the exercise gives the beneficial effect of exercise. This damage causes a host of reactions to occur: chemicals are released; secretions are discharged; neurological pathways are activated; genes become alive. In short, things happen; intense things happen. The benefit of the vibration platform makes the point: the damage is actually the cure.

We have known since 1892, when a German physician named Wolff discovered the phenomenon (known since as Wolff's Law), that bones gets stronger when episodic stress is applied to them. This is the specific benefit of the platform: it builds bone density. It was used by the Russian space program to help astronauts counteract the effects of zero gravity from being in space. Without the force of gravity pulling on the skeleton, astronauts lose bone at the rate of 0.2 percent per month. Conversely, a professional tennis player or baseball pitcher (on earth) can build 30 percent more bone on his playing arm.

To build bone, you not only have to use it, you have to beat it up a bit. High-impact activities, such as running and weightlifting, build bone. Shocks to bone (as long as the shock is not so great as to cause permanent damage) only make it stronger. Bone is living tissue, and it responds to activity. Mechanical stress—the impact of your feet pounding pavement, the weight of a barbell at the gym, or the shock that travels up the arm when you whack or throw a baseball—all these events—stressors—create microscopic fractures. Your bone not only repairs the tiny fractures, but it also responds by building more bone on top of them: the growth factor of the hormesis effect.

It is because of the hormesis effect that many health advisors now suggest high intensity exercise. If we were to run laboratory tests on someone who has just worked out intensely at the gym, the lab results would show that the person is in a dire physiological state: inflammatory markers would be elevated. If we didn't know he had been working out, we would assume he is ill: oxidative stress would be evident; cortisol—the stress hormone—would be high. The muscles and bones would be suffering from extensive microtrauma. But the meaning of those reactions to the trauma our athlete has induced is that they are a signal for his body to repair itself and come back stronger than before.

Unfortunately, most of us tend to simulate the life of an astronaut rather than the life of an athlete. If hormesis results in overcompensation in relation to a reaction to a stressor, then inverse hormesis must also be acknowledged. It results from undercompensation because of the absence of a stressor. When there is no challenge, there is no growth. There is just cruising. While low-impact activities such as walking, swimming, and cycling are good for your heart and muscle tone, they don't do much for your bones. Without the damage from the stress of intense, damaging use, and the consequent healing from the damage, as wear and tear sets in with age, we should expect to get increasingly weaker over time. It's a pleasant way to live—cruising along like a well-oiled car; but it doesn't build strength that is resilient and creates a reserve "bank" for when the tides turn, nor as we age.

BEING HORMETICALLY POISONED BY PLANTS SO THAT WE CAN LIVE LONGER

Exercise is one of the easiest examples with which to understand the broad concept of hormesis. But so is eating. One of the most highly documented hormesis effects relates to the consumption (and non-consumption) of food. Eating puts stress on the body because, like exercise, a host of biological activities rev into action to handle the digestion. But, in addition, we are used to thinking of eating vegetables in particular as producing benefits because of their vitamins and minerals. In fact, a main focus of the health movement has been centered around the concept of eating your daily requirements of vitamins through plants. Yet, there is a small body of research that suggests otherwise—that the benefits of eating vegetables is solidly hormetic.[5]

Plants, like all living entities, have defense systems. They protect themselves from harm by emitting poisonous substances that their predators will then ingest. These poisons will either harm the predator, or make the taste unpalatable so the predator is not likely to want to repeat the experience. When we humans, however, are the predators, we then similarly ingest these defensive poisons. But because we are often larger in size than plants, we ingesting a sufficiently small quantity of the poisonous chemicals that, rather than fatally poisoning us, we benefit hometically (or homeopathically) from the low-dose poisoning the plants are giving us.

Not eating—referred to as either intermittent fasting (IF) or calorie restriction (CR)—is also hormetic. Periodic and short fasts have been shown to promote optimal health, and, as well, to prevent and reverse disease processes in many chronic conditions including diabetes, cancers, and cardiovascular disease. As well, IF and CR are good for the brain and neurodegenerative brain disorders. Utilizing them is like exercising your brain muscles.

---

5. Taleb, p. 37.

Dr. Mark Mattson has been studying the effect of IF on the brain and describes the hormetic effect: "The cells of the brain are put under mild stress that is analogous to the effects of exercise on muscle cells. The overall effect is beneficial."[6] Mattson's research demonstrates that chemicals involved in the growth of brain cells are significantly boosted when food intake is dramatically reduced. Because of an uptake in proteins called neurotrophic factors, memory and learning are seen to improve. And, as a result of the intermittent stress, neurons become more resistant to later stress factors.

HORMESIS IS ANTI-FRAGILE

Nassim Nicholas Taleb, in his brilliant, funny and sometimes irreverent tome, *Antifragile*, has strengthened the connection between hormesis and health. Taleb creates specific categories to describe attributes of things.[7] If we drop a champagne glass on the floor, it will most likely break because it is, as Taleb terms it, *fragile*. It is fragile because its integrity as an unbroken glass depends on its being treated in exactly the same way each time (carefully), with no deviation. It must be treated as breakable. If, however, we drop a rubber ball onto the same floor, it won't break; it will bounce. It will remain virtually unchanged from the fall, and we could then describe it as *robust*. But there is a third category that Taleb feels doesn't have a name, and is largely ignored. He calls it *antifragile*, and its main attribute is that if you damage it (or, don't follow its prescribed rules of how it needs to be treated), it will only get stronger. It won't happen to a champagne glass, nor a rubber ball, but the systems within the human body fulfill this definition. They are all hormetic in nature. Damage heals.

Taleb's categorization of antifragile reminds me of Ruth

---

6. www.naturalnews.com/035166_intermittent_fasting_brain_health_calories.html.

7. Taleb, passim.

Sackman's category of a cancer-ridden body as *resilient*. Ruth was the founder and director of the Foundation for Advancement of Cancer Therapies, and I served as her assistant for many years in the 1970's and 80's. The organization disseminated information about non-toxic and biological treatments for cancer. Over the years that Ruth ran FACT, she communicated with and advised many thousands of cancer patients. She had as much experience with cancer as any oncologist at Sloan-Kettering, and she was a trusted voice for what worked and didn't work in terms of reversing cancer. I asked her once what the criteria were for successful reversal: was it severity or stage of disease; progression of the disease within the body; size of the tumor; placement of the cancer tumor? None of those were her answer. Her answer was *resiliency*—that is, the body's ability to recover. Or, as I understand it today: the body's ability to push toward a return to homeostasis in a changing environment: the very definition of hormesis.

Taleb emphasizes that antifragility exists specifically in complex systems (like the human body). He also broadens the meaning of the term to refer to urban planning, economic, technological and cultural, as well as biological systems. Taleb has found that most complex systems not only gain from small stressors, but they are designed to gain more when these stressors are distributed irregularly, or randomly. This point is counterintuitive to us because we tend to dislike disorder and randomness. We find disorder to be frightening because of its unpredictability. And when confronted with disorder, we attempt to either remove or control the phenomenon, thus eliminating the shocks, and making them follow a smooth line of evenness and order.

Taleb uses the specific example of the economy, and it's a good illustration. We try to take the boom and bust out of the economy, and instead aim for a gradual upward trend. Taleb makes clear that this effort is illusionary to create long-term correction and strength. Removing the small shocks in a complex system can only, at best, create stability for a time. The downside is that it makes the system prone to major shocks in the long term.

Again, I am reminded of Ruth's wise understanding about the nature of the human body. She would refer to the negative impact of the vaccinations that were preventing the childhood diseases in her day—the febrile diseases of chicken pox, measles and mumps, and thus the elimination of those diseases. (Unlike myself, who had all three of those diseases before I was seven, my daughter had only one day of chicken pox, with only five small red bumps.) Research documents that those adults who did not have these periodic activations of the immune system in childhood are more prone to get cancer as adults. When an attempt is made to remove the normal flow of events—whether biological or economic—then the system never gets a chance to make periodic self-corrections. Removing the small corrections doesn't create stability; it only creates the illusion of stability. And we then see the equivalent of a tsunami—ferocious attempts at self-correction, traumatic resetting to try to return to homeostasis. These major shocks are infinitely more damaging and destructive—cancer as opposed to periodic bouts with non-life threatening afflictions that help our bodies to recognize pathogens, respond to them, and detoxify through fevers and bodily discharges.

FEELING STRESS TO LIVE LONGER

As a psychoanalyst, I see the hormetic effect on the level of the psyche. Just as the body is primed to experience and deal successfully with stress, so too is the human psychological system. On the level of the psyche, we call these stressors "feelings."

The biological precursors of feelings are hormones. We are only at the beginning stages of understanding the relationships between feelings and hormones, but we do know a few. We know that cortisol is a hormone produced under acute stress conditions. We know that epinephrine and norepinephrine are produced under our primitive animal system of reaction: fight or flight. When we are faced with a stressful situation—such as a car barreling down the road right toward us—the production of these hormones can be life-saving. It allows us to have the heightened energy to jump out of the way. But when we imagine a situation to be stressful longer than it need be attended to for survival purposes—or when we "think" a situation is life-threatening when it is merely "feeling-threatening"—then we produce these crisis hormones, and their concomitant feelings, unnecessarily and sometimes for an unduly extended period of time.

Perhaps we decide, then, to go on a "medication" that promises to take away our disturbing feelings—pain, anger, disappointment, shame or guilt. But, if the medication does what we want it to do, if it takes away the emotional negativity we feel, if we are left with an emotional evenness, how then do we learn from our feelings? If, as parents, we do not help our children to feel sadness at the loss of a pet turtle, how do the children learn to use the intelligence of their emotions to cope with future losses of people they love? With the pervasive attitude in our country that normal (though painful) feelings need to be banished (through either medication or repression), how, then, have we been enabled to use our feelings as a source of information? With one in ten Americans post-high school age adults on some kind of anti-depressant, these questions are not insignificant.

Psychoanalyst and author Bruno Bettelheim, in his timeless book on myth and fairy tales, *The Uses of Enchantment*, addressed this issue of the importance of exposure to uncomfortable feelings as a step toward emotional maturity. He makes note that unlike the safe and pleasurable experience of the act of parents reading stories to children, the actual contents of fairy tales are never entirely "safe." They often begin with the death of a mother or father, or the kidnapping of a child. The protagonists in these tales must engage in Herculean struggles to resolve their predicaments. Their successes in meeting the challenges, in facing suffering with courage and determination, and emerging victoriously transform them into heroes and heroines from whom we can learn. These ancient tales, then, are not mere fluffy childhood stories; rather, they are lessons and inductions into psychological growth that reflect an essential aspect of life and life's ongoing difficulties. Bettelheim suggests that fairy tales serve the function of preparing children for the exigencies of later life.[8] Bettelheim is describing the hormesis effect.

POST-TRAUMATIC GROWTH SYNDROME

Hans Selye is credited with being the originator of the medical use of the term "stress." He defined stress as being any stimulus that provoked an organism into the emergency flight or flight response. As Selye's thinking developed, he came to understand (as Wolff had before him) that a healthy organism has the ability to rally from the insult, to recover and return to homeostasis, and to even get better. Selye gave us the term "eustress"—in contradistinction to "distress"—to indicate the hormetic effect of stress, a lose dose stress, a stress that has the effect of enhancing our functioning.

Recently, a cultural phenomenon has been created that seems to not honor Selye's differentiation between eustress and distress; as well, it represents the opposite of what Bettelheim says is necessary for emotional growth, and what Taleb would vehemently argue is creating fragility as opposed to antifragility. This phenomenon is called "trigger alerts," and consists of warnings that you are about to be exposed to something that may be a repetition of a formerly damaging event, and that is likely to induce a kind of re-damage. It is, in effect, a pre-emptive strike in order to avoid sparking symptoms of post-traumatic stress syndrome.

The precedent of these alerts seems to have originated with online forums, where trigger warnings have been used to flag

---

8. See Bettelheim, passim.

discussions of rape or other sexual violence. Recently, it has spread to college campuses. In early 2014, students at the University of California, Santa Barbara, passed a resolution that recommended that warnings be issued in instances where classroom materials might touch upon "rape, sexual assault, pornography, kidnapping, and graphic descriptions of gore." The attempt was to create a "safe" environment. But, we should ask ourselves: can any environment be really safe? And what price do we pay in our attempt to create such a utopian vision? Should childhood exist without the complicated lessons of danger and difficult challenges, and the ensuing growth from mastery, as is evidenced in fairy tales?

Critics of the practice of trigger alerts have wondered whether readers of *The Great Gatsby* should be forewarned about misogyny, or whether *The Merchant of Venice* should have an anti-Semitism warning attached. Yet, as Jessica Valenti mused: there is "no trigger warning for living your life."[9] Surely our cultural attempts to increasingly attempt to bend the world to accommodate each and every personal frailty does not help us to overcome them. Over-protecting the vulnerable doesn't empower them; rather, it disempowers them. Those who are advocating trigger warnings are arguing for reverse hormesis. They are suggesting that we build precedents based on fragility rather than recovery. And, as with fragility in economic systems, or technology, or the body/mind and health, supporting—even encouraging—fragility of the body/mind only weakens us as individuals and as a culture.

David Halpern, a government advisor for the U.K., has proposed a way of revisiting the antifragility factor. He calls it, "post-traumatic growth syndrome."[10] He is suggesting that rather than protect, or over-protect, ourselves from possible trauma and re-trauma, that we envision the possibility of growth from the

---

9. Jessica Valenti, *The Nation*. www.policymic.com/articles/87283/9-feminist-arguments-against-using-trigger-warnings-in-academia.
10. Taleb, p. 41.

stimulus. Within the popular culture, we embrace the idea. We have sayings like: "If it doesn't kill you, it makes you stronger;" "When life gives you a lemon, make lemonade;" "Don't fret, it will build character." We already know the principle intuitively. But having a term to describe it might help us to remember it as a principle to live by. Let's try calling it *Post-Traumatic Growth Syndrome*.

HORMESIS GONE WILD: NOT LIVING LONGER

Now that we don't live with the physical stressors of running through the woods to chase down a buffalo for dinner, or chopping down a tree to make shelter, we deliberately expose our bodies to stressors, as in exercise or IF and CR. But what about the stressors that we don't choose? What about disease and pathogens that cause disease?

Jay and I have both treated a large number of cancer patients. This is not surprising, given that it is about to out-run heart disease as the leading killer in our country. The question then becomes: how is hormesis, or its failure as a healing response, evident in cancer?

We know that organisms in a state of health have productive hormetic responses: adequate and growth-producing responses to loss, injury or irritation. (My left foot is stronger now than my right since I broke it three years ago.) There are three basic responses that all living entities have to damage, and these responses exist from the smallest protozoa to humans, and from the cellular level to the largest organ: they are *regeneration*, *isolation*, and *inflammation*.

Hormesis is most emphatically a regenerative response. As we travel down the evolutionary ladder, we find an increasing ability for *regeneration*, that is, to grow anew—tissue, organs or even parts of the body. Salamanders can regenerate a new tail; starfish can grow a new appendage. The ability to regenerate is related to dedifferentiation. The human, highest up on the evolutionary ladder, possesses only a limited capacity to regenerate because most of our cells have evolved to a high level of specialization. The more specialized the cell, the less its capacity to regenerate. Skin cells regenerate quickly; a wound that punctures the skin will heal quickly and entirely. Heart muscle is more specialized, and when it is damaged, it will die and be replaced by scar tissue. Nerve cells in the brain are the most specialized of all, and these have the least regenerative capacity.

Isolation, as a response to an injury or pathogenic condition, occurs when a partition is erected between a damaged area and the rest of the body. This cordoning off the area protects the rest of the body from infiltration by the diseased tissue. Tumors and cysts represent this defensive functioning of the body. Toxic and unnecessary waste matter is collected in one place, isolated by thick membrane walls, and this sequestered area lives on as a kind of internal garbage pail for the body.

Inflammation is the third line of defense. This is the defensive posture that we witness with our intrepid athlete who has worked out to the max. Redness, warmth, swelling and tenderness or pain around the injured tissue are the overt manifestations of injury, and this is what the overworked athlete experiences when he is rubbing his tired, aching legs. Inflammation can occur almost anywhere in the body, and as a hormetic response, to almost any kind of stimulus, with a wide range of diversity as wide as from a particle of dust to an atomic explosion. The presence of fever (warmth) is a clear indication that an inflammatory process has generalized within the body. Fever evolved at least three hundred million years ago in cold-blooded vertebrates as a means of fighting invading organisms. It changes the internal climate that makes the body inhospitable to the infecting agent. We can think of it as the body's natural chemotherapy.

Since the advent of antibiotics, immunizations and the wide world of pharmaceuticals that defines modern medicine today, we have become (as Taleb would say) biologically fragile, creating a reverse hormesis effect. Cancer is a disease where all three of the biological defense mechanisms have failed. The body is no longer sufficiently reactive to the pathogenic cells that we call cancer. After mounting reactive responses strenuously, and for an extended period of time, absolute fatigue finally sets in. We then see a condition of underreactivity. Medical histories of cancer patients often reveal that this condition of failed hormesis is historical for them. Proving Ruth's theory as correct, these patients often have a long-standing history of never having had the common childhood febrile diseases that most of us had a generation ago. In creating the vaccinations against these diseases, modern medicine has allowed us to bypass growth-producing hormetic effects from exposure to pathogens, and created a population pool of people who are destined to remain underreactive (reverse hormetic) for most of their lives.

But, it is not for lack of trying that hormesis doesn't assist us in healing from cancer. Hormesis becomes a last ditch effort to save the organism, the life of the patient. As in any hormetic response, growth occurs. This new growth—the neoplastic proliferation—represents a return to a once useful adaptive response to injury, the phylogenetic initial defensive maneuver of regeneration.

The statistics of cancer in light on the regenerative power of its various organs and tissues is suggestive of a vigorous attempt at hormesis in cancer conditions. The highly differentiated nervous system rarely gives rise to cancer. On the other hand, the digestive and reproductive organs, where regenerative capability is relatively strong, account for 75 percent of all cancers. The phenomenon of the "born-again" spleen is further evidence. It has been observed that in cases where the spleen has been surgically removed, there can be regenerative growth of the organ. Remnants of functioning splenic tissue have been found many years after removal of the organ. What makes this remarkable from the hormetic point of view is that the spleen is the only organ in the human body that is not susceptible to cancer.

Heart disease, like cancer, begins as a hormetic process. The arterial system is like an extraordinarily complex map. There is no place within the body that blood vessels do not reach. It is thought that that damage occurs because of the twisting and turning these vessels must make in order to accommodate the human body. We now know that tears and wounds in arteries develop after just a few years of life. Yet, hormesis is activated in a healthy body, and the tears are repaired without long-lasting damage. Yet, when the damage is stronger than the body's ability to repair, further growth is stimulated, the amount of cholesterol is heightened, and wild new growth of arterial cells in promoted. These cells form distorted scars—what we call arterial plaque. Ultimately, the plaque becomes so pervasive that the blood supply to the heart or brain is diminished, and the body is primed for a heart attack or stroke.

In both cancer and heart disease, the hormetic defense has become the disease.

WHAT TO DO

Radiation is only growth-producing when it is absorbed as a low-dose therapy. The human body is antifragile in relation to low-level radiation. We respond to it continuously, from the day we are born, as it rains down on us from the outer reaches of the cosmos, and seeps up from the bowels of the earth. Low-level radiation is everywhere on the planet, and from it, life once evolved, and we are still dependent on it. The body is primed to receive it, and to respond to it. If we increase our exposure to it—if we make it a "medicine"—as a low dose phenomenon—our bodies soak it up, and react to it, and get stronger, as in any hormetic effect.

Unfortunately, medical radiation (used for both diagnostic and therapy purposes) is high dose, and thus destructive to tissue. High level radiation leakage of damaged nuclear power plants is, similarly, high dose.

I have asked Jay how to protect ourselves from the radiation leaking from Fukushima. His answer would only surprise those not familiar with hormesis. He said exposing ourselves to low-dose radiation will increase our ability to withstand the stress of higher doses should they come our way from Japan.

My recommendation: if you have radon coming out of your basement, do what Bernie Cohen did after his second study showing the positive effects of exposure to radon (as discussed later in this book). Go down to your basement and turn off the radon eliminator. Or, open a spa in your basement to share the wealth with your friends and neighbors (as we mused merrily in the documentary—called *Because People Are Dying*—while we stood in Molly Cheshire's high radiation basement).

Alternatively, take a vacation to one of the hot springs around the world, and soak in pleasure as your body absorbs all that friendly low-dose of radiation. Or, wear Jay's stones. And put a water stone in your water and drink radiated water, as my sweet dog Lilly did (see the Introduction). She is still alive today, jumping around playfully like a young pup in spite of being 14 years old, six years after she was at death's door from an undiagnosed illness. And she is still happily drinking radiated water (as am I).

Jane G. Goldberg, Ph.D.
New York, NY
June 2014

The Hormesis Effect

The Miraculous Healing Power of Radioactive Stones

INTRODUCTION

Karma's Pit-Stop In Desolate Nature

IT HAS TAKEN US ELEVEN hours to get here from the hub of busyness—our point of departure: La Casa Day Spa; NYC. This has been the most interesting uninteresting journey I have ever taken. After we left civilization—at the Colorado Springs Airport, we drove for four unrelenting hours, through land that has only brown grass (presumably out-dated wheat plants) and leafless trees; no people, no cars. We watched an exquisite almost endless sunset that looked more like a part of the earth than the lower case of the sky, merging the two into one great orange streak that never wanted to die. And then the round full moon, at first hesitantly peaking over the horizon, and then shimmering in its radiant fullness as it encompassed the sky. Well—it is mid-November—and winter has arrived here. But—for sure, there is a wild barren beauty to this seemingly desolate part of the world.

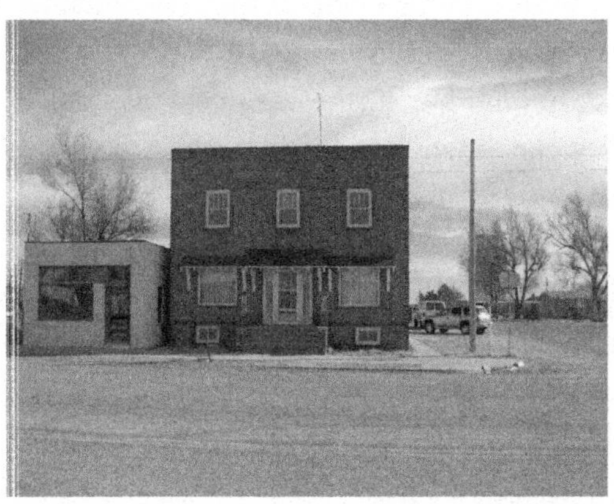

The (former) Mineral Palace in Pritchett, Colorado.

We are at the Mineral Palace—Jay Gutierrez's implementation of his vision of the next health jump in the

American—and dare I say—the world's health care system. It is a modest, eight room "hotel" (really more like a bed and breakfast) where "patients" will come to be treated for all variety of illnesses—from the minor afflictions like carpal tunnel syndrome to the life-threatening ones such as terminal cancers.

I am here because of my interest in the health revolution that Jay hopes to inaugurate. It all started—not with human health—but with my sweet dog Lilly. My daughter woke up one morning with Lilly's throw-up all over her bed. In spite of our coaxing, Lilly refused to eat or drink for the rest of the day. That day turned into the next day, and then the next. Over the next several days, Lilly visited four vets, who brought in three different specialists, including a homeopathic vet. They each saw from her blood chemistry that she was ill—dying even, as they all explained euphemistically to me that she was "very very sick." For that week, I kept little Lilly alive by bringing her to the vet every day to get her re-hydration fix. She went down from a hearty 6.5 pounds to a skeletal 3.5 pounds. She essentially stopped moving, too weak for the effort.

On the eighth day of Lilly's illness, and $3000 worth of vet bills later, one of my patients came to her psychoanalytic session and noticed how weak and ill Lilly had become. She told me about a woman, Donna, who had a pulsed magnetic machine (built for human health)—and how Donna had saved the lives of her two dogs by using the machine on them. Both dogs were now twenty—well into dog-old age, happily prancing around.

I called Donna immediately, and that evening Lilly and I went uptown to Donna's apartment to use the machine. Donna explained that she had the idea of exposing her dogs to the pulsed magnetic energy the machine emits only after the dogs kept throwing themselves at the machine whenever it was in use. She noticed how after each session on the machine, the dogs got more spry and energetic. We gave Lilly the treatment; afterwards, I put her on the floor and watched her energy and natural curiosity

(curiosity depends on energy to manifest it) return to her as she slowly made her way around the apartment, sniffing, looking, walking for the first time in a week.

Then Donna thought Lilly might be thirsty. She put out a bowl of water that had a small rock in the bottom of the bowl. Much to my surprise, Lilly drank from it. Donna explained that the rock was a "hormesis" rock—and that it was emitting a very small amount of radiation that would help Lilly to heal. I was skeptical, having never heard of this concept before—but Lilly seemed to have a mind of her own about this special water.

When I left for home, Donna made sure that I took a hormesis rock with me to continue Lilly's "water therapy" at home. Yet, I was still not convinced. When we got home, I placed five bowls of water out—each with a different kind of water. Lilly had available to her: 1) alkalized water, with a pH of 9.5 from added mineral salts; 2) honey water (honey has lots of natural minerals that would have been good for Lilly); 3) Pedialite (which the vets had all recommended); 4) filtered NYC tap water; and 5) the hormesis water. Like a homing pigeon drawn to his roost, Lilly, throughout the day, always dove straight for the hormesis water, ignoring all four other bowls.

Thus, I began my journey into this land of learning all about a healing technology that has turned my conceptual world topsy-turvy as I have embraced concepts that I have spent my life arguing with and fighting against.

Perhaps our guides are where we choose them. And sometimes they are in non-human form. Lilly's health crisis brought me to where I am now, and helped me to remember, once again, the lesson about health that has become like a repetitive mantra for me, returning at critical junctures of my life: this is, I think, the real meaning of the holistic health revolution. For most of us, even those of us who are ill, sometimes very ill, as Lilly was, our bodies still retain a resiliency for healing. However, the information and knowledge of how to heal ourselves remains, often, a long-ago, forgotten memory, a memory that exists only, at times, within our genetic structure. But we are able to access this memory if we look. The health revolution is not about new learning; it is about coming to remember what we already know. Lilly knew what she needed to get well. I was the one with the forgotten knowledge who was assigned the task of accurately reading Lilly's intuitive wisdom.

The writing of this book has been an unparalleled learning experience for me. Fear of all radiation is a feeling that most of us in the U.S. today share about radioactivity, radon and radium. This, too, was my understanding the day Lilly, started her descent into near-death. I myself have spent my life avoiding x-rays at all costs. I have been kicked out of dental offices because of my refusal to take dental x-rays. When there was no avoiding them, I would insist that I be completely covered in a lead apron. My obsession with avoiding radiation even went so far as my circumventing hospitals that do radioactive cancer treatments during my daily jog. And, of course, I was an avid opponent of nuclear energy. But, through my initial introduction to Jay, and from reading the relevant research in the preparation for the writing of this book, all of these formerly held beliefs have been challenged. I invite the reader to begin what may well be a journey as profoundly unexpected as my own.

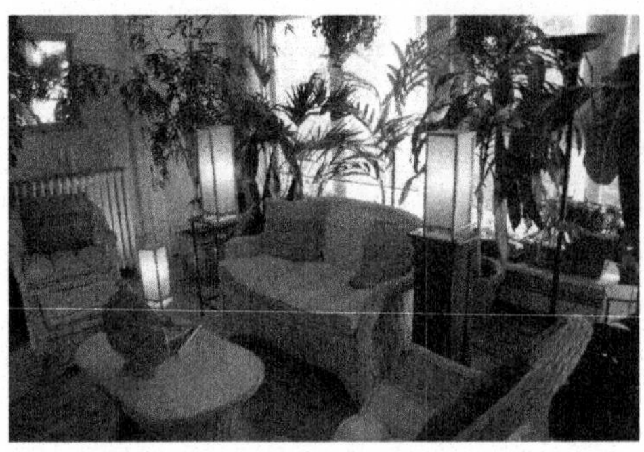

Dr. Goldberg's La Casa Day Spa, New York City.

Jane G. Goldberg, Ph.D.
New York, NY
March 2009

1

SERENDIPITY OR DIVINE GUIDANCE

Life began nearly four billions years ago under conditions of radioactivity far more intense than those that trouble the minds of certain present-day environmentalists. . . . We need to keep in mind the thought that these fierce energies flooded the very womb of life. The two relevant professional societies, the American Nuclear Society and the Health Physics Society, have also supported this stance in carefully considered Position Statements: It is the position of the American Nuclear Society that there is insufficient scientific evidence to support the Use of the Linear No Threshold Hypothesis in the projection of the health effects of low-level radiation. — Prof. James Lovelock, forward to Bruno Camby's *Environmentalists for Nuclear Energy, PS-41, June 2001*

ONE OF JAY'S FAVORITE SAYINGS is: "God doesn't call on the qualified, He qualifies the called." Jay has a strong belief that he was called upon to take on this responsibility of healing people. Several times he has tried to walk away from this calling, but he explains that somehow he has always been called back.

So the story goes: Jay was on a helicopter mission in Northern Wyoming. He was a helicopter repairman and was frequently sent out to retrieve downed helicopters in remote areas. On this particular fateful day, Jay found some green-blue stones on the ground. He knew a lot about turquoise and, he began to think that the stones he had found were, indeed, a form or blend of turquoise. The beauty of the stone captivated him. It was stunning in color, as deep as the ocean blues and as luscious as the green fields and the rain forests. It looked like the world map contained inside of a stone.

Jay decided to mine the area for more of those gorgeous stones to make jewelry. Originally he tried to pry the stone loose with generators and a jack hammer. It was inconvenient to get out there. He had no money. He went by himself, to the middle of nowhere—and he didn't even know why. But he felt like a homing pigeon—he just kept being drawn back. The work of trying to get the stone out, in sufficiently large pieces that he could work with, was proving to be frustrating. The material was so brittle that when he jack-hammered it free it would break up, rendering it useless for making jewelry.

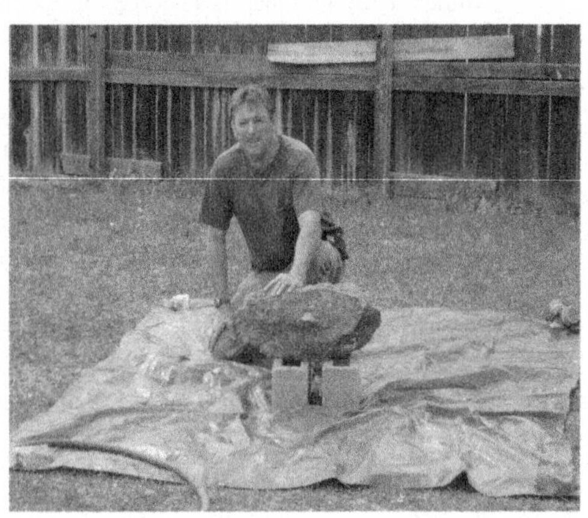

Jay Gutierrez with Eliat Stone.

After several unsuccessful trips to the site, Jay found some men near where he was working who had a quarry. Jay asked, cajoled, begged—it took him three years to get permission from the owners of the quarry to retrieve the stone. Fate is a funny thing. Jay had no idea why he was going to such lengths to get out a bit of stone to make little pieces of jewelry, and he had no idea what exactly he was going to do with the jewelry after it was made. But Jay and the stones seemed to have a destiny to fulfill, and so he remained diligent in his efforts to get to those stones. Ultimately, because the stone he wanted was embedded in limestone, it had to be dynamited out.

At first, Jay began to make jewelry himself, giving it to friends and selling some—but jewelry is a hard thing to sell. Good thing he had a day-job of repairing helicopters. Yet, he found himself deriving a lot of personal satisfaction that went into the fine crafting of the jewelry.

Eventually, there was a lot of Jay's jewelry out there: mostly gifts to friends and friends of friends. As time passed, Jay started getting reports back from people who had been wearing the jewelry. These people were claiming quite remarkable things. They were asserting that they were getting healings and pain relief from the stones. Arthritis was disappearing; inflammations were calming down; long-standing open wounds were healing after years—sometimes decades—of oozing; even some cancer tumors had disappeared. Jay thought, at first, that these people were making up their miraculous "cures" because, as he reasoned, they wanted to believe it. He assumed their beliefs about the extraordinary healing powers of the jewelry were just "in their heads"—a figment of their overly active imaginations. But eventually, there came to be too many reports to ignore or to assume that all of these people—hordes of people at this point—were making up this phenomenon.

Jay took the stone to a lab and had it analyzed. The lab result revealed that the stone contained several elements. This beautiful blue-green stone that he had spent years of his life chasing was, he learned, a mixture of malachite, chrysocolla, turquoise, and silver. Jay knew that malachite is not an uncommon stone. Once Jay knew the material that his stones were comprised of, he was able to do a search of the medical history of the stone. Malachite has an interesting history dating back to Egypt. Long ago, the Egyptians were battling cholera. Everyone was coming down with cholera; most were dying. There was one exception: the only people who were not being affected were the slaves who were mining malachite. Since that time, healers who believe in stones have postulated that malachite has enormous healing properties.

Generally malachite has either chrysocolla or turquoise mixed in with it. But, Jay's research led him to understand that the only other place in the world where you can find malachite with both chrysocolla and turquoise is in Israel. There, this stone is known as the King Solomon Stone, or the Eilat Stone. It is found in the mines from the times of King Solomon near the town of Eilat. It is the national stone of Israel. Eilat is the southernmost city of Israel, and the waters of the Red Sea were the passage of the Israelites from slavery to freedom in the Promised Land. King Solomon was a wealthy and wise king, and Eilat was the royal port from which he traded with Africa. His mines were famous and operational until approximately twenty years ago. Copper was being mined out of them until the price of copper dropped and it became no longer financially feasible to pump water out of the mine to get to the cooper. The mine has been flooded ever since. Unlike the King Solomon Stone, however, the stone Jay found has a high content of silver. The presence of silver gives this stone some of its unique power, as silver is a conductor for electricity and is, as well, a natural antibiotic.

And, finally, there is the secret ingredient that makes this stone more than magical: the lab report also showed that this magnificent stone was replete with thorium. As any Chemistry 101 student knows, thorium is a radioactive element.

RADIOACTIVITY 101

Since the beginning of time, at the very creation of the earth, life developed in a bath of radiation. All of life on our planet—both human and otherwise—has absorbed and used radiation to our benefit, and it remains as essential today for the continuation of all species as it was when life first developed. We live both under radiation—raining down on us from our atmosphere and beyond; and we live above radiation, as it spews out from the fiery inner core of our earth.

Radioactivity is a form of energy. It arises due to the presence of radium or radon. Radon, a gas, is a by-product of the decay of the element, radium. Radon is ubiquitous, seeping out from the earth's crust, and wherever there is water situated where the rays are coming out, the water itself becomes radioactive.

Radioactivity, whether from water, or from stones, rocks and ore that we find on the surface of our planet, is ubiquitous, found all over the earth. It is created by unstable isotopes of four elements: thorium, uranium, potassium, and rubidium. But like many things in the universe, elements are happiest when they are stable—which means on the cellular level that they have the same number of protons and neutrons. In this process of acquiring stability, the atoms of these radioactive isotopes begin a decay process in which electrically charged particles are emitted—alpha and beta particles and gamma rays. And, it is this decay, or disintegration, that throws off the specific form of energy that we call radiation. When atomic stability has been reached, there is no more decay, and thus, no more emission of radioactivity. This process of resolution can take between a few minutes and 13,500,000,000 years.

In the natural world, radiation is given off spontaneously and continuously without any external source of power. Once material becomes radioactive, it continuously gives off energy in small packets or "rays." These bundles of energy are called nuclear or atomic radiation, or, more generally, ionizing radiation. Everywhere on earth, we live in a sea of background radiation, weak or strong, depending on the location. The same radioactive rock can have a strong emission of radiation from one spot, and less than a centimeter away, it can register only a minor blip on a Geiger counter.

Yet, even though we live in, under, above and around radioactivity, a deep fear has developed in our country about all things radioactive. The fear stems from the common belief that any dose of radiation increases the likelihood of two dreaded diseases: cancer and congenital malformations.

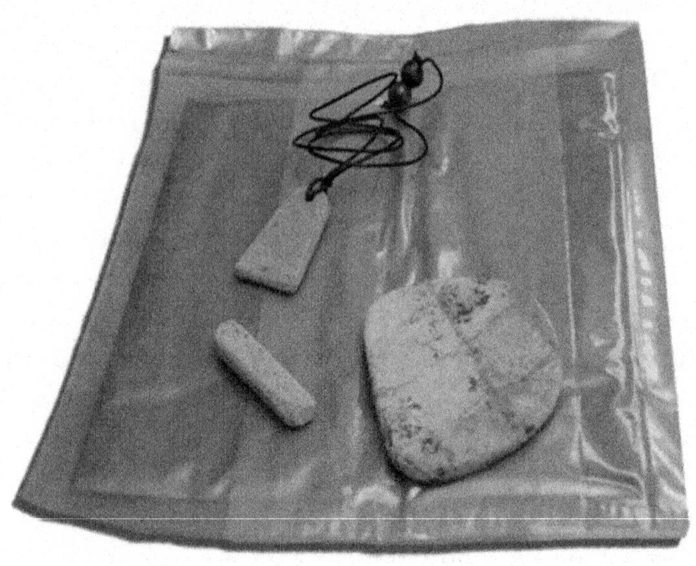

A radiation hormesis kit, comprised of a mud pack, water stone, stone pendant, and green stone.

BEYOND MAGIC

This stone that kept calling out to Jay had moved him from art (jewelry making), to spirituality (King Solomon's mines), to science (radioactivity). Yes, indeed: way beyond being a magical stone.

The saga of the search for stones didn't end, though, with that beautiful stone. After finding out that the stones were radioactive, Jay began to work with people in a more structured and careful way. He developed a robust reputation for being able to heal intractable illnesses.

And then, in the midst of gathering the stones, giving away the stones, and compiling anecdotal evidence of the value of the stones, a very fortuitous thing happened to Jay. He went to prison for a year. He willingly became the fall-guy for an elaborate scheme of his superiors that involved re-positioning (some would call it "stealing") helicopters. But Jay made good use of his time in prison: he devoted himself to doing research to find out why slightly radioactive stones would have the effect of healing people with such a wide array of afflictions. And, in his research, he came across a scientific and medical concept that was to change the direction of his life, as well as my own life, and the lives of the countless "patients" he has worked with, restoring them back to health, saving their lives.

One day, after his stint in prison, now armed with theoretical knowledge that supported his own experiences with the stones, Jay got a call from a man in Colombia, South America. This man had found out that Jay was working with radioactive stones, and he, too, had some "hot" stones that he had mined. He shipped Jay some of his Colombian hot stones—much hotter than anything Jay had worked with previously. Jay feared that the level of radiation these stones were emitting would overwhelm the immune system. He needed to find a way to reduce the emission.

He started adding water and crushing the stones into a muddy sludge, and then separating the material into small packets—each with a specific dosage of radiation. He was experimenting with different dosages—trying to get the dosage that would be maximally beneficial to the most number of people. He wanted the dosage to be strong enough to stimulate a response in the body, but weak enough to not overwhelm the body. He gave away a lot of these packs to people who used them for various afflictions—and he was impressed with the results. Then, he ran out of those Colombian rocks.

Jay was assigned another helicopter mission from his job—this time in the middle of Utah. From the air, as he was making a test flight, he saw some more of the beautiful blue-green stone. He went home, hopped into his truck, and drove back to the spot. He picked up a couple of hundred pounds of the green rock. On his way back, he had driven about 100 miles at this point, and he saw a huge mountain of rock. He stopped, stretched, looked around, admired the scenery, and then stooped down to pick up a single stone that had caught his eye. A nice stone. Not as beautiful as the Eilat stones; but still a nice stone. One mere stone he took, for no apparent reason, and tossed it in the truck. Then he took all of his wares to his shop.

He laboriously, tediously measured all of the hundreds of pounds of rock. Not a single ounce of those hundreds of pounds he had lugged home were stones that had any radioactive elements in them. Feeling discouraged and impatient, almost as an afterthought, he remembered that one stone. He went to his truck, reached in and took out that one lone stone that had been sitting there. He measured that stone. It was perfect—precisely the amount of radiation that he had determined was necessary to heal most afflictions.

That night Jay got call from a doctor in Illinois who he had been working with. She had six stage-4 cancer patients. Jay knew he needed to find stones for them. He got up early the next morning. There was a blizzard brewing. In this blazing snow storm, it took Jay 14 hours to make a normal four-hour trip to get back to that place where he had thoughtlessly, serendipitously thrown that one stone into his truck. He went to the hillside where he had found the rock. He spent three hours looking, and couldn't find a single stone. He couldn't accept that he was going to go back empty-handed.

He went into the near-by town, not quite knowing what his next move would be, but determined to stay until he found the stones he needed. He met an old man who had lived around those parts for decades, and this old guy knew everything there was to know about the land and the history of the land. He told Jay that there used to be uranium mine close to the area that Jay had been looking. But he told Jay that it was senseless to go back there because the area had already been had been picked clean for uranium ore.

Nevertheless, Jay followed his nose and intuition, refusing to go back without stones. He turned right, he turned left, he turned right again, he went over railroad tracks. He had no idea where he was nor where he was going. And then, he found himself at a loading dock. He got on his hands and knees, and crawled under the loading dock. And—voila—there was a big heap of stones that his Geiger counter was registering as the perfect level of radiation—the same as the original stone he had found. Every stone he found under that loading dock was hot. The trip back was just as bad as the trip coming; it was still snowing. It took the same fourteen hours to get back. But those stones saved the lives of the six stage 4-cancer patients.

And this is how the whole journey has been for Jay. If he hadn't found that first stone that was an afterthought, he wouldn't have ever gone back to that place; six people would have died who could have been saved; and he found a supply of stones that lasted him well into his next few years of saving peoples' lives and curing other intractable diseases.

THE IMMORTAL APPLE

Jay's work is not limited to humans. His hotel-spa, the Mineral Palace, is in the middle of cattle country. While Colorado scores low on the national average of cancer prevalence, the cattle ranching area is the highest in the state. The near-by ranchers have not only asked Jay for his help with their own cancers, they have asked for help with their cattle too.

So the story goes, as Jay tells it: "There was a man down here who owned a burro. He had this burro for about twenty years and was very fond of it. Because of its age, it was having a hard time walking. It also had worms and its ribs were showing. We

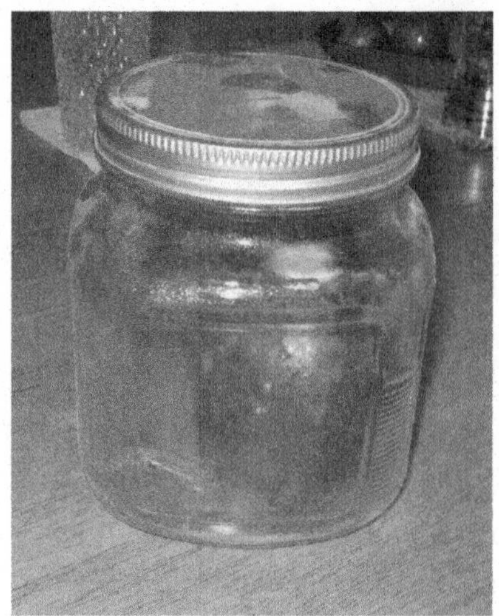
"Immortal apple" - with stone.

put some hot stones in its water, and before you knew it, the burro was gaining weight and the man was riding it again. We knew the water is good for cats and dogs, but now we are starting to work with the bigger animals."

Jay continues with his story: "A rancher came to me one morning and asked if my rocks could help his cattle. The calves that they had weaned off the mothers were getting sick because of the rapid temperature changes. It was fall and the weather was getting hot and then cold. The ranchers try their best to keep their cattle organic, but even with this good intention, they still feel they need to vaccinate them and give them antibiotics. This rancher had eighty head of cattle in one range, and another eighty head in another range. We decided to try a little experiment. With one herd, we put hot stones in the water tanks; we left the other herd without the water stones as a control group. The result of our experiment was clear: the cattle with the stones in the water stayed healthy. Cattle in the other herd continued getting sick.

"One of the problems the ranchers have is the build up of algae in the water tanks. The stones kept down the algae, and alleviated the need for vaccinations and antibiotics. Without those medications, the ranchers were able to promote a better weight gain. The cattle drinking the hormesis water are healthier, and the ranchers are putting out less money for their care, as they are saving the costs in vaccinations, medicine, and vet bills. Both cows and humans are happy with this solution."

And, then there is the apple. In another little home-devised experiment, Jay put an apple in a sealed glass jar with a stone in the jar. The control apple was in a glass jar with no stone. This little experiment has been going on now for over a year. The control apple has long since passed its prime. It is slick from mold and fungal overgrowth. The "stoned apple," however, looks almost as fresh as the day it was born.

On the previous pages compare the pictures of the rotten apple and our prize, possibly immortal apple.

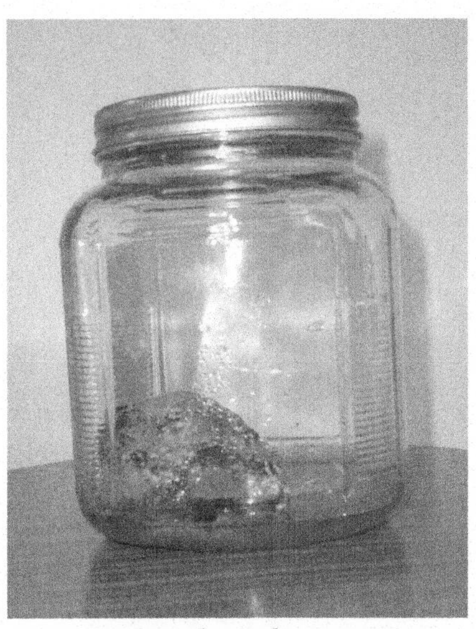

Rotten apple - without stone.

Over the course of Jay's work with patients, one of the people he helped was a Nemenhah Native American tribe Chief and Medicine Man. Chief Cloudpiler encouraged Jay to become, himself, a Medicine Man. Jay, who is one quarter Choctaw, found this idea of going back to his own heritage appealing, and studied the curriculum, went through the paces of learning, and was, indeed, awarded the distinction of becoming a certified Medicine Man of the Nemenhah Band and Native American Traditional Organization. As such, his work with patients is covered under NAFERA (Native American Free Exercise of Religion Act, 1993). NAFERA allows Medicine Men to work with plants, feathers and stones.

2

WHAT YOU THINK YOU KNOW

The unjustified excessive concern with radiation at any level, however, precludes beneficial uses of radiation and radioactivity in medicine, science and industry. — *Mayo Clinic Proc 69:436-440, 1994*

IT WAS HORRIBLE ENOUGH THAT we developed a weapon—an atomic bomb—that could kill so many people and so instantly. But, what made it even worse was that the killing didn't stop at the moment of the explosion. The expectation was that the fall-out would fan out, continuing on, for months and years, to the initial victims and to their progeny, presumably—killing on a sliding scale. We were told (and some of us witnessed) that with nuclear energy, high doses kill quickly and horribly, burning off skin and destroying intestines and other internal organs; and we were told (and all of us believed) that lower doses, to those who were far enough away that they survived the initial explosion, kill more slowly by triggering leukemia and other cancers.

From this understanding, scientists deduced the rough formula that underlies virtually all nuclear safeguards written since 1945. The formula is woefully inaccurate, but nevertheless, it is the formula that holds sway: it is postulated by most scientists that even the smallest exposure to nuclear radiation is harmful, and as the exposure increases, so do cancers and deaths. Scientists explain that the effect is linear: the more exposure, the greater the toxic effect; the less exposure, the less effect—but, be forewarned (we are told): there is always some toxic effect. This effect is called in the scientific literature, appropriately enough, the "linear-no-threshold theory"—LNT—of radiation, referring to the notion that there is no threshold over which radiation is not harmful.

It seems, though, that the actual hard data suggest otherwise.

First, we need to distinguish between the concept of nuclear and atomic energy, and radioactivity. The words "nuclear" and "atomic" are used interchangeably. They are both adjectives, referring to the nucleus of the atom. We have nuclear reactors or nuclear bombs, or nuclear medicine. Or, you can put the word "atomic" in for all those "nuclears."

Atoms that are undergoing nuclear transformation or decay are said to be radioactive (an adjective) because they give off radiation. Radioactivity refers to a quantity (large or small) of radioactive atoms. Radiation can also come from outer space (cosmic rays), but it still results from atomic or nuclear reactions at the atomic level. Nuclear reactors control the rate of nuclear fissions, whereas a bomb is designed to produce the energy rapidly

And while it may seem far afield to discuss nuclear power plants, and nuclear warfare in a book about healing stones, the perception that most of us have about radioactivity derive from events within the last sixty years involving bombs and the building, and failures of nuclear power plants.

CHOOSE: TODAY'S FULL-BODY SCAN OR YESTERDAY'S FALL-OUT FROM NAGASAKI-HIROSHIMA?

Let's establish what everyone agrees on: There were two

nuclear bombs that exploded in the air above the Japanese cities of Nagasaki and Hiroshima. Each bomb created large fireballs that shot into the air, and the heat from them was scorching. Many thousands died of being burned alive (though these figures are inexact: some families perished altogether, and in situations like this, record-gathering was difficult). Many also died of subsequent cancers that developed from being exposed to high-intensity radioactivity spurned by the bombs (though these records, too, show wide variability in terms of exact numbers).

This is where the agreement stops. Over a billion dollars have been spent to-date on figuring out the rest.

We first need to know that there are essentially four different types of radiologic rays, and they affect biological organisms differently. In the order of their ability to penetrate, they are alpha, beta, x-rays and gamma.

Alpha rays are big fat particles (think of an obese person who has trouble walking). Alpha rays have the least penetrating power of the rays, and deposit all their energy into the skin because they don't have enough energy to get past the skin barrier (think of an obese person who has trouble walking). Alpha particles are the main constituent of radon gas, which is colorless and odorless. Radon gas itself is not dangerous. Radon is merely the vehicle by which products of the radioactive decay chain can enter the lungs, and then later be absorbed by the sensitive cells of the bones and liver.

Beta rays are photons. They can travel a few feet in air but can usually be stopped by clothing or a few centimeters of wood. They are considered hazardous mainly if ingested or inhaled, but can cause radiation damage to the skin if the exposure is large enough. Unlike alpha rays, Beta rays begin to show mass. By the time we move up the ladder of radiation energy to x-rays, there is sufficient power to penetrate through one side of the human body and come out the other side.

X-rays were chosen to be the ray used in medical diagnoses

and therapies because their penetration power allows them to get past the skin barrier, thus enabling us to "see" into the body, and, as well, because they are not as destructive as the more penetrating gamma ray.

Gamma rays are pure electromagnetic waves, and they can penetrate more deeply than any other ray. They can cause irreparable damage to the interior of the body—to organs, tissues, and bones. Gamma rays are used in industry to see into structures that are denser than the human body, like metal. Neutrons are another form of radioactive rays produced specifically in nuclear fission and fusion.

The body does not know or care where radiation comes from. It registers the radiation the same whether the rays come from a man-made x-ray machine, an atomic bomb, or a stone lying in a park. However, the amount of energy emitted from the source changes.

The distinction between kinds of rays and their properties is important because it helps us to understand the true nature of the destruction wrought from Hiroshima and Nagasaki.

According to Myron Pollycove, Chairman of Radiation, Science and Health, after the nuclear bombs were dropped on Japan, there were, in fact, no deaths from radiologic burns. He has described it as a biochemical impossibility. The rays that were emitted from the bombs were almost exclusively gamma rays and neutrons. Neither causes burns. They penetrate much too deeply to stop at the skin and damage the skin through a burn. Rather, both gamma rays and neutrons, when hitting human skin, are absorbed *into* the skin (as opposed to being deposited *on* the skin) and then penetrate and distribute fairly evenly throughout the body. They do terrible, lethal damage to the interior of a body; however, burning the skin is not one of the damages they inflict.

It is true that there were many people in Japan who died a horrible death from being burned by the aftermath of the bombs. But, it is important to understand accurately the origin of what caused the burns. The unfortunate victims of burns did not suffer from radioactive burning. If the U.S. had decided to not drop the atomic bombs, and to continue fire-bombing Japanese cities as it had already done, the number of burn injuries and burn deaths would not have been significantly different, and the manner of suffering from these injuries would have been the same.

It is also true that there were large numbers of people who subsequently developed radiologically-induced cancer. This data is invaluable because it is compelling evidence to the destructive power of exposure to high-level radiation. The scientific advances in high-level radiation have moved so rapidly that yesterday's technology of atomic bombs has caught up with the today's practice of everyday medicine. Today, in the U.S., we deliberately expose a large part of our population to roughly the same amount of high-dose radiation as the bomb. Christopher Windham points out that the radiation dose from a full-body scan today can be almost as high as the dose received by the survivors of the bomb who were exposed to high-level radiation. Data from the Radiological Society of North America shows that 68.7 million CT exams were performed in the U.S. in 2008. And, as the survivors close to the bomb experienced increased levels of cancers, a new study published in the April 2009 issue of *Radiology* has the sobering conclusion that people who undergo numerous CT scans over their lifetime, similarly, are at a significantly increased risk of cancer. Some data show that this effect may be as high as 12 percent.

THE HEALTH BENEFITS OF THE ATOMIC BOMB

In spite of the fact that were radiologically-induced cancers from the bombs, it is also true that there were large numbers of people who did not develop radiologically-induced cancers. The size of this latter group has been a surprise to most scientists. Yet, according to a United Nations Scientific Committee on the Effects of Atomic Radiation (UNSCEAR) report, among A-bomb survivors from Hiroshima and Nagasaki who received "some" low-level radiologic exposure, there was no increase in the number of total cancer deaths. The operative word in the research findings is "some"—as opposed to "no exposure" or "lots of exposure." Quite to the contrary of the anticipated predicted deaths of those who had any level of exposure, the incidence of leukemia (generally thought of as a radiation-induced cancer) was lower in these low-level exposed survivors than in age-matched survivors who received no radiation exposure.

There are other detailed studies of those living near atomic bomb blasts. The findings are consistent: at points distant from the blasts where radiation was minimal but existent, leukemia deaths among A-bomb survivors was below normal, while as expected, closer to the blast where radiation was high, leukemia deaths rose well above normal. But, and here is where it gets really interesting: the exposed survivors haven't just not died of leukemia or other cancers; they haven't been dying for any reason. They're healthier than a comparison group of, shall we call them, "radioactive virgins"—people who have received no radioactive exposure. Dr. Sohei Kondo, in 1993, published *Health Effects of Low-Level Radiation*, in which he reported findings of a significantly lower death rate for those who had been exposed to low levels of the radiation fall-out than for those who had no exposure at all. Specifically, those who were a moderate distance from the epicenters, in the outlying areas of Nagasaki and Hiroshima, have outlived their contemporaries who received no exposure. And, among the survivors exposed who have not died of cancers, no adverse genetic effects in their progeny have been detected during fifty years of study.

The scientists involved in creating the atomic bomb considered the explosions over Nagasaki and Hiroshima to be, from a non-political, exclusively technical point of view, hugely successful. Ted Rockwell, who was part of the Manhattan Project which was instrumental in building the bomb, as well as being former technical director of U.S. Naval Reactors, says "the U.S.

government did *not* want to radiologically poison the Japanese populace." He explains that they wanted, planned, and executed the bomb to explode in the air—far away from people. Radioactive measurements were taken from the first day, and subsequent days, of the bomb explosion.

After just two days, the level of radioactive particles had already dropped to what would constitute low-level, close to normal background radiation. As cited in the Townsend Report:

> Some people went into Hiroshima the first day after dropping of the A-bomb when much but not all of the radiation contaminants had dissipated through wind currents. These persons suffered less cancer, had better lifetime immunity, and enjoyed longer lives than people who visited Hiroshima two or more days after the mushroom cloud, when radiation particles had even further dissipated.

It is not surprising that the Japanese, who were subjected to these nuclear bomb blasts would then become world leaders in measuring and understanding the actual health effects of radiation. As well as the effects of high-dosage radiation, they have become especially interested in the effects of low doses of radiation. Because their investigations have clearly shown that low doses of radiation are beneficial to health and that medicinal treatments with low-dose radiation can be used to cure diseases, including cancer, they are no longer afraid of radiation.

And, consequently, they are not afraid of nuclear power. Japan now has the largest nuclear power program in the world. The Japanese recognize nuclear power as an essential energy source because of the stable supply of uranium fuel and its ability to resolve a variety of environmental problems. There are now fifty-one nuclear power reactors in operation, supplying 35 percent of the electricity generated in Japan.

A study by M. Delpha, was entitled, "*Fear of nuclear power could be met with data from Hiroshima.*" The author was hoping to convince the rest of the world that low-level nuclear power and low-level radioactivity from the atomic bomb are not as fearful as most of us believe. Most Japanese scientists, and a large amount of the Japanese public, are now aware that those who were exposed to the low-level nuclear fall-out have better health and longer life than those who were not so fortunate. Yet, almost no one outside of Japan is aware of the data documenting this effect.

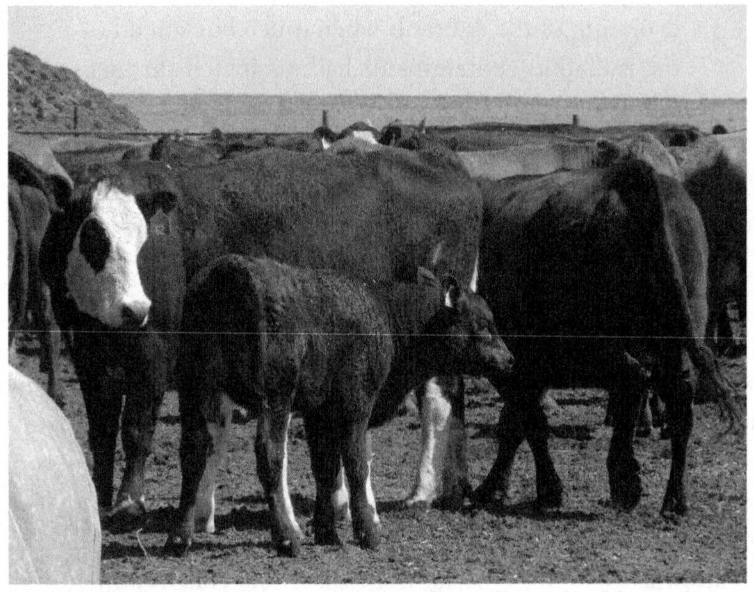

Jay added "hot" (radiation hormesis) stones to the water troughs of these sick cows and they all fully recovered.

The bombing of Japan has had a profound effect on our world. It also moved many of the scientists who had assisted in the development of the bomb. Some, to their moral credit, began to agonize over their roles in developing the A-bomb. Nuclear researcher Jerry Cuttler feels that it is not an accident that soon after the bomb was dropped, the hypothesis began to circulate within scientific and governmental circles that there is no level of radiation that is not harmful. The hypothesis contradicted known science with close to 100 years of research behind it; but perhaps it did not contradict the moral dilemmas that had been aroused by creating a force of such sheer destructive magnitude. Intense political activity was applied to stop bomb development, testing and production.

BUT WHAT ABOUT THE MILK?

On April 26, 1986, roughly forty years after the atomic bomb was dropped, a violent explosion occurred in the fourth unit of the Chernobyl nuclear power plant in Russia. Large quantities of radioactive material were ejected into the atmosphere. Russia panicked. Within eleven days, 116,000 people were evacuated, forced to change their place of residence, never to be allowed back to their homes again.

After the mass evacuation, fear of the radioactive particles being dumped across Europe and Asia came, and then the rest of the world, too, panicked. The headlines in the Western press shouted: "Chernobyl hecatomb," "Hiroshima, Nagasaki, Chernobyl," "Death from Chernobyl." Respectable newspapers and weeklies announced: "Thousands of bodies are being buried in Chernobyl." For a long time after, there were concerns about the radioactive material contaminating grass, waterways, rainwater and milk.

In fact, however, the explosion at the Chernobyl nuclear reactor did not kill thousands of people. Indeed, thirty plant workers and firefighters were killed. Twenty-eight died within four months. But these deaths were either from the explosion itself, or exposure to very high intensity radioactive material within the reactor rather than the delayed aftermath of free-floating radioactive particles falling around (fall-out), infecting the populace. The number of clean-up people exposed to high-dose radiation was 106. Of those, nineteen died during the following eighteen years. This figure conforms to normal mortality of ~1 percent/yr.

About 381,000 people engaged in the accident clean-up were exposed to lower levels of radiation. According to Professor Zbigniew Jaworowski from Central Laboratory for Radiological Protection, studies have documented that, like the Japanese populace who were exposed to low doses of the atomic bomb, these clean-up people, too, subsequently proved to have even better health than the non-exposed segments of the population.

Ultimately, the radiation doses to which the populations in Russia, Ukraine and Belarus were exposed had nearly no negative impact on their health: these people did not and still do not suffer more frequently from leukemia; nor do they give birth to more children with genetic defects. These are the conclusions from the UNSCEAR report, which was prepared over a sixteen-year investigation, by 142 of the most prominent experts from twenty-one countries. To the scientists familiar with prior studies on low-dose radiation, these findings are not surprising. According to the Chernobyl Forum, the surrounding population and most of the cleanup workers received doses comparable to doses many people receive from normal background radiation.

After the explosion, there was grave concern all over the world for infant health, as milk is known to concentrate radioactive particulates, and specifically iodine 131. Iodine 131 was released in the explosion. When babies and pregnant women drink milk, they expose the fetal and infant thyroids to potential thyroid cancer. Milk was carefully monitored for weeks and months after the explosion. Indeed, iodine 131 showed up in the milk of parts of Russia, as well as Washington, D.C., Baltimore, Philadelphia and New York City. Iodine 131 is not a naturally occurring substance. It is created only through man-made effort. Thus, there was no doubt that the tainted milk was related to failure of a nuclear power plant.

In Russia, one year after the explosion, as expected, cases of childhood thyroid cancers began to be reported. Yet, as there was no record-keeping of the prevalence of thyroid cancers before the explosion, it is difficult to form meaningful conclusions derived from this data. Because radiation induced thyroid cancer develops unrevealed for six to nine years, most researchers find this data—showing a pathogenic response as early as a year after exposure—to be suspect. As well, no correlation was found between the children's exposure to various radiation doses and the thyroid cancer incidence. UNSCEAR experts surmise that this increase in thyroid cancer incidence was likely to be caused by a factor unrelated to the Chernobyl radiation leakage. And, if they were induced by fall-out radiation, it is a comfort to know that except for nine cases, they were successfully treated.

Nor did the radioactive release heavily contaminate enormous areas of land in Russia for hundreds of years, as was predicted. Today, the land around the failed Chernobyl power station, this once highly radioactive land, is now rich in wildlife, much more so even than neighboring populated areas.

Chernobyl's failure spurred environmental activists to promote even more fear about nuclear energy. Since Chernobyl, the anti-nuclear activity has expanded to encompass opposition to nuclear energy and nuclear medicine. The fear of radioactivity has been witnessed most profoundly in peoples' attitudes toward nuclear energy plants. Citizens of Sacramento had the city close down its nuclear power plant for fear of what the radiation might do. Instead, the district put up windmills. On a windy day, these windmills are capable of producing 1 percent of what the power plant did. In addition to the windmill, a photovoltaic solar plant was built, which has generated one-third of 1 percent of that power. Since 1990, eight other nuclear power plants have been shut down in the United States.

An estimated 251 nuclear power plants are in various stages of planning and construction throughout the world, but the industry has ceased to exist in the U.S. And, back to the milk situation: while the milk in the U.S. was found to be contaminated with iodine 131, the high readings occurred in May, a full month after the explosion. Washington, D.C.'s milk continued to have high radioactive readings through August—three months after the Chernobyl radioactive fall-out had passed this part of the world; neighboring Virginia had no high readings. Here is the mystery: iodine 131 has a short half-life of seven days. Half of the ionizing radiation had disappeared by the end of seven days. Whatever happened to the U.S. milk, we can't blame the Russians.

THE SCHIZOID-PARANOID POSITION ABOUT JEWELRY, KITCHENS AND BASEMENTS

In this country, our schizophrenic paranoia about radiation has reached disproportionate and unreasonable heights. The fear of radiation has brought us to the point where we are afraid in our own homes, as we are chopping up the veggies in the kitchen for the dinner soup, or watching TV in the downstairs finished-basement den, or wearing our favorite Christmas present, a beautiful new piece of jewelry—a ring or a bracelet—from our spouse.

In 1998, it was found that hundreds of very rare chrysoberyl gems, commonly known as cat's eyes, were highly radioactive. Tests in Bangkok, where many of these stones originated, showed that the radiation levels in some stones were more than fifty times above safety limits. Many of these stones were imported into the U.S., and we were warned that wearing these stones in a ring or a bracelet could be lethal.

Then, nearly ten years later, in 2007, *Consumer Reports* published an article on kitchen countertops entitled "Countertops, The Hottest Rocks." We are led to wonder, from the article, if we are putting ourselves and our families at risk by choosing to have beautiful, natural stone countertops in our kitchens. This stone (most often granite) is mined from the earth's crust in quarries, and then made available to home builders, throughout the world. The earth's crust contains elements that were originally produced in the supernova explosions of stars in our galaxy over the billions of years that the earth has existed.

Some of these elements are radioactive, and therefore any building materials extracted from the earth's crust can be potentially radioactive too. And, indeed, following the *Consumer Reports*' concern, W. J. Llope documented his measurements of various kitchen countertops. He found "hot" spots in some of the stone countertops he visited in homes, and concluded that pregnant women and children who live in these homes need to safeguard against danger. But, even more disturbing, he warned us, was that some of the counters were made from uranium ore, and, as he says, "Where there is uranium, there is radon."

Until the 1980s, the concept of radon as a dangerous gas found in the basements of homes did not exist in our collective psyche. For many years, any apparent concern was side-stepped by regulators. But, then, excess radiation was discovered by accident. Nuclear power plant workers had been routinely monitored for their exposure levels to radiation. In December, 1984, a nuclear power plant worker set off the alarm for radioactivity on his way *into* the Pennsylvania Limerick power plant. This was odd! His reading should have been higher on his way out, after having been exposed to the radiation in the plant, not on his way in.

Subsequent investigation found that areas around Reading Prong, Pennsylvania and various locales in New Jersey had residential readings for presence of radon that were exceptionally high. This was all the evidence the Environmental Protection Agency (EPA) needed to step in and make a sudden and remarkable turn-around in its formerly disinterested position on residential radon. They decided that they could, should, and would regulate nature. Overnight, our perception of the natural world changed from being a fragile and defenseless virginity that our environmental watchdogs were sworn to protect, into the idea that we live in a hostile environment that invades our very homes through the emission of a dangerous gas, radon, that will poison and kill us all.

Because radon is a gas, its point of entry into our bodies is through our lungs. Our lungs, then, are the most vulnerable, and lung cancer was proposed to be the potential after-effect from breathing in the dangerous radon as it accumulated in our basements, seeping up from the rock formations and cracks in the earth. With no scientific proof whatsoever, with mere speculation, the EPA took these indisputable facts and announced a highly disputable conclusion: so they said, as many 20,000 lung cancers a year were being caused by residential radon inhalation.

In the mid-1980s, the EPA ran with that ball—and launched an aggressive campaign against radon in peoples' houses. Almost overnight, a hundred-million-dollar industry was created around the radon-abatement industry as basements in houses were ventilated to banish the radon from all spaces it might collect in.

Bernard Cohen, Professor Emeritus at Pittsburgh University, had a particular interest in the phenomenon of radon gas because his own residential stomping grounds were in the area of the highest radon readings. Cohen's intent in his original research study was to prove the connection between radon inhalation and lung cancer that the EPA had suggested.

But, there was a hitch in the plan to declare basements (as well as kitchen counters) as the most dangerous place in our homes. In 1990, Cohen published the results of his first study, and then in 1995, he published results of an up-dated investigation. His research had taken five years, cost millions of dollars and involved accumulating data from 1,760 U.S. counties, 90 percent of the U.S. population. Cohen had performed what may be heralded as the largest epidemiological study ever conducted in the U.S.

The results of Cohen's study were entirely unanticipated. He found that the areas with the highest radon levels had the lowest lung cancer rates. In other words: yes, there is, indeed, a correlation between radon gas and lung cancer; but the correlation is negative. Less radon, more lung cancer. And, the effect is not limited to reduction of lung cancer specifically. The highest levels of radon found in homes yielded lower incidences of other cancers, better immune systems, and longer life.

No one believed the data at first, including Cohen. He re-analyzed his data, correcting for variables that may have skewed the results. No matter how he examined the data to try to find confounding variables, he continued to find a negative relationship between radon levels and lung cancer death rates. If you take two maps of the U.S.—one highlighting the places of high incidence of radon and the other highlighting the places of high incidence of cancer, and overlay the maps on top of one other, you will see the exact inverse correspondence that exists. (Based on his findings, we should all be making plans to be Bernie Cohen's neighbor in order to take advantage of the high radon rates in his vicinity.)

Prior to his study, Professor Cohen had had a ventilation system installed in his basement to reduce the radon entering his home. After the study he turned the ventilation system off. Yet, in spite of the unequivocal data, still today, many companies promote the fear of a basement-induced death in your own home.

Dr. Arthur Robinson, President and Research Professor at the Oregon Institute of Science and Medicine, declares not only should we forego attempting to eliminate radon from our homes, we should be finding ways of bringing more in. "At least 20,000 people are dying of lung cancer each year in the U.S. who could have been saved by raising the radon concentration of the air in their homes." And, in what would seem to be a stunning tour-de-force suggestion to most people, he recommends a novel approach to the persistent problem of nuclear waste disposal:

> The most sensible use of low-level radioactive waste is as a concrete and insulation additive in residential homes—especially in areas where there is insufficient natural radiation for optimum health.

3

SAVING THE PENGUINS BUT KILLING THE CARS

> The current mode of extrapolating high-dose to low-dose effects is erroneous for both chemicals and radiation. Safe levels of exposure exist. The public has been needlessly frightened and deceived, and hundreds of billions of dollars wasted. A hard-headed, rapid examination of phenomena occurring at low exposures should have a high priority. — Philip Abelson, Editor Emeritus of *Science*; Editorial in *Science* 265, 9 Sept 1996

TO UNDERSTAND THE ORIGIN OF the nature of Jay's work and the stones, we need to go back in time. We need to know something about the history of radiation—and how it came to pass that the knowledge of the therapeutic use of low-level radiation became forgotten, or ignored, or deliberately misrepresented, and why the use of damaging high-level radiation became the prevailing diagnostic tool and treatment modality for cancer. And, finally, we need to understand why radiation therapy was ultimately placed under the exclusive rubric of medicine.

Long before the discovery of radiation, long before radioactive gas itself had been identified, ancient peoples understood intuitively and through experience that certain waters contained healing properties. For thousands of years, the ill and infirm journeyed long distances seeking cures at waters wherever water was bubbling up from the interior of the earth. In Europe, the use of hot springs with high radon content dates back some 6,000 years. For over eight centuries, numerous radioactive hot springs such as those found at Misasa and Tamagawa in Japan have been enjoyed. We know, too, that the Romans loved to go to what we now call radon spas.

In 1903, the discoverer of the electron, J. J. Thompson, discovered the presence of radioactivity in well water. This led to the discovery by others that the waters in many of the world's most famous health springs were also radioactive, due to the presence of radium emanation—what we now call radon gas—produced by radium in the ground through which the waters flow.

Most of the healing waters at famous health springs around the world emit low levels of radiation. Still today we have healing springs, with radioactive water, at Bath in England, Bad Gastein in Austria, Joachimstal in the Czech Republic, and two hours from Jay's Pritchett, Colorado, hotel and spa, in the little town of Canon City, Colorado. In fact, throughout Colorado there are several naturally occurring hot springs that bring radioactive sizzling hot water to the surface of earth.

The waters at Hot Springs, Arkansas, similarly, are radioactive, and are the most famous radioactive spring in the U.S. The properties of the waters in Hot Springs have been valued so highly in the past that in 1832 Congress established the Arkansas Hot Springs as the first federal reservation, a forerunner of the national park system. Even the military recognized their importance and established the Army and Navy General Hospital there in 1879. United States' Surgeon General Dr. George H. Tomey wrote at the time that

> Relief may be reasonably expected at the Hot Springs in . . . various forms of gout and rheumatism, neuralgia; metallic poisoning, chronic Brights disease, gastric dyspepsia, chronic diarrhea,

chronic skin lesions, etc.

JUST ANOTHER FORM OF ENERGY

The simplest understanding of radiation is that it is energy. Radiation "dose" or "exposure" is a measure of energy absorbed.

We humans, from the beginning of time, have been looking for forms of energy in our environment. There are many forms of environmental energy: sound, heat, light, gas and oil are the ones that are most easily recognized. On the most basic foundational level of what we are comprised of, we ourselves are energy. We generate our own energy, and, as well, we are able to absorb energy from energy sources outside ourselves. To the extent that we can find external energy sources, our bodies don't have to work as hard to stimulate our own energetic reserves. So, if we are outside on a cold night, and we can build a fire and use its heat to stay warm, we have saved ourselves the task of shivering and creating our own internal warmth. Thus, our energies can go elsewhere. We can put our energies, for instance, into enjoying the star-studded sky.

Every activity that we perform—from thinking about lifting a finger to actually running a marathon—each and every activity both creates energy and uses energy. Digestion creates energy; it also uses energy. Our bodies convert the energy of food from either plant life or lower animal life. This food energy comes originally from the sun; it is then absorbed by the plants through the process of plant digestion—which we call photosynthesis. The energy from the plant life is then either absorbed directly by us (if we like vegetables), or absorbed into lower animal life (cows, lambs) which we then eat (if we like meat).

THE CHEAPEST POPULIST CURE EVER

The scientific history of radiation begins in 1895, when Roentgen first published his x-ray paper. A few months after Roentgen's discovery, the health benefits of low-dose x-rays were demonstrated. In 1896, Henri Becquerel discovered the spontaneous emission of radiation from uranium, a phenomenon he called "radioactivity." And, in 1898, Marie Curie discovered radium. Because of these findings, the concepts of radiation and the health benefits of low-level radiation became widely known all over the world.

For instance, in the U.S., a news item was reported in 1896 stating that experiments by Dr. William Shrader prove unequivocally and "conclusively that the rays are invaluable" in the treatment of diseases. Two guinea pigs were inoculated with a diphtheria culture; then one pig was exposed to the rays for four hours and remained alive eight weeks later; the other pig, not exposed to the rays, died within twenty-eight hours after the injection of the diphtheria.

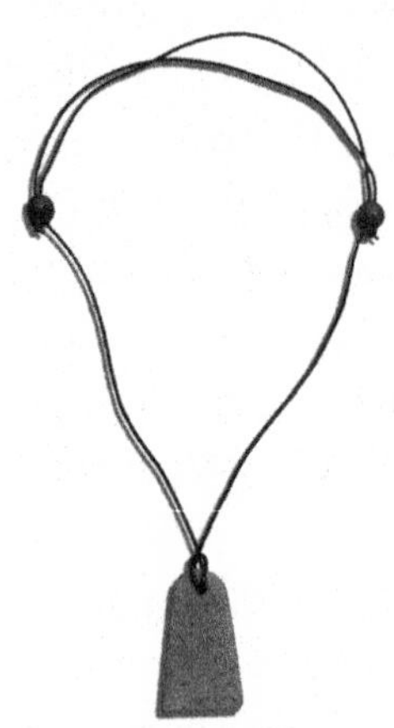
Stone Pendant Necklace.

Initially, the difference between low-dose and high-dose radiation was seen as an all-important distinction. In1908, Gager summarized the state of knowledge at that time by differentiating between overstimulation, which is destructive and can lead to death, and constructive stimulation, which increases metabolism and proves to be beneficial to the organism.

The beneficial effects of low-level radiation were repeatedly confirmed by scientists over many years. They led successful applications of low-dose radiation in stimulating the body to reject infections and inflammatory diseases.

The field of nuclear medicine had its origins in 1923 when Georg de Hevesy proposed using radioactive tracers in biomedical research. Following de Hevesy's lead, other physicians embraced and demonstrated the notion of the benefits of radioactivity. In the 1920s and '30s, the Mayo Clinic was using whole-body radiation to treat people with both gangrene and suppurating wounds with great success. Amputation rates went down by 80 percent.

Following the lead of the scientific discoveries, ever-enterprising entrepreneurs, especially in America, lead home to the entrepreneurial spirit, put the new rays to more mundane uses. Low-dose radium-infused products were created which became big business. Thomas Edison introduced a home fluoroscopy unit in 1896.

In the 1920s, x-ray units were used in beauty parlors to remove unwanted facial and body hair. Beginning in the twenties, but going well into the 1950s, fluoroscopes were used to measure the fit of children's shoes. Radium laced water was bottled and sold in the twenties and thirties. Devices were invented that could be used in the home to add radon to drinking water, such as the popular Revigator, a "radioactive water crock" made of radium-containing ore which held several gallons of water. It came with its own spigot, and had the following instructions on the side: "Fill jar every night. Drink freely."

Radium-laced water was called "liquid sunshine" and was considered to be more valuable than either gold or platinum. Entrepreneurs cleverly figured out how to infuse a host of products other than water with radium. Radium was added to toothpaste, hair tonic, beauty creams, soaps and candy. Ladies' corsets contained radium. One could play "radium roulette"—the wheel, balls, and chips were painted with radium. Or, how about purchasing a glowing radium-painted crucifix? Even suppositories and contraceptives contained radium—all with no apparent ill-effect, and with what many believed to be health-inducing benefits.

In 1949, Wade V. Lewis discovered radioactivity in a Montana mine that originally had been a silver and lead mine. Two years later, a Los Angeles woman was visiting with her miner husband and noticed that her bursitis disappeared after several visits underground. She convinced a friend of hers to come from California, too, for her bursitis. And, the friend, too was helped.

And then there was a stampede.

In using the radioactive mines, the general populace was putting to use the early scientific finding that low-level radiation gave many health benefits. They found, too, a way of using radioactivity for cures of a variety of afflictions, bypassing the medical system which was, at that time, just beginning to dig its nationwide foothold into health care. Thousands of people—most of them with bursitis, arthritis or other rheumatologic complaints—some in wheelchairs, some carried into the mine on stretchers—made the trip to Boulder, Montana to what became known as the Free Enterprise Radon Health Mine.

In 1952, *Life* magazine wrote a story about this mine and even more people flocked to the area to sit in the mines, breathing in the fumes of radioactive air. The idea caught on, and eventually sixteen radon health mines were operating within a thirty mile radius in Montana. By 1954, tens of thousands of people had traveled to Montana to visit either the Free Enterprise Mine, or one of the other local mines that had opened their tunnels to the arthritic public.

Until a few years after the end of World War II, ionizing radiation was considered and documented to be an effective way of combating diseases. However, several factors converged that eventually came to give radiation a bad name. First, as products were flooding the market promoting the various health benefits, there was insufficient regulation of the claims being made, and of the products themselves. Radioactive quack cures became available, and continued to be manufactured into the 1940s and 50s. Soon, all radioactive products, fake and real, fell under suspicion.

As well, there were a few cases of negative consequences from overuse of low-level radiation. Most notably were the radium painters. In 1917, the U.S. Radium Corporation in New Jersey hired seventy women. These women felt lucky to have a well-paying job in which they sat at tables in a dusty room, mixing up glue, water and radium powder, creating a glowing greenish-white concoction that they then painstakingly applied to the hands and faces of clocks, watches, altimeters and other instrument dials.

The painting was done with a camel hair brush. After several strokes, the brushes would lose their shape. In order to paint neat and sharp numbers on the dials, the girls were encouraged to frequently "sharpen" the fine brushes by using their lips and teeth to straighten the bristles. In fact, some girls painted their teeth or applied glowing "makeup" as a novelty to show their friends. Naturally, some of the paint was ingested.

In the late 1920s, some dentists began to notice jawbone deterioration in five of these young women. Later, cancers of the head and neck, anemias, and other disorders were found in these five women. They sued the company before they subsequently died. These girls' suit and deaths were well-publicized, and, as a result, fear of radium was instilled in most of the country. It wasn't until actual studies were done, later, that it was documented that none of the other dial painters showed effects that could be attributed to "radium poisoning."

In spite of the early deaths of these women, dial painting continued because of the advent of World War II and the need for aircraft instruments that could be seen in the dark. At this point, however, the work was carried on with strict attention to the protection of the painters. The management of the dial painting plants issued a warning to the dial painters not to tip their brushes with their lips.

Data analyst shows, interestingly, that this added layer of protection did not mean that these later dial painters did not acquire radium within their bodies. Almost all of the dial painters who were measured in these later phases of the work were found to have measurable radium within their bodies, but at a lower level than was found in their predecessors. No dial painter who started in this industry after the warning was issued, in spite of having measurable amounts of radium in their bodies, ever developed any radium-induced malignancies nor showed any adverse effects that could be attributed to exposure to radium. The suggestion is: even when our bodies register exposure to increased levels of radiation, this is not necessarily a bad thing. (In fact, it can be a good thing.) It appears that the dose is the critical variable: too much of a good thing can become a bad thing; a little amount of a bad thing can become a good thing.

Another factor that changed public opinion about radiation was a notorious radium poisoning case in 1932. Eben Byers, a well-known Philadelphia socialite who was a millionaire steel tycoon, as well as a strapping sportsman and U.S. amateur golf champion, believed, as many did, in the health-inducing benefits of radium water. He consumed massive amounts—over 2,000,000 times the current EPA limits, a 5,480,000-year dose over a three year period. He, like the radium-painters, died an early death from ingesting an overdose of radium. Even though Ebers' death parallels a drug-overdose death from over-consumption of a substance, the fear of radium-induced cancer became widespread. *Time* ran a full page obituary, further fueling the fear of low-level radiation that had begun to take hold.

Although these early radium-induced deaths were tragic, ultimately, the lesson of their deaths is clear: rather than supporting the notion that low-level radiation is harmful, the evidence supports the idea that moderate and low-level exposure causes no harm.

The advent of antibiotics in the late 1930s and early 1940s changed the entire application of modern medicine, and also contributed to the negative perception of low-level radiation. Following World War II, drug companies in the U.S. conducted worldwide searches to find molds and soil bacteria that could be synthesized in the laboratory and made into antibiotics. The mechanism of the efficacy of antibiotics is that they work by blocking the formation of the bacterial cell wall, thus killing the bacteria.

Antibiotics were released to agricultural chemists. During the 1950s, T. D. Luckey, a biochemist at the University of Missouri School of Medicine, and his colleagues were feeding antibiotics to livestock, expecting that the suppression of intestinal flora would decrease growth of the animals. Instead, the researchers discovered the opposite effect: low-dose dietary antibiotics caused a surge in growth; poultry, pigs and cattle fattened enormously on a diet containing low doses of antibiotics. Since this research, feeding antibiotics has become standard practice for these, as well as other animals. In surveying the literature, Luckey found that this phenomenon of "reversal of effect" depending on dosage was common. He termed it "hormesis."

After antibiotics were discovered, penicillin became available for widespread use in humans, as well as animals, and it was hailed as the new wonder drug. Antibiotics took over as the main medicine, dwarfing all other forms of medicine in spite of the fact that there were many others that were equally effective.

As well, the similarity of theory and concept between the newly named hormesis effect and the bourgeoning medicine of homeopathy coupled homesis with the same disadvantage that homeopathy suffered. (After all, the names of both share the same etymon.) When homeopathy was first introduced into this country, it was met with great hostility from the practitioners of the opposing school of allopathic medicine. Many of the first homeopaths were charged with malpractice, and subjected to both persecution and prosecution. The hormetic effect was, then, thrown into this mix of being seen as disreputable medicine.

The final death knell, and perhaps the most important, for the continued usage of low-level radiation for health purposes came after the dropping of the atomic bombs on Hiroshima and Nagasaki. After the war, our country engaged in subsequent development, testing, and stockpiling of nuclear weapons—all representing sources of high-level radiation. Some scientists became fearful of the damaging effects of high-level radiation. They worked aggressively to stop further weapons testing, and their efforts had the side-effect of promoting fear of all radiation—and, as had already happened with hormesis and homeopathy—the effect of low-level stimulation got mixed in and confused with high-level stimulation, with no distinction made between the two.

AND THEN CAME THE FEAR: CALL IT AN OUTRIGHT PHOBIA; CALL IT RADIOPHOBIA

Over the years of usage of low-level radiation in this country, there had been thousands of radium users and workers who enjoyed exceptional health. By the mid-1940s, there had been ample evidence amongst those who were regularly exposed to low-level radiation of longer life, faster wound healing, improved fertility, as well as reduced cancer rates and reductions of other chronic and fatal diseases. Already "cures" in the radon mines had been plentiful; and because of the large numbers of animals that had been brought in with various afflictions as well, and were then seen to be jumping and frolicking as they had in their younger years, the placebo effect seemed to be an unlikely cause of the positive responses.

Yet, in spite of these positive outcomes, low-level exposure to natural sources of radon and radiation lost favor as a therapeutic modality. The politics of the winds of radiation therapy had shifted. The initial embracing of the radium cure had become transformed into radiophobia. People became afraid of even very small doses of ionizing radiation. The Federal Drug Administration (FDA) obtained authority over radiation, and the use of therapeutic radiation became limited to high-dose radiation and to regulation under the auspices of the medical-pharmaceutical industry.

More recently than the radiophobia generated by the dropping of the bombs at the conclusion of WW II, a fear of radon was stimulated by epidemiological studies on miners. These men have prolonged exposure to radon and an early study showed a correlation with lung cancer. Re-examination of the data, however, suggests that there are other cancer-inducing factors that could have accounted for the correlation: specifically, particulates suspended in the air of all mines as well as fumes from diesel engines. The data on the effect of radon gas on people who do not spend their lives underground, as Bernie Cohen's studies indicate, tell quite a different story.

In the 1970s, nuclear power was going through an explosive growth period. Simultaneously, environmental activism was developing that led to the formation of numerous politically oriented environmental groups. According to Bernard Cohen, nuclear power became a target for activists for several reasons: 1) it was a new industry; 2) it was an industry sponsored by very large corporations which were being heavily accused of putting profits ahead of public safety; 3) it was related to the development of nuclear weapons, around which had developed an intense fear. Still today, even with our current energy crisis, there remains much negative opinion about nuclear power, and it is generally considered to be a health hazard to reside near a nuclear power plant.

The fear of radiation is fueled by the popular idea that being hit by a single particle of radiation can cause cancer. Yet, as Bernard Cohen points out, every one of us is hit by 15,000 of these particles every second, and a typical diagnostic x-ray hits us with about a trillion. The reason we survive is that the probability for one of these radioactive hits causing cancer is just one chance in 30,000,000,000,000,000 (30 quadrillion). It's hard to get better odds than these. (Thirty quadrillion is thirty times the number of hairs on all the heads of the current human population of the earth.)

In spite of the fact that much of the rest of the world has embraced nuclear power, no new nuclear power plants have been ordered in the U.S. since 1974, and the last attempt to build another power plant here was in 1978. In spite of the fact that we have created an industry that attempts to banish radon from our homes, the prevalence of lung cancer has not dropped in these areas where remediation has been most intense (to the contrary, lung cancer rises as radon presence falls). In spite of the fact that there is overwhelming evidence that survivors of Hiroshima and Nagasaki exposed to low-level radiation are enjoying longer and healthier lives than those who were not exposed to any radiation at all, much of the world and most of our own country remains deeply ignorant of the health benefits of low-level radiation.

There is an interesting little anecdote to be told about Roslyn Yalow, Nobel Laureate and the woman who is credited with being the founder of nuclear medicine. In 1992, she was attending a conference in Chicago celebrating the anniversary of Fermi's first demonstration of an atomic chain reaction. The reaction was created fifty years earlier, in 1942, in the Staggs Athletic Field with a pile of graphite and uranium chunks. At some point during the course of the conference, the other participants realized that Dr. Yalow was nowhere to be found.

The Nobel Laureate had wandered outside to the place where the environmental non-profit organization, Green Peace, was demonstrating peacefully against nuclear power. Just as peacefully, Dr. Yalow approached the crowd and asked them if they would be willing to sign a paper attesting to the fact that they were willing to give up all nuclear medicine. She pointed out that if you shut down all nuclear reactors, you shut down all creation of radioactive isotopes. Upwards of 40 percent of all medical procedures involve radiation in one form or another; a large number of these involve radioactive isotopes. Seventy percent of all medical research involves the use of radioactive isotopes. Dr. Yalow wanted the protestors to understand that if any of their grandfathers had a disease that needed to be accurately diagnosed, he would probably be availing himself of a medical technology that involved the use of nuclear power.

WE ARE ALONE IN OUR FEAR

In spite of the phobia that has developed, in spite of the regulations that have now been put into place, The Free Enterprise Radon Health Mine in Montana still operates today. The state of Montana was once the only place in the U.S. where one could go for supplemental radon exposure; that is, until December, 2008. It was at that time that the Mineral Palace (in Pritchett, Colorado) and La Casa Day Spa (in New York City), began to make radon steam baths and float baths available.

Most of the world, however, does not agree with the radiophobia that exists in this country. Various spas and clinics around the world offer the therapeutic use of radon. The treatment may involve the intake of radon gas (in mines or caves), or the radiation may be acquired through the transcutaneous resorption of radon dissolved in water—the "taking the waters" as it has been called at the world's various radioactive hot springs.

Some 75,000 people a year seek treatment for arthritic and other complaints at a dozen radon spas in Germany and the government accepts these therapies as effective. Throughout the rest of Europe—in Austria, the Czech Republic, Poland and Armenia, low-level radiation therapy is offered at medically supervised clinics (also called spas) where the therapy is prescribed by physicians. Japan has clinics, as well, and therapeutic low-level radiation is now an official therapeutic modality there. The best estimate of the usage in Russia is that they treat a million patients a year with radon. The Russian application of low-level radiation is performed in hospitals. In each of these countries, insurance generally covers 90 percent of the cost of the treatment.

SAVING THE PENGUINS BUT KILLING THE CARS: THE POLITICS OF RADIATION

Americans began creating radioactive wastes shortly after 1896, but no special precautions were taken for handling such wastes until 1954 when the federal Atomic Energy Commission began licensing all radioactive materials. During this period of time, many places, including large sections of whole states—for example, New Mexico and Colorado, where uranium mining occurred—were dumped with lots of radioactive trash.

Rod Adams, editor of *Atomic Energy Insights*, reports on a story that illustrates the inconsistency of the thinking that has gone into the notion of radiation "poisoning." There is a nuclear reactor at McMurdo Sound in Antarctica. It was decided that the soil near the reactor was contaminated and had to be removed. It was shipped to the U.S., and used as parking lot fill in Port Hueneme, California, where it was doubtless much safer. And so were the cars parked on it. Perhaps those who regularly park in that particular lot should give a prayer of gratitude for their unexpected good fortune for having this supplemental radioactive exposure (though we did all pay for it—through our tax dollars). But those of us who are not yet aware of the health benefits of low-level radiation exposure surely may have a difficult conflict to resolve in wondering whether it was better to irradiate the vast numbers of people using that parking lot in California vs. the vast numbers of people who were walking on that particular piece of earth down in Antarctica.

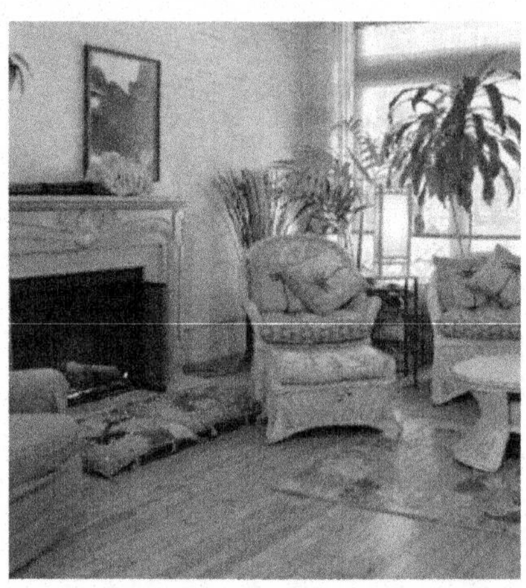

La Casa Day Spa, New York City.

And while Chernobyl may have begun as a localized Russian disaster, its long arms did reach over to both our own country and Europe—and not just in the milk. Like the radon industry that was created in this country, the "Chernobyl business-plan" has been a financial boon for many. Soviet authorities granted pensions and social privileges to 600,000 people who were counted as victims of the explosion. It is estimated that, at present, over 3 million people are entitled to some monetary privileges on the account of "permanent health detriment caused by Chernobyl radiation." Russian politicians are reluctant to even begin talks about taking away these privileges. Up to the year 2015, in impoverished Byelorussia, the "Chernobyl relief payments" alone will equal $86 billion.

The U.S. and Western Europe have transferred $800 million for the elimination of accident consequences; the European Bank for Development and Reconstruction plans to contribute another 2.3 billion Euros. Kiev claims that during the next twenty years, coping with the accident consequences will cost upwards of $5 billion. It has been speculated that the urgency for funds for the disaster consequences has its roots in the fact that some part of this money will go for patching up the holes in the state budget. This is a lot of financial hullabaloo for thirty initial deaths, and no further evidence of any lingering health problems anywhere in the country.

In the U.S., from 1946 to 1977, practically all federal matters relating to ionizing radiation were handled through the Joint Committee on Atomic Energy. The Joint Committee, with a stable membership from both the House and the Senate, was dedicated to developing facts and an understanding of atomic energy. In its place, currently, there are two dozen congressional committees. Unlike the Joint Committee, these sub-committees lack a stable composition of membership, their staff lacks in-depth knowledge on ionizing radiation, and the committees are without an overview power.

An irradiated organism can distinguish dosage of radiation, but it cannot distinguish whether the radiation is of natural or human (man-made) origin. In both cases the nuclear particles arise from the same processes and have the same characteristics. And our bodies are impacted by over a billion nuclear rays everyday from these natural sources.

There are now many regulations and standards that set permissible levels of radiation emission. Yet, paradoxically, and non-sensibly, the magnitude permissible for human-origin material is lower than the permissible level for the very same materials from natural sources.

Ironically, hearings on the topic of radiation standards may well be held in rooms in the national Capitol, where natural radiation from the granite walls measures at a level above that of a nuclear power plant. This same level of emission from any nuclear power plant on U.S. land would bring immediate and intense regulatory action accompanied with heavy fines.

There are other glaring discrepancies in the regulation of exposure to radiation. Many people work at jobs that expose them to natural radiation that is above the background radiation that we are all exposed to just by virtue of being on our radioactive planet. Those who spent time both above the earth—e.g., pilots and stewardesses—and those who spend time below the surface of the earth—e.g., miners—are exposed to more radiation than most of us. This exposure is not regulated or controlled. By contrast, workers with human-made radiation sources such as uranium mining, industrial radiography, nuclear medicine and some defense activities, receive a much lower level of exposure and yet, there is continual regulatory pressure to reduce their permitted exposure level.

The impact of nuclear power radiation on the world population at large, from many decades of world-wide nuclear power, is estimated to be less than one ten-thousandth of the average natural radiation background. We receive much more radiation by merely walking on earth—anywhere on earth—than by living near a nuclear power plant.

In spite of many attempts, no government can regulate or eliminate exposure to radiation from natural sources. To do so, with some fantastic, bizarre Super Hero invention, we would have to block out both the sun and our atmosphere's cosmic rays from reaching earth. We would have to suspend our bodies above earth in order to escape from all the radioactive dirt, stones, bricks, food and grasses that, ubiquitously, cover the surface of the earth.

But we couldn't go out too far in our bodily levitation, because then we would be entering into the atmosphere which is filled with radioactive cosmic rays. If we decided to pragmatically prolong our stay here on good old mother earth, we would have to declare entire states off-limits—especially Colorado—and we would have to re-locate the entire city of Denver because both city and state register as particularly high in naturally occurring background-radiation (even though the cancer rate in Colorado is low).

We could all move to the low background-radiation states, in the southeast and eastern gulf coastal regions, but, according to epidemiological data, doing so would significantly increase our chances of contracting cancer. We would have to destroy a great many of our buildings that are made from bricks, plaster and concrete that hold isotopes of uranium, thorium and radioactive potassium. The U.S. Capitol building and Grand Central Station would have to be vacated immediately because they emit among the highest levels of radiation of any man-made structures—more, in fact, than is legal for any nuclear power plant to emit. We would have to remove all smoke detectors and television receivers from houses.

Perhaps we would be best served by cancelling our trips to foreign countries where radiation is inherently high. Most notable are areas in China, India, Brazil and Iran. We would need to especially avoid the fabulous black sand beaches in those countries, because the black sand is actually monazite—in which the principle radioisotopes are from the decay of thorium 232 and radium 226.

Perhaps most importantly, we would have to stop sleeping with our partners-spouses, and we would have to stop eating bananas (and we really couldn't do both at the same time—eat a banana in bed while watching TV, simultaneous to snuggling up to our loved one—that would knock us out of the radioactive ball-field). What does sharing a bed with someone and eating a banana have in common? Both of them—the human and the fruit—emit radiation on a continuous basis from potassium (from the blood in the case of the human, from the banana in the case of the fruit). Potassium is essential for life, but it contains a radioactive isotope. As Dale Klein, the Nuclear Regulatory Commission Chairman, said in a policy speech:

> The Customs agents told me about one particular port that receives nothing but bananas—and virtually every shipment sets off the detectors. That struck a chord with me, because some of my fellow Commissioners have joked for some time about creating the 'standard banana' as a harmless unit of radioactivity. The public needs to understand there is such a thing as harmless exposure—which I think most people would grasp if you explain it in terms they can understand . . . like a 'standard banana.'

In spite of technical shortcomings in the political arena, both federal and state legislatures exert strong influences on the development of radiation protection standards. There is some evidence, however, that the winds of politics of low-level radiation may be changing again. The U.S. Department of Energy (DOE), the EPA, the Air Force and other government agencies, have started a $20 million program to study the effects of low-level radiation.

In addition, the National Cancer Research Institute and the National Institute of Radiological Science have joined forces with institutions in Japan, including several universities as well as the Central Research Institute of Electric Power Industry (CRIEPI), to study the effects of low-level radiation.

4

THE UP-SIDE OF RADIOACTIVITY

In a surprise move, leading U.S. and international scientific experts agreed in an historic accord that an increase in cancer has not been observed at radiation exposures below 10,000 millirem given to the whole body in a short time. — The "Wingspread Conference"; August 1-3, 1997

AFTER THE EARLY 1950S, THE U.S. government made it virtually impossible to get low-level radiation products. But research into the specifics of the properties of the reverse effect depending on dosage continued to intrigue Don Luckey. He noticed that the reversal effect was particularly strong when the "dose" was of ionizing radiation.

As he looked at the evidence showing the stimulation of low doses of physical, chemical and biological agents, he was overwhelmed by the extensive literature on the specific stimulation by ionizing radiation. Luckey began to do his own research, and observed that the effects included the growth of algae under irradiation, the growth of peas under irradiation, an increase in life span of invertebrates and insects, and seedling stimulation by x-rays.

One study showed that the increased growth rate was

directly proportional to the log of added radiation. Luckey did not under-estimate the importance of exposure of all humans, plants and animal life to low-level radiation. As he says: the biologic effects of low-dose irradiation is a "leitmotif (that) runs throughout the 20th century (medical) literature . . ." Luckey is the man who is rightly credited with propelling the science of low-level radiation into its next generation of thought, research, and application.

In 1980 and 1982, after years of research, Luckey wrote the two definitive books on the benefits of low-level radiation, compiling the research that had been done world-wide for decades. He presents data compiled on thousands of people working in jobs that exposed them to low-dose radiation. Luckey reviews the data from studies that followed workers in nuclear power plants, research facilities, bomb factories and submarines. When comparing the number of deaths per 1,000 workers, those exposed to radiation consistently had fewer deaths. Combined data from 7 million person-years show those exposed to low-level radiation had 52 percent the risk of dying as unexposed control groups. Lucky references over 2,000 studies to support his view.

IF YOU DRINK COFFEE, IF YOU EXERCISE, THEN YOU ARE GUILTY OF USING HORMESIS

To understand the nature of how low-level radiation works, we need to understand the concept of hormesis. Hormesis is used by most of us in everyday life—in better and worse applications. Anyone who drinks coffee in the morning uses a hormesis effect; anyone who smokes or drinks alcohol uses hormesis; anyone who walks or runs or lifts weights for exercise uses hormesis; anyone who avails themselves of vigorous exercise that gives a slight stress to bones or muscles, such as running, or playing tennis uses hormesis. Each of those activities can have stimulating, pleasurable effects. None of them are dangerous in mild doses, but they each can be destructive when the quantity of activity reaches a certain critical tipping point.

If, for instance, we reach that dangerous tipping point in exercise, we can come to physical exhaustion where our bodily systems begin to shut down; we can push ourselves to a point that is 100 percent fatal to 100 percent of humans. But, at smaller doses, exercise is a stressor that our bodies adapt to, that helps our bodies to become healthier, and that becomes a highly beneficial and essential part of a health regimen.

The word "hormesis" is derived from the Greek word "hormaein" which means "to excite." In 1943, two researchers, C. Southam and J. Erlich, found the effective concentration of phenolic compounds in wood which protects trees from fungi decay. Despite the fact that high concentrations of oak bark extract inhibited fungi growth, low doses of this agent stimulated fungi growth. They modified the word "hormone" to "hormesis" to describe stimulation induced by low doses of agents which are harmful or even lethal at high doses.

Generally, hormesis is any stimulatory or beneficial effect, induced by low doses of an agent that are in contrast to a detrimental or even lethal effect induced by high doses of the same agent. Hormesis is, then, an adaptive response of living organisms, and it may be to chemical, biologic or radiologic agents. It is a modest overcompensation to a disruption, and it leads to improved fitness. The phenomenon has been reported in biomedical literature since the 1880s, and forms the basis for all immunology, vaccines and homeopathic treatment.

There is a long history throughout science and medicine, even before the hormesis effect was scientifically demonstrated, that suggests that large and small doses evoke opposite effects. In the late 1400s, physician Paracelsus understood that dose is the difference between cure and danger: "The dose makes the poison." In the 1880s, Rudolf Arndt and Hugo Schultz showed that substances vary in action depending on whether the concentration is high, medium, or low.

According to the Arndt-Schultz Law: high concentrations

kill; medium concentrations suppress or inhibit; and low, or minute concentrations stimulate. "Poisons are stimulants in small doses" is the general understanding of the Law, and Arndt and Schultz demonstrated that this principle seems to be universally applicable to all inorganic toxins. They demonstrated the phenomenon with mercury, chromium, arsenic and iodine in yeast cultures. In fact, a more literal translation of the Arndt-Shultz Law is: *sufficiently diluted toxicants should have a beneficial effect on the organism*.

The distinction is important; the phrase "sufficiently diluted" is ambiguous, yet means the difference between lethal poisoning and therapeutic benefit. (This too, is one of the issues in hormesis' cousin, homeopathy: it has been demonstrated in a lab that even when the dilution of a substance is so powerful that there is not a single molecule of the original substance remaining, the vibrational frequency is sustained.)

The Arndt-Schultz Law demonstrating the hormesis effect was widely accepted at the time it was formulated, and was referred to extensively in the pharmacological literature for over thirty years.

After the demonstration of the effect by Southam and Ehrlich, at the close of World War II, physicians observed the effect in their use of penicillin. Supplies of penicillin were limited. Researchers Miller et al. (1945) explained why reducing the dose to make short supplies of the new drug go further sometimes had the reverse of the desired effect. At low doses, penicillin actually stimulated the growth of Staphylococcus.

Still today, the work of Miller is regarded as the gold standard of the use of antibiotics—that if the dosage is too small or application too short, the intended therapeutic effect will not be achieved. As well, the hormetic effect is widely accepted automatically today, as we know the stimulatory effects of many substances that are part of our everyday life. A peg of whiskey, a whiff of nicotine from a cigarette, caffeine in a cup of coffee—all these stimulate, as all alcoholics, coffee drinkers and smokers know. Yet, a single intake of a few liters of alcohol, or as little as half a gram of nicotine or caffeine will kill. These substances, along with many others, stimulate at low doses and kill at high doses.

FROM GOD-GIVEN TO MAN-MANIPULATED

In 1896, it was discovered that the nucleus of an atom could be manipulated to be made unstable (reflecting the same instability found in nature in uranium and thorium) and, thus, become radioactive. We had discovered a method for artificially manufacturing radioactivity. Because naturally occurring radiation had been shown to have various health benefits, it was a logical extension to assume that this man-made form of radioactivity could be found to be useful for medical purposes, as well.

Today, man-made radiation has come to be considered to be one of humanity's proudest achievements. The ionizing radiation produced by a high-energy electric source has been found to have many useful characteristics: for example, it can pass through the human body and thus allow shadowy "x-ray" pictures of our bones to be created on sensitized film. Some of us, who are old enough, remember the special occasions when we went to our local shoe-store as children. Obligingly, we would place our feet on an x-ray scanner, and voila! We would gaze at our feet bones with great fascination. Today, nearly everyone in the U.S. has benefitted from the medical use of diagnostic x-rays at one time or another, whether for a broken bone, to evaluate dental dilemmas, or to detect certain cancers.

The penetrating power of man-made high-level radiation makes it useful, but also makes it dangerous. In 1927, Nobel Prize winner, Herman J. Muller, found that x-rays are mutagenic; they create changes in cells. He proposed that mutations that are induced by radiation are mostly detrimental. When it became generally accepted that excessive radiation is harmful, the first regulations for dose limits were introduced.

When radiation penetrates human tissue—which is composed of billions of cells—the radiation pierces the cells like a tiny but powerful bullet, disrupting the structure of any cells that take a direct hit. If the dosage is sufficiently high, some of these disrupted cells start multiplying without limit. Sufficient multiplication is a condition we call cancer.

A FORTUITOUS MARRIAGE OF CONCEPTS

In a paper Luckey presented in 1998, he stated that his purpose was to promote harmony with nature and to improve the quality of our lives with the knowledge that cancer mortality rates decrease following exposure to low-dose irradiation. He explains the term he chose: Hormology is the study of excitation. As he says:

> Low doses of many agents evoke a bio-positive effect; large doses produce a bio-negative effect. The message is simple: small and large doses induce opposite physiologic results.

The hormetic principle is then: *low-dose stimulation and high dose inhibition*.

Calebrese and Baldwin agree with Luckey, and report that thousands of scientific studies have demonstrated that hormesis is a universal concept, and that it is seen across the whole plant and animal kingdoms. As they say: "the hormetic model is not the exception to the rule, it is the rule."

Luckey named the specific reverse-effect of radiation, "radiation hormesis." He supported his conclusion by demonstrating that while radiation in high doses exerted only adverse effects, radiation in low doses, on the contrary, resulted in anti-aging effects, cancer suppression, improvement of immune function, promotion of growth and an increase in defense against disease.

Similarly, Roslyn Yalow states without equivocation that no reproducible evidence exists of harmful effects from increases in background radiation three to ten times the usual levels. She points out that there is no increase in leukemia or other cancers among American participants in nuclear testing, no increase in leukemia or thyroid cancer among medical patients receiving Iodine-131 for diagnosis or treatment of hyperthyroidism, and no increase in lung cancer among non-smokers exposed to increased radon in the home.

When asked whether people living near nuclear waste grounds have reason to be afraid, she countered with asking whether or not pilots, who receive more radiation exposure on aircrafts than one would get from living near a radioactive waste disposal site, should be afraid. Finally she stated that scientists have never, for the most part, accepted the validity of the hypothesis that exposure to low-level radiation is harmful.

In his book, *Radiation Hormesis*, Luckey reviews the myriad of benefits from increased levels of ionizing radiation: fertility, early physical development, immune competence, radiation resistance, mental acuity, and mean life-span. He documented that supplementation with low-dose irradiation provides decreased heart disease, sterility, infections, lung diseases, cancer deaths, and premature deaths.

Luckey argues that low-dose radiation is needed to maintain health, and that we suffer from a chronic state of radiation deficiency. He suggests that these benefits would accumulate if we lived with twenty times more ambient radiation than we have now. The optimum appears to be many times our present background. Such evidence indicates additional irradiation would provide a new plateau of health for most people.

We should think of the concept of radiation hormesis as being comparable to those essential nutrients that are not present in adequate quantities in certain environments. Modern life has rendered us deficient in a number of materials important for health and long life, including, for instance, vitamin A and selenium. While an excess is harmful, the converse is also true: small amounts are needed for essential physiologic functions.

Supplementation of deficiency is now standard practice for the increasing numbers of people who avail themselves of vitamins, minerals, herbs, even specific foods. This supplementation is done for both vitamin A and selenium. It has been extensively and consistently confirmed that supplemental radiation, above the natural background level, stimulates organisms, enhancing their growth and increasing their life-spans. It is now clear that additional supplementation of low-level radiation creates significant therapeutic responses.

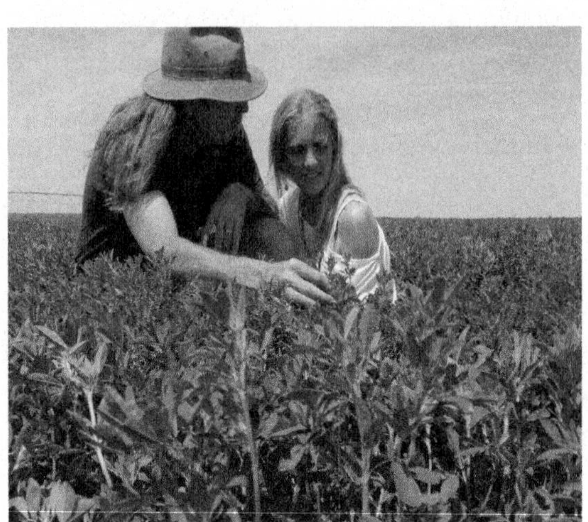

Jay and Faye in a crop field treated with hormesis water.

Ted Rockwell specifies that the immune system's responses to low-level vs. high-level radiation are entirely different phenomena. He describes what is comparable to a black and white switch in the body that distinguishes between the two: they have different genomes, and they form different proteins.

> Low-dose initiates the type of response that is essentially error-free—a healing response. High-dose is a survival mechanism—it is a much less effective protection.

5

THE HEALTHY CELL IS A SUICIDAL COMMUNIST

In reference to the misconceptions of risks of low-dose radiation, the situation is "the greatest scientific scandal of the century" — Prof. Gunnar Walinder, former Chair, Swedish Radiobiology Society

SCIENTIFIC RESEARCH POSITS AN ELEGANTLY simple theory that explains why exposure to low-level radiation is curative, and curative for so many diverse ailments: low doses of radiation slightly damage the body's cells and DNA, thus causing the immune system to react. Science has documented a number of other factors that serve, similarly, as challenges, or stressors that induce positive effects. Stresses that have been reported to delay aging and prolong longevity include temperature shock, heavy metals, pro-oxidants, alcohols, exercise and calorie restriction.

Even the prevailing explanation for aging related to oxidative stress has been recently shown to have a hormesis effect. For more than forty years, leading researchers postulated that when free radicals, oxygen ions and peroxides build up in cells, they overwhelm the cells' ability to repair the damage they cause, and the cells age. A whole industry of alternative antioxidant therapies—such as Vitamin E or CoQ10 supplements—has sprung up as the result of this theory.

Irradiation is just one more of any number of possible stressors on this list of what Hans Selye originally called eu-stress—good stress, stress that ultimately benefits the organism. In the case of low-level radiation, the challenge to the immune system increases production of stronger, healthier cells—cells that are able to fight off all manner of pathogens. Thus, it is not the radiation that is killing the pathogens that are causing the illness; it is the body's response to the radiation.

Since the first reports on the benefits of low doses of ionizing radiation, thousands of medical and research papers have been published documenting its therapeutic benefits. Despite the fact that high doses of ionizing radiation (as in x-rays and radiation therapy for cancer) are detrimental, substantial data from both humans and experimental animals show that biologic functions are stimulated by low-dose radiation.

Low-level ionizing radiation is an essential trace energy for life, analogous to essential trace elements. Irradiation supplementation promises increased quality of life and a new plane of health for people in the 21st century. It is likely, as indicated by numerous research studies, that a large number of cancer deaths are preventable by increasing our daily exposure to low-dose radiation.

THEORIES 1-10

Although still we may not know the entire mechanisms of radiation hormesis, the following theories are explanative of this process:

1) Increases Apoptosis

Apoptosis is the event of cellular suicide. It is a natural, health-inducing process whereby cells, for the sake of the overall good of the many, obligingly commit suicide. It occurs spontaneously in healthy tissues when a cell has reached the end of its life span or in embryos when a selected cell is no longer needed. (Apparently, healthy cells are suicidal communists. They do have, as Freud proclaimed 100 years ago and has been roundly criticized for ever since, a death instinct.)

This cellular suicide is a kind of programmed cell death that cells in the body undergo either in the normal course of growth and development or when something goes wrong with them. In the case of a damaged cell, "garbage" is able to be removed before the decay spreads uncontrolled, infecting other areas. Just as we want to remove our trash because rotting garbage becomes a health risk, and just as we need to bury our dead because having dead bodies lying around becomes a health risk, so too do cells need to remove their sick, dying and dead compatriots to avoid health risks. A body that allows damaged cells to continue to inhabit its space will ultimately become polluted and damaged itself. Once damaged cells are eliminated by the apoptosis police guard, healthy cell replacement is stimulated.

Apoptosis is important in health, but it is especially important in cancer. One of the specific problems with cancer is that the cancer cell, left to its own devices, is immortal. Cancer blocks the cell-signaling pathway that allows apoptosis; this is how cancerous conditions keep the defenses of the body at bay. The cancer cells just don't want to die, and provided with the right circumstances, a cancer cell colony can replenish itself indefinitely. And, it's really hard to kill a cancer cell by other than extraordinary means.

Chemotherapy and high-dose radiation are, of course, extraordinary means. They are so extraordinary—they are so strong in their power—that the body, on a cellular level, begins to look like a battlefield when the war is over—and all you see is dead bodies—bodies of men who were only an instant before young and vigorous, as well as bodies of those who had been previously wounded and infirm. It's a wholesale slaughter—both war, on a societal level, and, as well, the war on cancer—medical treatments of cancer on a cellular level.

And, according to one study, even chemotherapy can't keep a good cancer cell down. The study showed that cancer cells were able to recover even after exposure to a chemical cocktail which triggers suicide in normal cells. Researchers conclude that this mechanism helps cancer cells to block the effect of chemotherapy drugs. This refusal to die, or shall we call it, the power of resurrection, helps to explain why cancer patients treated with chemotherapy and high-level radiation are told initially by their doctors, "we got it all," only to find out later that they "didn't really get it all." Maybe they got it all; but the same old cancer cell that was killed decided to be born again.

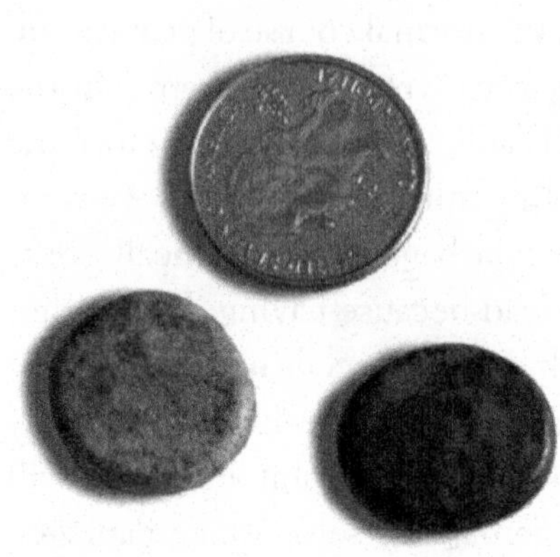

Mouth Stones.

It has been shown, however, that cancer cells can be tricked into apoptosis. Radiation hormesis induces cellular death of cancer cells and other pathogens. Dr. Sohei Kondo showed that radiation hormesis increased cellular apoptosis, thus cleaning up the body on the cellular level from damaged and sick cells.

2) Promotes Cellular Detoxification

Cancer cells, however, may not be the only cells that have immortality as, at least, a possibility. Nobel Prize winner, Alexis Carrel, kept cells from the heart of a chicken embryo alive by simply immersing the cells in a nutrient solution and changing the solution. Each day new nutrients were added and waste was cleaned out. The experiment continued for twenty-nine years without a hitch. It was beginning to seem as though with the right nutrients and with proper waste elimination, the cells would go on living forever. And then a fatal mistake was made! Carrel's lab technician accidentally forgot to change the solution. The cells became toxic from being immersed in their own waste products. The cells died from being lethally auto-intoxicated.

There are over 70 trillion cells in the body. Continuous detoxification is essential for health. Maybe with proper detoxification, any cell can be prompted to live forever.

Professor Bertram Boltwood of Yale explains how radiation hormesis aids in the detoxification process: the radioactivity carries electrical energy into the depths of the body, and there subjects the juices, protoplasm, and nuclei of the cells "to an immediate bombardment by explosions of electrical atoms." These electrical explosions stimulate cellular activity, "arousing all secretory and excretory organs, causing the system to throw off waste products." Low-level radiation is, thus, an agent for the destruction of bacteria and other pathogens on the cellular level. Fungus has been a specific pathogen that appears to be especially vulnerable to exposure to low-level radiation.

3) Stimulates DNA Repair

The human body undergoes roughly 200,000 DNA repairs every day in every cell. Ted Rockwell has said that "it is the repair and removal process (or lack of it) that kills us." Low doses of ionizing radiation induce the production of special proteins that are involved in DNA repair processes. Studies using two-dimensional gel electrophoresis indicated the formation of new proteins in cells irradiated with low doses of radiation. Also, it was further shown that cycloheximide, a protein synthesis inhibitor, blocks this hormetic effect.

The beauty of the DNA-Repair theory is that it resolves the leading contradiction about the effect of low-level radiation: whether it heals you or makes you sick, cures you or kills you. The theory explains both why people exposed to radiation both live longer but also could die sooner. Exposure to radiation can do either. If the DNA repairs itself, you live longer. If the DNA fails to repair itself, it kills you sooner. And, those who are most susceptible to the repair not occurring are the infants, the children and those whose health was already compromised, before the exposure, in some significant way.

4) Loosens DNA Coil

In 1953, James Watson and Francis Crick discovered that DNA is coiled. In fact, DNA is not just coiled, it is super-coiled: coils of coils allow all of the DNA molecules to fit into an infinitesimally small area of each cell. The particular nature of the wrapping is an important diagnostic indicator of the health of the cell. According to research conducted by Philip Lipetz, the coils become looser as we get older.

However, in cancer conditions, the opposite effect is witnessed: coils become too tightly wrapped. Chemical treatment of the cancer cells has the effect of re-loosening the coils. And, according to Lipetz's research, so does low-level radiation. After the application of the treatment—either chemical or radioactive—the cells return to normal. This loosening of the coils is, in fact, another mechanism of DNA repair that is in response to the challenge of the low-level radiation.

5) Allows Rest-Recovery from Damage

We know that there is some process of repair or recovery of cells, on both a genetic and biochemical level, if for no reason other than that based on modern radiation therapy techniques. It has been known for at least fifty years that the total amount of radiation delivered to a tumor and surrounding tissues can be enormously increased by the simple expedient of introducing "rest periods" between each treatment. Without some sort of recovery phenomenon in play, there would be no radiation therapy today, because all patients would be suffering from gross and immediate overexposure. This, of course, is not the case.

6) Promotes Free-Radical Detoxification

Feinendengen and his co-workers indicated that low doses of ionizing radiation cause a temporary inhibition in DNA synthesis. The maximum inhibition was at five hours after irradiation. This temporary inhibition of DNA synthesis would provide a longer time for irradiated cells to recover. This inhibition also may induce the production of free radical scavengers, so irradiated cells would be more resistant to any further exposures. There is also evidence that there is stimulation of super-oxide dismutase, a powerful antioxidant that blocks free radical damage, and ATP, the source of energy for all cells.

7) Stimulates the Immune System

Despite the fact that high doses of ionizing radiation are immunosuppressive, many studies have indicated that low-dose radiation stimulates the function of the immune system. It has been known for almost a century that exposure to low-level radiation stimulates an increase in the production of lymphocytes (white blood cells).

In 1909, Russ first showed that mice treated with low-level radiation were more resistant against bacterial disease. Luckey's 1982 book compiled a large collection of references supporting immuno-stimulatory effects of low doses of ionizing radiation. Specifically, it has been demonstrated that radiation hormesis:

- increases the number of immune system helper T cells
- decreases the number of immune system suppressor T cells
- increases the activity of p53 protein, a material that has been described by scientists as decreasing the incidence of many cancers

8) Increases Production of Enzymes

According to Bernard Cohen, enzymes have the capability of repairing the DNA damage that can initiate development of cancer. Low-level radiation increases the time available for this DNA repair, thus stimulating the immune system to resist the growth of tumors, and establishing yet another way by which potential cancer cells are enabled to altruistically commit suicide (apoptosis).

9) Rejuvenates Cells; Confers an Anti-Aging Effect

Lipid peroxide is decreased. This diminution is important because lipid peroxide is the process whereby free radicals "steal" electrons from the lipids in cell membranes, resulting in cell damage. Because of this decrease, beneficial effects to cell membrane permeability occur. According to research by Yamaoka, stimulatory radiation creates high permeability of cell membranes.

This contribution to cellular health gives relief for ailments—the ailments that the radon mines in Montana were so successful in eliminating: arthritis, bursitis, inflammations. But, improvement in cell permeability also confers a powerful anti-aging effect. Exposure to low-level radiation may be the most effective anti-wrinkle therapy available on the market.

10) Has Beneficial Effects on Neuro-Transmitting and Thinking Systems

Key enzymes and hormones are increased. Scientists at several top medical centers reported increased levels of insulin as well as endorphins and enkephalins. These are the feel-good hormones: beta-endorphins are a pain-reliever; m-enkephalins create a feeling of well-being. The increase in enzymes and hormones explains some of the "rejuvenating" effects observed. Improvement has been seen in both hypertension and diabetes. As well, there is increased brain cell membrane permeability.

THE BROAD STROKE THEORY

The research points to two essential theories of why exposure to low-level radiation confers better health and longer life. First, we no longer live in harmony with nature, and while radioactivity is prolific in nature, a deficiency is created as soon as we move away from living in nature.

In the same way that most of us are deficient in Vitamin D because we are no longer exposed to sufficient sunlight, we are, similarly, deficient in exposure to the level of radioactivity that is necessary for optimal health. Exposure to low-level sources of radiation corrects that deficiency.

The second broad theory involves the various mechanisms that the body has available to it to repair itself. Because the protective and reparative mechanisms have been challenged, working at a higher level than they would in the absence of radiation exposure, mutations (both those caused by radiation and those that occur spontaneously) are found and repaired or destroyed. Thus, the whole-organism response to low-level radiation exposure in the radiation hormesis paradigm is a state of improved health when compared with that in the absence of radiation exposure. This leads to the decrease in the death rate that has been observed in thousands of studies—both human and animal.

DISAPPEARANCE; RAPID DISAPPEARANCE; RAPID DISAPPEARANCE WITH LITTLE OUTLAY OF MONEY

Jay read the research. As a helicopter mechanic, Jay had learned to think analytically and logically. He was able to understand complicated scientific concepts by breaking them down into their component parts, and putting them back together in the most basic terms, just as he was able to break down an engine from a downed helicopter and understand how to put it together again to make it work.

But, ultimately, all the research in the world was not what

was important to Jay. What was important was that he was saving lives. For him, the proof was what he was seeing before his very eyes: stage-4 cancers (and other diseases) disappearing; stage-4 cancers (and other diseases) disappearing rapidly; and stage-4 cancers (and other diseases) disappearing rapidly with very little outlay of money by the patients.

But, as Jay says, the documentation that low-level radiation works is extensive. Nobody who takes the time to read the research can argue with the fact that this phenomenon is real. But, what had not been accomplished, until Jay figured out how to do it, was a delivery system. The mines work; the water spas work; the effect lingers for a period of time. But then you go home, and eventually the effect wears off. It gets expensive to continue going back to the location of where the radioactivity is naturally present.

Jay figured out a way to bring natural radiation home to the patient. It's simple; it's cheap, and it works. It works as effectively as drugs, without the toxic side-effects of drugs.

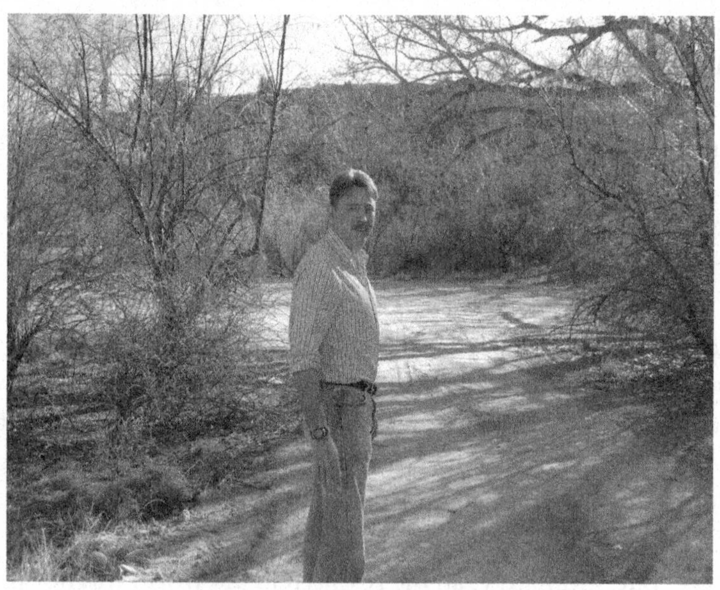

Jay Gutierrez at Two Buttes, Colorado.

6

WHO'S HUNGRY? (AND THE CANCER CONNECTION)

> The hypothesis of the risks of cancer induced by low doses and dose-rates is founded on the extrapolation of data of highly-exposed human groups, applying the risk as being constantly proportional to the received dose without being limited by a threshold, the linear no-threshold (LNT) assumption. This hypothesis conflicts with itself and has many scientific objections; and it is contradicted by experimental data and epidemiology . . . [the Academy] denounces utilization of the linear no-threshold (LNT) relation to estimate the effect of low doses. — The French Academy of Medicine, Dec 2001

HERE'S WHAT JAY SAYS WHEN a cancer patient calls: "Oh, can't you give me something harder to work with?" Yes—hard as it is to believe, Jay finds cancer to be one of the easiest diseases to reverse with radiation hormesis. He has seen the stones eliminate solid tumors in four months. He considers colon, breast and brain cancers to be often a "piece of cake to treat."

But Jay's sense of how the stones impact on cancer has been a gradual deepening of understanding. For a long time, Jay thought the success he was having with his cancer patients was due to the phenomenon that he had read about in the research material—the main theory that underlies the effectiveness of radiation hormesis: the activation of the immune system. This theory suggests that it is the person's own body that is fighting off the cancer. Given the vast extent of research on radiation hormesis that had arrived at this conclusion, such an explanation for Jay's own success seemed reasonable as well as sufficient at the time.

A fortuitous phone call one day changed his understanding. A group of women who he had spoken to some weeks earlier called him; they were all crying. They told him that their friend, Cindy, who they were sitting with, was going into a grand mal seizure. One of the women taking care of her grabbed one of the stones that Jay had sent, and put it on the back of Cindy's head. Instantly, the seizure stopped. As Jay was to find out, the seizure was the least of Cindy's problems. She was on oxygen twenty-four hours a day, couldn't use her hands, could barely talk, was in a wheelchair and was in so much pain that morphine had ceased to be useful as a pain-killer. Cindy had been like this for seventeen years. When she had last seen her doctor, who had been her physician for twenty years, he told her that this was as good as it was going to be. Seemingly parenthetically, the physician had diagnosed the patient as having an extreme amount of systemic aspergillus, a specific form of fungus. This reference to aspergillus was the first time Jay had heard of this form of fungus, but as fate would have it, it was nowhere near the last.

Jay's stone that stopped Cindy's seizure had been a gift from a friend, but until that day, Cindy had never used it. After that initial phone call, Jay worked closely with her, using the stones in a variety of ways for the next thirty days. When Cindy next walked into her doctor's office, she stood there, with her hand out and said, "Hi Doc, how are you doing." Needless to say, her physician stood there, absolutely stunned, for quite some time.

AND NOW, FOR CANCER

Jay's first cancer patient came from a physician who Jay had been working with and who was using the stones with her patients for pain relief and other minor problems. The physician called Jay late at night in an absolute panic because she had just been informed that her own daughter had been diagnosed with brainstem gliomas, and had been given just a few years to live. She asked Jay, in desperation, if he thought there was anything he could do.

Jay describes that he found himself, at 3 a.m. in his shop, digging through a pile of stones that he had recently mined. He had an eerie sense that there had to be one right and perfect stone for the young girl's condition. And then, seemingly miraculously, the stone appeared. Jay felt confident that this was the stone that he needed to help the girl. He took the stone into the shop, sliced it up, and rounded it out until it was in a condition that made it ready and easy to be used.

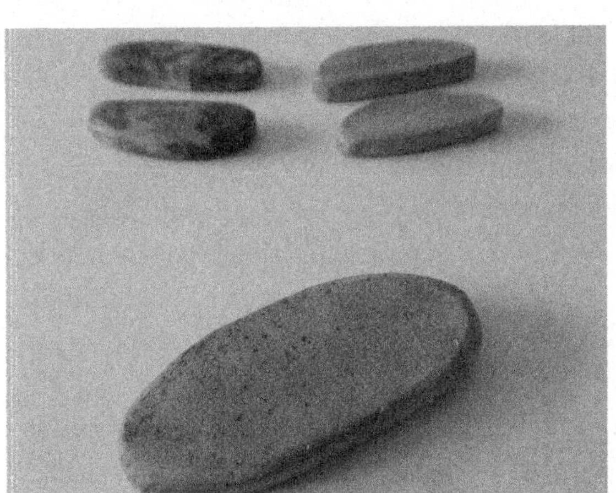

A sample of some of Jay's radiation hormesis stones.

The next morning Jay sent the cut stone to the physician. He instructed her to place it right over the tumors that were at the base of her daughter's brain. And then he, and the physician, and the young girl waited. All they could do was wait. But, after a nerve-racking month and a half, the girl had a Pet-scan to re-evaluate her condition. It's hard to say who was more surprised and overjoyed—Jay, the mother, or the girl. The tumors were completely gone!

At that point, Jay got more confident in working specifically with cancer, and started working consistently with other cancer patients. He found that he was having great success with even terminal cases.

And then, the aspergillus word appeared again. Jay researched aspergillus, learning more about fungi in general as well as this fungus. Fungi are single cell living forms of life which inhabit the land, air and waters of the earth. They occupy a kind of twilight zone, falling somewhere between plant and animal. They are everywhere, and have been here on earth several billion years.

Quite remarkably, fungi have had little genetic change over that period of time. They are survivalists. They can change their form from rapidly growing to no growth for thousands of years, such as seen in their living spores which have been found in Egyptian tombs. They have the ability to endlessly and creatively modify their metabolism to overcome the defenses of their host. They are exceptionally aggressive, attacking plants, animal tissue, food supplies, as well as other fungi and protozoa, amoebas and nematodes.

There are over 500,000 different species of fungi. They are more highly developed than bacteria and viruses—and also harder to get rid of once they have established a foothold in the body. The fungus that most of us are familiar with—we see it growing on food that we keep too long—is mold. Molds reproduce by releasing spores into the air.

The main route of entry of mold spores is through inhalation of dust particles contaminated with the fungi. Immune responses to inhaled spores is a natural defense against infection. The immune response, however, can induce inflammation in the lungs and lead to chronic and sometimes lethal infections that are difficult to diagnose.

From learning about fungus, Jay's whole understanding of how the radiation hormesis operated changed.

Jay's next case was when a doctor he had worked with in

Pennsylvania called about a patient who was dying of breast cancer. She told Jay that the woman's breast had a tumor that had been seeping for some time, and that the material oozing out had a foul smell. The doctor wanted to use an escharotic on the tumor. Escharotics, sometimes called black salve, are a mixture of bloodroot and zinc chloride, and have a long history of use with cancer tumors. But escharotics are corrosive agents and are generally exceedingly painful to the patient. The physician wasn't sure that her patient could bear the pain.

Jay was specifically interested in the physician's description that the oozing material was foul-smelling. Jay was aware that of all pathogenic agents, fungus has the most distinctive and most foul odor. As he says: "If you can smell it, it is a fungus." Jay suspects that the recent success of using dogs to smell cancer has to do with the distinct smell of fungus.

Jay sent the physician an especially hot stone—a stone with a higher than usual level of radiation, and instructed the physician to tell her patient to put the stone directly on the tumor. Within twenty-four hours, the tumor stopped seeping. In two weeks, the tumor was completely gone.

Jay's insight came to him as an epiphany: he remembered that the theory postulated by research scientists of the successful effect of radiation hormesis is that the radiation is slightly damaging to cells. Cells in the body are normally in a constant state of duplication and repair. This duplication, or renewal, occurs in practically every cell of the body. Healthy cells excel at this task of continuous repair in response to repetitive injury. For example,

- you get a whole new stomach lining every ten days.
- you get new skin every thirty days.
- you get a new liver every six weeks.
- you get new lungs, new arteries, and new blood cells every three months.
- and you get new bone cells every six months.

When there is damage, the body goes into action to repair itself in the most efficient way possible. When you get a bruise, your body heals it. When you get a cut on your skin, your body heals it. When you get a broken bone, your body heals it. It's all part of your body's cycle of renewal, where old cells die and new ones are born.

What Jay understood, at the moment of his epiphany, was that the process of repair when fungus is involved is more complicated than the normal process of cellular and tissue repair. What is also happening with the use of radiation hormesis is that the radiation is damaging not just the healthy cells but the cells of the fungus as well. And here is the crux of Jay's insight: the fungus can't repair itself as rapidly as the healthy human cells can. The fungus ends up dying. And consequently, because the healthier cells are now no longer being stressed by the presence of the fungus, nor by the accompanying pathologic complications of the fungus, the healthy cells end up being restored to their normal, vigorous functioning.

WHO'S HUNGRY?

When you have a fungus in the body, the fungus demands to be fed. Who's really hungry when you feel a craving for food, especially for sweet food? Is it you? Or, is it the fungus? The answer most often is that it is the fungus who is hungry. Fungi, like viruses and bacteria, are living organisms. They do not exist without a daily menu of the food they like to eat. We know that cancer specifically feeds on sugar. Research has shown that fungi, bacteria, viruses—all pathogens, in fact, feed on sugar.

Physician Max Gerson, who cured countless cancer patients in the 1940s and 50s, and whose protocol is still being used today to cure cancer, noticed that several diseases were common to his cancer patients. He stated:

I found cancer frequently combined with chronic

osteoarthritis, high or low blood pressure, chronic sinus trouble, or other chronic infections . . .

What is interesting about this list is the concordance of these diseases with known fungal infestations. Chronic sinusitis is caused by a fungus—even orthodox medicine admits this. Osteoarthritis is an inflammatory disease. The foods most suspected of creating this inflammation are rich in fungi, molds and yeasts.

The natural foods used to treat or prevent hypertension are very similar to the natural foods used to treat or prevent cancer, suggesting that these two diseases have a common correlative, if not causative factor. Furthermore, these two diseases both have a high correlation with smoking: tobacco is heavily loaded with fungi and yeasts.

Fungus is like an internal vulture: it eats dead tissue in the body. Once we have fungus in our bodies, we become microbial chemical factories that support the growth of the fungus. Fungi are masters at producing a wide array of biologically active substances that serve the producing fungus extremely well.

While there are many thousands of fungi that have been identified, most of them are harmless and cause no disruption in our healthy functioning. But, after its meal, fungus expels a byproduct. We call this waste product "mycotoxins," and these mycotoxins are excreted within the body, and then absorbed by the body's cells, tissues and bloodstream. While the fungus itself may be harmless, the mycotoxins are capable of causing disease and death in humans and other animals. All molds and yeast are mycotoxins.

It is the mycotoxins that are the ultimate cause of many health problems and the main culprit behind most diseases. Fungi and their mycotoxins manipulate their hosts on the cellular level, and prevent us from defending ourselves by subverting the immune system. Fungi perform around 350 different hormone conversions.

As with most waste products, they are poisonous. The mycotoxins kill healthy tissue, thus creating more food for the fungus. The immune system then falls behind in repairing the damage the mycotoxins have created. In its attempt to kill the fungus, the defenses of the body are often fighting a losing battle.

Over 1,000 mycotoxins were studied in the 1930s and 1940s by the pharmacology industry as potential antibiotics. They were discarded as being too toxic for use. Yet, some have survived the test of medical safety and are currently used in medication. In order to understand the level of toxicity mycotoxins emit, one has only to look at what some of these mycotoxin medications cause in humans. For instance, the mycotoxin cyclosporine, used for organ transplantation, causes cancer and atherosclerosis. It also causes hyperlipidemia—elevation of lipids, including cholesterol and triglycerides—in *all* humans who have received it. Many develop gout and other diseases as well.

Several researchers and clinicians have indicated the specific correlation between cancer and fungi. Italian oncologist Tulio Simoncini says in his book, *Cancer is a Fungus*, that a fungus infection forms the basis of every neoplastic occurrence, and this formation tries to spread within the whole organism without stopping. Further, he says that the growth of the fungus colonies, together with the reaction of the tissue that tries to defend itself against the invasion, causes the tumor.

Similarly, Constantini, Wieland and Qvick, in their book, *Prevention of Breast Cancer: Hope at Last*, say that all major types of cancers found in humans have been documented to be correlated with the presence of aflatoxin, a specific mycotoxin from fungus. Their position on the role of mycotoxins in cancer is particularly compelling because of the weight of authority they bring to their research with their respective qualifications. A.V. Costantini, M.D. is the head of the World Health Organization (WHO), as well as Professor and Medical Director in Clinical Chemistry, Department of Internal Medicine, School of Medicine, Albert

Ludwigs University, Freiburg, Germany. Heinrich Wieland, M.D. is Medical Director for WHO, and Professor at the Collaborating Center For Mycotoxins in Food, Division of Clinical Chemistry in the Department of Internal Medicine, School of Medicine, Albert Ludwigs University, Freiburg, Germany. Lars I. Qvick, M.D., Ph.D. is Co-Medical Director of WHO as well as Professor at the Collaborating Center For Mycotoxins In Food, Division of Clinical Chemistry, Department of Internal Medicine, School of Medicine, Albert Ludwigs University, Freiburg, Germany and Medical Director, Pharmacia AB Stockholm, Sweden.

Researcher and clinician Robert Young goes so far as to say that there is no such thing as a cancer cell: there are only cells that become fungalized as a result of an overly acidic condition in which microorganisms can grow speedily and happily.

The forms of cancers that have been shown to be caused by fungi-mycotoxins are: adrenal cancer; angioma; brain tumor; breast cancer; colon cancer; esophogeal cancer; gallbladder cancer; intestinal cancer; kidney cancer; laryngeal cancer; leukemia; liver cancer; lung cancer; lymphoma; nasal cancer; nerve cancer; oral cancer; osteogenic cancer; ovarian cancer; pancreas cancer; parathyroid cancer; pituitary cancer; prostate cancer; rectal cancer; salivary cancer; sarcoma; skeletal; skin cancer; stomach cancer; testicular cancer; thyroid cancer; tracheal cancer; urinary cancer; urogenital cancer; uterine cancer; vaginal cancer.

GETTING WORSE BEFORE GETTING BETTER

Jay noticed, as many holistic healers before him have noticed, that when someone has been ill, if they take a natural path toward cure, before they get better, often they get worse. This is known as the "Herxheimer's reaction." Dr. Carl Herxheimer, a German dermatologist, first described the body's reaction to the massive killing of microorganisms. This massive killing results in a sudden load of toxins that is released into the bloodstream. Nutritionist Bernard Jensen called this stage of recovery the "healing crisis." As the body begins to heal, it needs to detoxify from the toxic poisons and wastes that have accumulated. This process of detoxification releases waste and pathogenic products from cells and tissues, and as these toxic wastes are being circulated in the body, on their way toward being eliminated from the body through the various eliminative channels, the person can experience symptoms of temporary toxicity. Symptoms such as headache, nausea, even a worsening of the same symptoms that made the person feel ill, might occur in the first days of detoxification from use of the stones. Jay, like all other holistic healers, considers these good reactions to the stones, indicating that the body is mounting a response. Jay's understanding of why radiation hormesis works is consonant with this holistic theory of waste removal and death of pathogenic material: by constantly damaging and killing the fungus through the application of the low-level radiation, the fungus eventually dies. As it is dying, it will drop more mycotoxins than normal.

This is what most holistic practitioners call "die off" or, as Jensen called it, a healing crisis. Jay refers to it as the "aggravation period." After this detoxification process happens, the body begins the process of repair that most of the theories of radiation hormesis have posited as the healing mechanism: the immune system is stimulated, and in its activation, it is enabled to speed up the repair from the damage caused by the mycotoxins.

Jay's understanding, then, is that the stones create a five-stage process: 1) the pathogens, including fungus and mycotoxins, are killed from the stress effect of the low-level radiation; 2) because of the death of these cells, the progression of growth of the pathogenic material is thwarted; 3) the normal cells, however, remain unaffected by the radiation because they are stronger and not as easy to kill; 4) the mess from the mycotoxins is cleaned up by the still healthy cells from the body's various mechanisms of detoxification; and 5) because of the first four stages, the damage from the pathogenic material is able to be repaired by the body's natural defense and immune mechanisms.

Otto Warburg won a Nobel Prize in 1931 for his understanding that cancer is a disease of an oxygen-deficient environment. He found that in reducing the oxygen supply to normal healthy tissue, the tissue then became cancerous. Perhaps Warburg was witnessing the effect of fungal spores. These spores can stay hidden in most living tissue, and, like cancer, they are able to grow aneorobically, without oxygen and using sugar as their primary source of energy for growth. Often they grow so steadily and prolifically that they then became the dominant life form.

In effect, Jay came to the conclusion that if your illness is caused by a fungus, then the effect of the radiation will be stronger. Because cancer has been shown to be generally intimately involved with fungal overgrowth, Jay has had great success with treating and curing many forms of cancer.

Over the fifteen years that Jay has been actively working with patients, and the wide range of health issues he has encountered in his patients, the more he is convinced that fungus, mainly candida, is the main culprit when dealing with ill health and all diseases. Because fungus presents itself in a myriad of ways in the body, Jay has seen many diverse illnesses, but always with the common thread being that they were fungus related.

The diseases that have been commonly associated with fungal overgrowth is as long as a list of diseases can be: anxiety; AIDS; Alzheimer's; arthritis; asthma; atherosclerosis; autoimmune disease; bladder disease; boils on neck; brain disorders; brain fog; casein-induced amyloidosis; chronic fatigue; Crohn's Disease; Cushing's Disease; depression; diabetes; digestive disorders; muscular dystrophy; ear, nose and throat illnesses; eye diseases; eczema; fertility problems; fibromyalgia; gout; hair loss; heart disease; hormone problems; hyperactivity; hyperaldosteronism; hyperlipidemia; hypertension; inflammatory bowel disease; intestinal disorders; joint pain; kidney stones; memory loss; mental dysfunction; Mollaret's Meningitis; multiple sclerosis; muscle stiffness; nail fungus; obesity; pain; postpartum depression; psoriasis; Raynaud's Syndrome/Disease; respiratory disorders; rheumatoid arthritis; sarcoid arthritis; sarcoidosis; sick building syndrome; sinusitis; skin disease; swollen lymph nodes; systemic sclerosis; thrombocytopenic purpura; weakened immune system; weight problems; yeast-related health problems.

Jay's impression is that it seems as though civilization has been gradually losing its ability to fend off these encroaching parasites. Yet, he has demonstrated that the use of the hormesis stones is an effective, fast and economical way of killing fungus and all other pathogens, and restoring the body to good health.

7

LETHALLY EXPOSED OR LIVING LONGER

In reference to the misconceptions of risks of low-dose radiation, such practices are "deeply immoral uses of our scientific heritage."
— Lauriston Taylor, chief of the Biophysics Branch in the Division of Biology and Medicine of the Atomic Energy Division; Chairman of the National Council on Radiation Protection and Measurements (NCRP)

THE RESEARCH DATA ON RADIATION hormesis come from a variety of sources and from laboratories and researchers all around the world. Ed Hiserodt, author of *Under-Exposed: What If Radiation is Actually Good for You*, organizes the data around four different research approaches:

1) animal tests: most of these are on mice. Mice have essentially the same genes as humans, only rearranged;
2) human studies of radiation exposure;
3) statistics of workers in nuclear power plants;
4) statistics on populations that live in high-background radiation areas.

Here are the results of only a few of the more than 3,000

studies documenting the effect of radiation hormesis:

ANIMAL STUDIES

- According to a letter written by Marshall Brucer, M.D. to *Time* magazine, mice exposed to modest amounts of uranium dust lived longer than controls.
- In 1963, the Atomic Energy Commission confirmed that morbidity rates were lower and longevity was greater in mice, rats, guinea pigs and hamsters that had received low-dose irradiation.
- Cows had been exposed to radiation after a Trinity A-Bomb test in New Mexico. They were seven to eight years old at the time of the test. They lived another eighteen years, and were finally euthanized because the humans got tired of waiting to see when they would die from radiation poisoning. Most cattle rarely live longer than fifteen years.
- Many studies have seen this effect: pregnant rats exposed to low-dose radiation became more fecund, producing more offspring per litter, an effect that persisted through twelve generations.
- One mouse study demonstrated that low-dose pre-exposure protected the brain from subsequent high-dose exposure.
- In an intensive analysis of immune cell populations in mice exposed to low-level radiation, immune stimulation was found.
- Irradiated mice showed a 20 percent decrease in ovarian cancer, a 46 percent decrease in mammary cancer, a 13 percent decrease in uterine cancer. Many other studies confirm the effect that low-level irradiation protects mice from cancers.
- Mice receiving 1,000 times their normal background dose of radiation lived longer than their non-irradiated cohorts.
- Mice were deliberately infected with a virus: those exposed to radiation recovered while the control mice all died within forty days.

- Daphnia magna is an aquatic animal whose population consists almost entirely of females. Interestingly, males are not required for reproduction. Females produce eggs in a transparent pouch found on the top of their bodies. The eggs develop into young and are released from the mother approximately every three days. In the study, females were irradiated with gamma rays from a Cobalt-60 source, to total doses of 250, 500, 1,000, 2,000, and 5,000 rads. Each brood of young was watched carefully so that the effects of the radiation exposure could be determined and documented. Relative to the "control" population, which received no radiation dose other than that from the ambient background, increased life-span, reproduction, and survival were noted in all of the dose groups except for those irradiated to 2,000 and 5,000 rads. At those higher doses, detrimental effects began to appear including reduced life-span and aborted young.

HUMAN STUDIES

- Dr. Sohei Kondo, in his 1993 book, *Health Effects of Low-Level Radiation*, documented that survivors of Nagasaki and Hiroshima who received some radioactive exposure live longer and healthier than those who had no exposure to the post-bomb radiation.
- A thirty-year follow-up of 1,155 low-dose radium dial painters showed that they had significantly fewer cancers than the general population and also lived much longer.
- Research on the health effects of plutonium inhaled and ingested by the Manhattan Project workers at Los Alamos was started in 1952 to determine the delayed effects. Workers at Rocky Flats and the Mound Laboratory were also studied. Although plutonium has been called "the most toxic substance known to man," the exposed group has remained in surprisingly good health ever since. Dire

predictions of catastrophic increases of lung cancers have not occurred. In fact, mortality has been significantly lower than the non-plutonium workers.

- A Japanese study reported on a twenty-five year follow-up study of Japanese fishermen who were heavily contaminated by plutonium from the hydrogen bomb test at the Bikini Atoll. So far none of the fishermen have died from cancer.
- Double-blind studies performed on patients at Japan's Misasa Radon Springs have confirmed the ability of its radioactive water to relieve rheumatism, neuralgia and other complaints. Similar results were obtained in studies conducted in conjunction with Radon Therapy Hospital specialists at Austria's Bad Gastein spa.

BACKGROUND RADIATION STUDIES

- In a large scale Chinese study, it was shown that the mortality rate due to cancer was lower in an area with a relatively high background radiation (74,000 people), while the control group (78,000 people) who lived in an area with low background radiation had a higher rate of mortality.
- In an area in Japan with a high average indoor radon level, the lung cancer incidence was about 50 percent less than the incidence in a low-level radon region. Researchers Mifune and Mifune also showed that in this high background radiation area, the mortality rate caused by all types of cancer was 37 percent lower.
- In the U.S., Bernard Cohen's large scale study indicated that the total cancer mortality is inversely correlated with background radiation dose.
- In another large scale study by Frigerio in the U.S., it was found that the mortality rate due to all malignancies was lower in states with higher annual radiation dose.
- In India, Nambi and Soman observed that in areas with a high background radiation level, the incidence of cancer and also

the mortality rate due to cancer was significantly less than similar areas with a low background radiation level.

- A study of people living in Ramsar, Iran, who are exposed to natural high levels of background radiation, have not shown increased cases of cancer.
- Rates of leukemia and lymphocytic lymphoma were studied in relation to altitude. Higher altitudes have higher radiation. The finding, however, was the higher the altitude, the lower the incidence of leukemia.
- In Brazil, the radiation level is five to ten times the "normal" amount. In a study by Freire-Maya and Kreiger of 44,000 pregnancies, no abnormalities or stillbirths were to be found.
- In China, as reported by Blot, a study compared background radiation levels from homes of women suffering from lung cancer. Those who lived in high-level radon homes had an 80 percent lower lung cancer risk than those living in a low-radon home.
- Auxier shows that in Kerala, India, there is 400-800 percent more background radiation than neighboring areas, yet the people there have the highest fertility rate with the lowest neonatal deaths of any other Indian state.
- In Germany, women living near uranium mining areas of Saxony, Germany, with high radon levels, have significantly lower lung cancer rates than a control group from East Germany where the radon levels are lower.
- In England, the towns of Cornwall and Devon have high background radon levels, yet have a cancer incidence well below the national average.
- 1,700 Taiwan apartments were constructed with steel girders accidentally contaminated with Cobalt-60, one of the more dreaded radioactive substances. Over a period of sixteen years, 10,000 occupants were exposed to levels of radiation that, according to traditional theories of the damaging

effect of all radiation, should have induced cancers many times in excess of background expectations. Taiwan health statistics predicted 170 cancers among an age-matched population of this size. But only five were observed. Describing this "incredible radiological incident," Y. C. Luan suggested that this might point to "effective immunity from cancer" from the very source thought most likely to give rise to it. In spite of the research findings showing that living in these radioactive apartments conferred protection against cancer, today, many years later, the building remains empty.

NUCLEAR POWER PLANT STUDIES

- In a Canadian study by Abbat et al., it was shown that the mortality caused by cancer at nuclear power plants was 58 percent lower than the national average.
- In the UK, Kendall et al. show that cancer frequency among nuclear power plant workers was lower than the national average.
- Luckey summarized the major nuclear worker vs. non-nuclear-worker studies and showed that the nuclear workers have 52 percent of the cancer rate in comparable non-exposed workers.
- Los Alamos workers had 58 percent as much total cancer mortality as the rest of the U.S. population.
- Gilbert et al., in studies of plutonium workers at Rocky Flats in Colorado, showed cancer deaths to be 64 percent of the average in the general population.
- One of the largest and most thorough studies of the effects of low-level radiation on nuclear industry workers is the Nuclear Shipyard Workers Study, funded by the U.S. Department of Energy, but never published. This ten-year, $10-million study matched 39,004 nuclear workers with 33,352 non-nuclear workers. The study was completed in

1987. In spite of the extensiveness of the study, results were released in 1991 only after pressure on the DOE, and it was in the form of a contractor's report, consisting of a brief two-page press release. The radiation workers in the study were exposed to external Cobalt-60. Myron Pollycove of the Nuclear Regulatory Commission documented that the cancer mortality is significantly lower among nuclear workers than among the non-nuclear workers.

- Kendall found that workers at Los Alamos who worked in factories generating radioactive substances, and who followed appropriate safe-handling practices received, on average, a three-fold higher exposure to plutonium than the maximum recommended by the National Council on Radiation Protection. People who worked at Los Alamos in factories generating radioactive substances have had less cancer and better immunity, and have lived longer.
- According to Voelz et al., the proportion of the total number of Los Alamos exposed workers who have died has been 57 percent lower than in the general population, and 43 percent lower than among Los Alamos workers who were not exposed.

HOW RADIATION CAUSES HARM

It is important to remember that high-level radiation is destructive to all living tissue. The studies cited here, showing positive effects, are not studying high-radiation exposure. They are studying low-level radiation exposure. The hormesis effect is the difference of a toxin depending on the dose. In the study on plutonium, for instance, the Rocky Flats workers had a lower cancer rate. But, the fact is: all heavy metals are toxic. In larger doses, they are extremely dangerous. Radiation, too, in large doses, is highly destructive.

It is useful to discuss how high-level radiation causes harm to the body. When radiation enters the body and hits a cell, one of four things can happen:

(1) radiation may pass through the cell without doing damage;
(2) it may damage the cell, but the cell may be able to repair the damage before producing new cells;
(3) it may damage the cell in such a way that the damage is passed on when new cells are formed; or
(4) it may kill a healthy cell.

If the radiation passes through the cell without doing damage or the cell repairs itself successfully (numbers 1 and 2), there is no lasting damage or health effect.

If the damage is passed on when new cells are formed (number 3), there may be a delayed health effect, such as cancer or genetic effects. Delayed effects from high-level radiation exposure may occur months, years, or decades later. If the damage to a cell is not repaired and is passed on to new cells (number 3), a cancer can begin to grow. There is a latent period during which time the cancer is growing to a size where it is large enough to be detected. The time of this latent period varies for different types of health effects and different types of radiation doses.

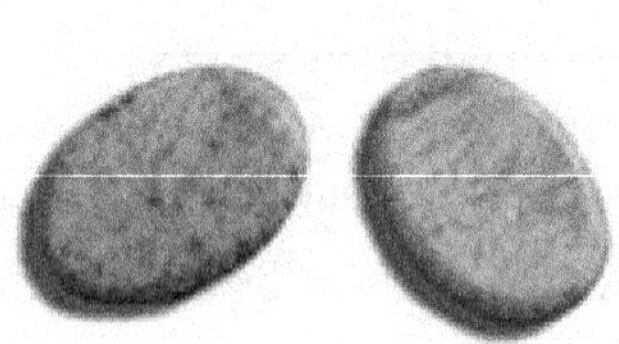

A set of Eye Stones.

When radiation kills a healthy cell (number 4), there will be acute and immediate health effects if the dose is high and many cells die. Death may occur within days or weeks from radiation sickness. Other acute effects include vomiting and loss of hair.

Radiation is also dangerous when used inappropriately to kill pathogens unnecessarily. Irradiating food has been an attempt to kill off pathogenic microorganisms before the food even reaches human mouths. The purpose of this practice is to prolong the shelf life of the food, and at this task, radiation excels.

The very success, however, of radiation's ability to kill microorganisms is also why it can be destructive to human health when used to "sanitize" food. While it is true that microorganisms can be destructive to our health by stealing nutrients, it is also true that they can contribute to the healthy functioning of an organism. For instance, some parasites pre-digest the food of the host organism into a form which the host can then use, thereby providing more effective and efficient assimilation of nutrients from one's diet. As well, parasites are effective in removing waste products which, without this function, would attract other toxic and deadly parasites.

An FDA report from 1968 found significant adverse effects produced in animals fed irradiated food, including:

- a decrease of 21 percent in surviving weaned rats
- a 32 percent decrease in surviving progeny of dogs
- dogs weighing 11 percent less than animals on the control diets
- carcinomas of the pituitary gland, a particularly disturbing finding since this is an extremely rare type of malignant tumor

In addition, a 1959 study in the *Journal of Nutrition* found that a statistically significant number of rats fed irradiated beef died from internal hemorrhage within 46 days. In 2000, another study in *Food Irradiation* concluded that food irradiation will increase the incidence of cancer. However, the article proposed that it will take between four to six decades to demonstrate a statistically significant increase in cancer due to mutagens introduced into food by irradiation. If food irradiation is finally prohibited, several decades worth of people with a susceptibility for cancer would then be in the cancer pipeline.

According to the Organic Consumers Association, irradiation of food breaks up cell walls, slices and dices chromosomes, kills enzymes, destroys vitamins, disrupts the chemical composition of food, and creates free radicals. These free radicals then recombine to form other stable compounds, continuing on their destructive path. Some of the compounds created are known carcinogens, including formaldehyde, benzene, lipid peroxides. Others of these compounds have never been seen or studied before.

In a study published in the *Proceedings of the National Academy of Sciences*, scientists from the University of Wisconsin-Madison report on cats developing severe neurological symptoms due to a degradation of myelin, the fatty insulator of nerve fibers called axons. The cats developed neurological problems only after they started being fed irradiated food. When they were taken off the irradiated diet, the animals' nervous systems began healing.

According to the Center for Disease Control and Prevention, "If the food still has living cells, they will be damaged or killed just as microbes are." Their website continues: food irradiation practices "inhibit sprouting . . ." And therein lays the problem. A food that has been stripped of its living cells, and is no longer capable of continuing the on-going life process of sprouting, is a food that can no longer transfer its living energy to our own bodies. Irradiated food no longer fits into the definition of the substance we call "food."

Water, too, is severely impacted by irradiation. We know from nuclear testing that profound malignant changes can occur in both people and animals exposed to high-level radiation. A primary cause may be the effect on water. When the explosion occurs, waves are formed which die quickly in the ground. But water continues to fluctuate for another 30 days. Swinging like a pendulum, these waves create a new and pathological ordering in the water. This change in the structure of water covers an area many miles away from the testing grounds. It makes no difference whether the test has been conducted in the atmosphere, on the ground, or underground.

People and animals then drink the water, and terrible

changes in them can occur. It has been noted that the number of suicides rises abruptly after such testing by a factor of two or three. Victor Inyushin, Head of the Biophysics Department of Kazakhstan University, explains this phenomenon: "The brain is made of water—about 85 percent. So these changes take place in the brain, and a conflict between the water structures arises. The bioplasma of the brain is disrupted, and the result is that the person is deprived of such an extremely important incentive as the drive to live."

OUR BEST PROTECTION AGAINST A NUCLEAR ATTACK

If our country were bombed, it would kill hundreds of thousands. The bombs would cause a large number of immediate deaths from the blasts themselves, and then yet more deaths from radiation poisoning. There would also be many subsequent radiological-induced cancers. And, as with the nuclear testing, water would change its structure, and thus, our brains would be affected.

There is, however, an interesting phenomenon to understand about how therapeutic low-level radiation protects against later exposure to potentially dangerous high-level radiation. The point being: if we are unfortunate enough to be attacked by a nuclear bomb, those who have been using Jay's hormesis stones will fare better in tolerating the high-level radiation that close proximity to the explosion will emit.

The phenomenon is called the "adaptive response." It is an important type of biological defense mechanism against all stressing agents, including but not limited to radiation. Here, living organisms (as small as cells, or as large as human beings) are exposed to a stress. This initial stress protects the organism against subsequent further and stronger stresses.

In terms of radiation hormesis, this is most easily studied by exposing cells to a low dose of radiation, thus priming the cell for its adaptive response. Then the cell is exposed to a high dose of radiation, a much more challenging dose. The adaptive response is observed when the effect of the high-dose is lower than when a similar challenge exposure has been administered, but without the initial priming dose.

Chromosome aberrations, the simplest tool for detecting genetic damage, have been studied in relation to adaptive response to low-dose radiation. It has been long known that radiation increases the number of genetic aberrations. Shadley's study on human lymphocyte cells shows that gene aberration is beneficially affected if the high dose is preceded a few hours before by a low dose: the number of chromosome aberrations caused by the high dose is substantially reduced.

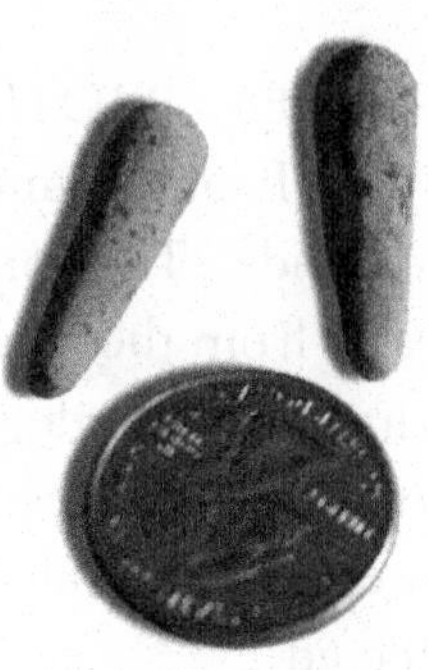

Ear Stones.

In another experiment, it was found that exposure of mouse cells to high dosage radiation caused chromosome aberrations in 38 percent of bone marrow cells and in 12.6 percent of spermatocytes. When these exposures were preceded three hours earlier by an exposure to low-dose radiation, the percentages were reduced to 19.5 percent and 8.4 percent respectively. There are many other examples of animal experiments, and the results are usually explained as stimulated production of repair enzymes by low-level radiation.

There are also many studies on humans that demonstrate the adaptive response after low-level radiation exposure. Studies have been done using various methods of testing the comparative effects, including detection of genetic mutations as well as detection of mutations in offspring. Also, the time of repair of DNA damage has been shown to be substantially reduced from initial low-level radiation exposure.

Brenda Rodgers from Texas Tech University left mice in cages in a Ukrainian forest a mile from where the Chernobyl nuclear accident had occurred eighteen years earlier. She left them there until they got a low-level radiation dose. She then moved them to her lab and quickly bombarded them with a high level of radiation exposure. This big dose created only about half the number of chromosome breaks in the mice pre-exposed to low-dose radiation, as compared to the mice without the pre-exposure.

Tanya Day, of Flinders University in Australia, gave mice a large dose of radiation. Four hours later, some mice received a second, far smaller dose. Rodents getting both doses developed only half as much DNA damage as mice that had just gotten the first dose. In fact, the mice that got the low dose had less damage than the control group of mice receiving no radiation at all.

The protection accrued from the adaptive response is long-lasting. Zaichkina has shown in mouse experiments that the effect lasts to the end of the life of the animal—up to twenty months.

The adaptive response has also been shown to protect an organism from transformation to malignancy. In Azzam's mouse study, after exposure to low-dose radiation, the rate of spontaneous cancer was reduced by 78 percent. In a similar study with human cells, Redpath saw the reduction to be 55 percent. Hashimoto's study in rats showed that total body low-level irradiation reduced the rate of metastasis.

Another study comparing low-level and high-level radiation doses on metastasis of tumors showed that when tumor cells were transplanted into the groins of mice, the rate of their metastasis into the lung was cut in half by total body irradiation with low-level radiation. Sakamoto showed that high doses, however, reduced the immune response, leading to increased rates of metastasis.

Because of these studies, Jay encourages people who have a history of cancer in their family to use the stones prophylactically. He also encourages cancer patients who decide to undergo either chemotherapy or radiation as a treatment for their existing cancer to use the stones first—before the administration of the high-dose therapies, thus priming the body into the adaptive response.

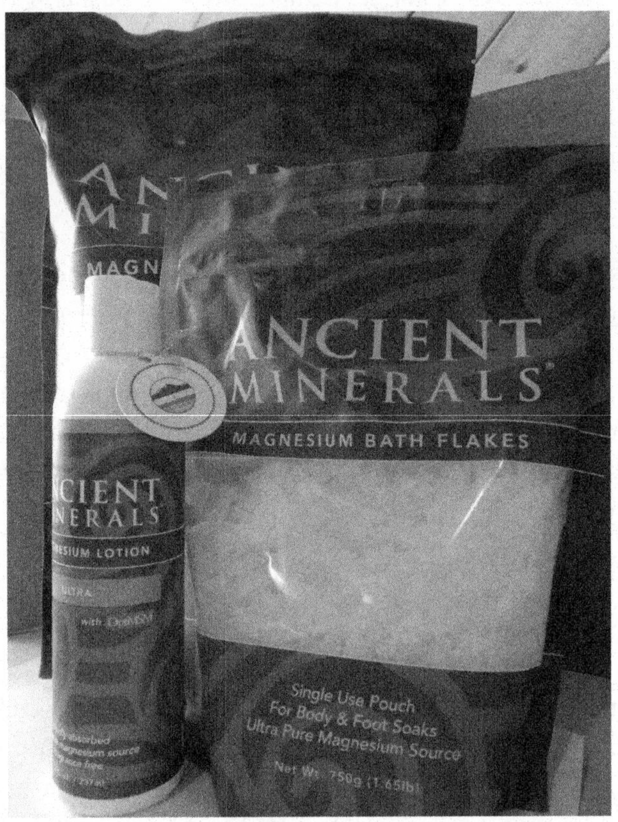

Along with low-dose radiation, Jay puts great emphasis on magnesium, which is an essential component in detoxifying and healing the body, as well as building up the immune system, protecting cells, relieving pain, and insuring proper muscle and hormonal functions. As such, magnesium works hand in hand with Jay's radiation hormesis program. Above are examples of magnesium flakes, oil, gel, and lotion, all which are carried by Night Hawk Minerals.

8

BECAUSE PEOPLE ARE DYING

A significant and growing amount of experimental information indicates that the overall effects of chronic exposure (at low levels) are not harmful. . . . The preponderance of data better supports the hypothesis that low chronic exposures result in an increased longevity . . . Increased vitality at low exposures to materials that are markedly toxic at high exposures is a well-recognized phenomenon. — Hugh F. Henry, *JAMA, 176, 27 May 1961*

ABOVE JAY'S SHOP IN DENVER, where he cuts and polishes the stones, is etched into a wood plague the words: "Because People Are Dying."

Jay is not a researcher. His work would not be seriously considered by any medical review board. They would see his successes as anecdotal (as opposed to double-blind)—a description that is always an insult to any medical methodology that purports to have scientific validity.

Jay doesn't care. He doesn't care because the medical research for the last 100 years has already validated the efficacy of low-level radiation. He doesn't care because he witnesses first-hand that the technique he recommends, of using stones that are slightly radioactive, works. He has witnessed this from over 3,000 cases he has helped. As well, he doesn't care about scientific validity of his work because people are dying.

Until Jay starting mining the stones, the problem with radiation hormesis was that low-level radiation was a scientifically documented phenomenon with no way to implement it into therapeutic activity. No one had figured out a consistent, reliable, easy-to-use on a continuous basis delivery system for the radiation. As Jay says:

> They are constantly doing more experiments, in fact more and more aggressively. They find out it works; they have known for over 100 years that it works. Then it ends. No individual is receiving the benefits of the results of the research. Another thirty years of radiating mice and then curing them of the induced cancers is not going to help the person laying in bed praying for a miracle. We have the method, dosage, and means to help these people. That's why I do this.

Jay believes that everyone breathing, everywhere on the planet should have a kit and a necklace of the stones he mines.

Although radiation hormesis is not a new concept, the therapeutic application of it to humans is. New concepts inevitably raise new questions. What is an optimal level of radon, alpha, beta, gamma and X rays for babies, children, teens, young adults, pregnant females, old people and sick people? How can the art of medicine best use low-dose irradiation? Is ionizing radiation essential for optimal physiologic functions? For life? Should whole populations be supplemented? How? Should control of the usage be given to health professionals, physicians, public health officials, or politicians?

Part of the problem in even thinking about these questions is that there is no consistent way of measuring dosage of radiation emission or exposure. There are generally four different measurement terms: Rads, Rems, Grays, Servs. There is also a different measurement for radiation vs. radon. The mRem/hr. number is the relevant quantity for the absorbed dose from external radiation, while the picoCurie per liter number (pCi/L) is the relevant quantity for the radon in the air we breathe. One country uses one term; another country, another term; one researcher uses one term; another researcher, another term. No one bothers to make a measurement method conversion simple. There is no website that converts all the different measurements back to one.

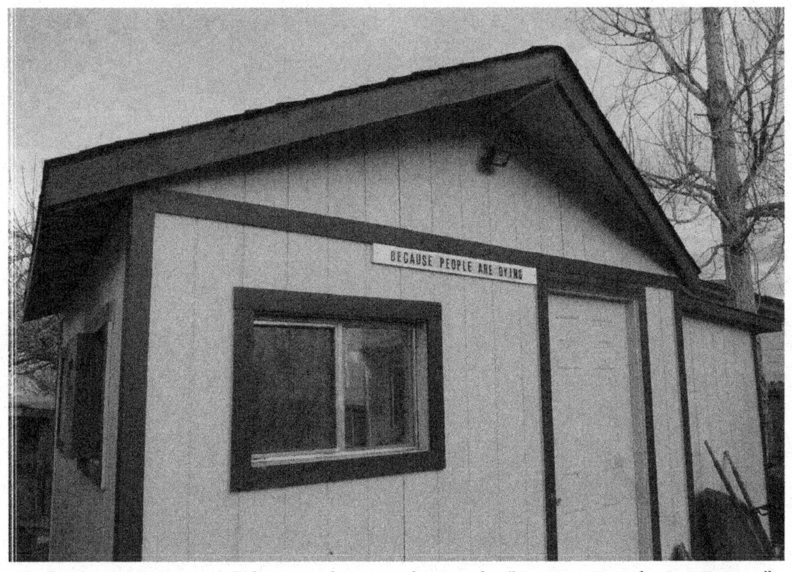

Jay's stone-cutting workshop, with a sign that reads: "Because People Are Dying."

Jay has spent many hours making the conversions so that he can talk to doctors and researchers from all over the world. For instance, one physician he works with from Colombia talks in terms of servs. Everything Jay does with him has to be multiplied times ten. It took some figuring out, but Jay finally understood that one cGy equals one Rem. And, one Rem equals 1,000 mRems.

For the sake of simplicity, Jay uses the measurement of millirems, or mRems. To put Rems and mRems in a context, at the elevation of his spa-hotel in Pritchett, there are about 300 mRems from background radiation a year. Most of us receive between 200 and 300 mRems per year (0.04 mRem/hr.) with background radiation. Flying on a commercial airplane results in approximately 1 mRems per 1,000 miles traveled, so every round trip from New York to Los Angeles results in about 6 mRems of additional exposure.

Sleeping next to another person for eight hours results in approximately 2 mRems per year due to the natural levels of radioactive potassium in our bodies. People that work in Grand Central Station in New York City are exposed to 120 mRems/year from the high uranium content in the granite walls. Brazil nuts have 1,000 times the radioactivity of most foods due to their radium content.

Typical members of the U.S. population receive the following types of radiation exposures (chart posted by Bernard Cohen):

- 650 mRem per nuclear medicine examination of the brain
- 509 mRem per nuclear medicine examination of the thyroid
- 405 mRem per barium enema
- 245 mRem per upper gastrointestinal tract series
- 150 mRem per nuclear medicine examination of the lung
- 110 mRem per computerized tomography of the head and body
- 7.5 mRem per year to spouses of recipients of certain cardiac pacemakers
- 6 mRem per dental x-ray
- 5 mRem per year from foods grown with phosphate fertilizer
- 4 mRem per year from highway and road construction materials
- 1.5 mRem from each cross-country airline trip (one way)
- 1 - 6 mRem per year from domestic water supplies
- 1 mRem per year from television receivers
- 0.5 mRem em from eating one-half pound of Brazil nuts
- 0.3 mRem per year from combustible fuels (coal, natural gas,

liquefied petroleum)
- 0.2 mRem from drinking a quart of Gatorade
- 0.1 mRem per year from sharing a bed with someone

If you used one of Jay's products—the mud pack—and had it next to your body twenty-four hours a day, 365 days a year, the dose you would be receiving would be less than half of what a nuclear worker is allowed per year. As of now, a nuclear worker can receive 30,000 mRems a year and this number is expected to be increased to 60,000 mRems a year. Jay wants his clients to receive 40,000 mRems per year.

Since research has documented that nuclear workers have better health than non-nuclear workers, if anything can be said about the dose Jay is using, it may be that most of us could easily tolerate and benefit from an even higher dose. (And, indeed, for certain afflictions, including most cancers, Jay increases the dosage.)

The other part of the problem with administering low-level radiation therapy has to do with getting it to the people, as opposed to making the people get to it. All of the low-level radiation products that were available in the 1920s and 30s—the radium-laced toothpastes, hair tonics, beauty creams, soaps and candies—are no longer available. The old mines in Montana proved to be then—and are now still—useful—and a lot of people get better from going in them.

But, without continuous exposure to the radiation, the afflictions that lead people to go there in the first place may return. The mines have a repeat clientele—for that very reason. Also, the dosage of the mines is not as strong as research indicates gives the maximum benefits. And, as well, the mines are all in—well—they are all in Montana. That's a long way to go for most people.

Alternatively, you might think to go to a doctor and ask for low-level radiation—after all, short of the few remaining nuclear power plants we have in the U.S., and dismissing those empowered individuals who have their thumbs on the red button of nuclear bombs, physicians have the largest supply of handily available radiation in the country. The problem with this idea of your local physician being your radiation supplier is that it is unlikely that you could find a doctor who would give you low-dose radiation treatments. There is no diagnostic category of affliction that low-dose radiation is recommended as a treatment. Thus, there is no medical protocol for its usage.

And, finally, the radiation would be x-rays, which are a fragmentation of the whole radioactive spectrum of natural Alpha, Beta, and Gamma rays. The stones, unlike medical X rays, are still in their natural state, and are always putting out a different amount and type of energy depending on their state of decay. Since the material is in different states of decay throughout its life, you always get a mixture—which makes the energy emitted whole as opposed to fragmented. It's like the difference between eating a healthy food, say broccoli, which has all the necessary vitamins in the balance that Mother Nature intended, or pulling out one specific vitamin, say vitamin E, and using that as extra supplementation. You can use derivative elements, and you can do it effectively, but whenever you do, you risk creating a systemic imbalance because the other elements may have lost the proportionate ratios in which they naturally occur.

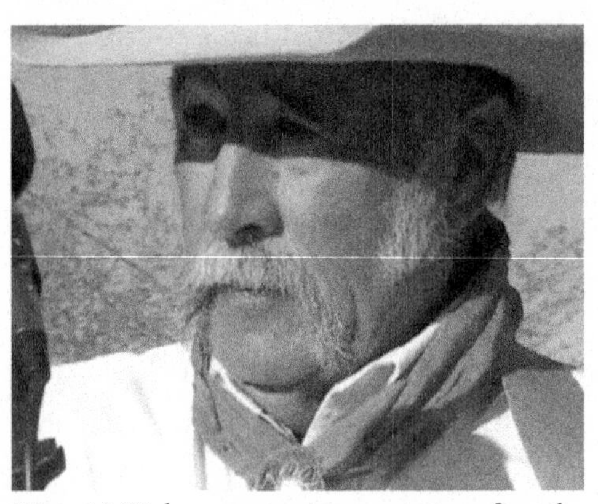

Wes McKinley, state representative for the hi-altitude, lo-cancer-rate, fine state of Colorado. At the grand opening of the Mineral Palace, Wes pronounced these punchy words: "Anywhere you want to go, you can get there from right here. So that makes us the center of the universe."

The other difficulty for Jay in bringing this healing technology to us was in the difficult act of finding and securing the stones. It was Jay's position as a helicopter repairman that led him to be able to go into hard-to-reach parts of the wilderness where the stones live. And, even if one was lucky enough to, similarly, find radioactive stones, there is still the task of cutting and slicing them to insure that they are kept at low doses.

The way in which Jay determined the proper dosage was through observation of the effects with the first people he worked with. They were, in effect, his laboratory experimental subjects, but he had done sufficient initial research to know that the specific doses he was using could, in no way, harm people. He started using a very low radiation emission. He increased the emission .2 mRems each time by sending out new, increasingly "hotter" stones, until the dosage created a noticeable biological response in the individual. There were times when he pushed too hard, and the body's response was uncomfortable for the patient to tolerate. This was the "die-off," or the healing crisis. Jay would then back off, and reduce the dosage.

It didn't take long before Jay was able to perfect a dosage that he found was easily tolerated by most people, yet still stimulated a response. Jay has observed that some people are more sensitive than others, and their response is stronger. He encourages these people to start slower. He may advise someone with known chemical or electromagnetic sensitivities to take only one sip a day of hormesis water, and to build up to higher dosages very slowly.

Jay is confident that no stone that leaves his shop has the ability to harm anyone. The gray stones put out about 0.05 to 0.07 mRems per hour. The mud packs put out about 0.4 mRems per hour. The highest dose comes from the cancer stones—at 30 m/Rems per hour. If Jay is told that someone has only a couple of weeks to live, his approach will be more aggressive, and he will risk an uncomfortable healing reaction with the patient in a final attempt to save the person's life.

The system Jay has developed for getting his stones ready for people to use is elaborate and careful. Jay mines in two different areas: north Wyoming and Utah. He is rarely without a Geiger counter. He uses a digital radiation detector to measure first the radiation level of the stones he finds. Then, after the stones have been made into his products, he measures the level of radiation of each and every stone, as well as the mud packs. As well, every stone Jay finds has to be taken to a lab to have the components analyzed. Many of the stones have arsenic; most malachite has a high level of arsenic. He needs to make sure that he is not having people drinking arsenic.

The products Jay has developed are natural, inexpensive, and simple to use. There are five different choices of application: gray water stones, mud packs, green stones, and pendants to be worn around the neck. For the seriously ill cancer patient, Jay uses what he calls a "hot tumor stone," or alternatively, referred to simply as the "gray stone."

THE GREEN STONE

This stone—also known as the Eilat stone—is quite remarkable because it is both radioactive as well as electric. The stone's unique properties have to do with the fact that it, like the human body, is electric.

All the tissues of our bodies are made of cells. Every function that occurs in the body is due to the activity of cells. Each cell has a waterproof membrane surrounding and protecting it. Because of IONS within the cell that hold an electrical charge, the cell membranes, too, have an electrical charge. A young and healthy cell has a membrane charge of around 70 millivolts.

The body's overall electromagnetic field is naturally at a higher intensity than all pathogenic cells, including bacterial, viral, cancer and fungal cells. An aged cell, similarly, has a membrane charge that is lower than a healthy cell. A cancer tumor cell has a charge as low as 15 millivolts. When the membrane charge becomes critically low, the cell has too little energy. In order for the cell to become healthy again, energy must be given to the cell.

Stones that emit electricity can be either piezoelectric or pyroelectric: the electric energy from a piezo source is derived from torsion or tension; the electric property of a pyro source is from thermal (temperature) change. The green stones work off pyroelectric: thus, a temperature change in the stone increases or decreases the electric output. The electric output increases from 260 to 380 milivolts when the stone is heated up. Jay suggests that before applying the green stone, it should be run under hot water for two to three minutes until it is warm or comfortably hot to the touch.

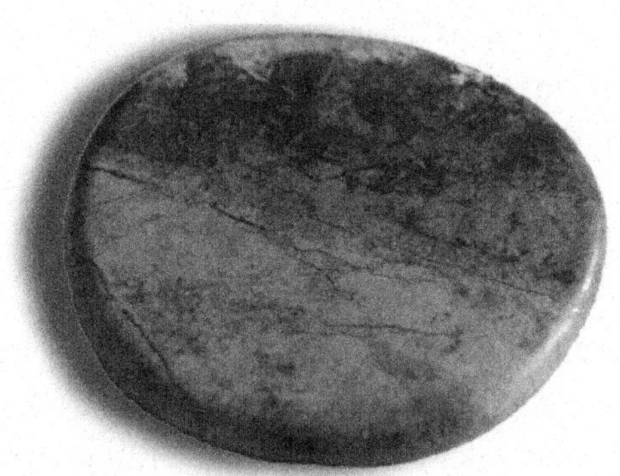
The Green Stone.

Because of these specific properties, the green stone, uniquely, can draw toxicities out of the body. And, because of the confluence of these properties, Jay has found that the stone is an effective pain-reliever, and has been used with good success on localized painful areas, and on tumors and lesions. The green stone, therefore, has four tasks it is capable of accomplishing:

1) it feeds us a minute dose of needed radiation (lower than the gray stone);
2) it feeds us a dose of needed electricity: it both absorbs and puts out a small DC (electric) current;
3) it draws out toxicities;
4) it reduces pain.

The electric property of the green stone is due to the fact that it's held together with silica, also known as quartz. When the green stone is held next to any place on the body, it confers electrical energy to the cells all over the body. Some people say that they can feel the electrical discharge of the stone.

Doubtless, the Arndt-Schultz Law, specifying that weak stimuli increase physiological activity, applies here: the sub-sensory electrical current of the green stone normalizes the ordinary activity taking place within the cell if it has been injured or otherwise compromised. This micro-current will increase the production of ATP, protein synthesis, oxygenation, ion exchange, absorption of nutrients, elimination of waste products, and neutralizes the oscillating polarity of deficient cells.

The biologically sensitive stimulation effect of the micro-current picks up where the body's own electrical current fails, as the human body must adhere to the natural law of electricity which is: "electricity must take the path of least resistance." Therefore, the electrical current emitted by the stone is destined to move around an injury or deficiency, rather than through it. By normalizing cell activity, inflammation is reduced while collagen producing cells are increased. Healthy cell metabolism creates a healthy, pain-free internal environment. Homeostasis is restored.

Jay talks about the green stone as though it were the workhorse of the kit. Although the dosage of radioactivity it emits is less than the other stones, its electrical emission makes it a doubly powerful healing tool. Jay believes that the two energies—electrical and radioactive—work in unison with each other, multiplying its healing power.

THE MUD PACKS

Jay saw people getting better with the radioactive stone (the original stone) which he kept at a steady 0.05 mRems per hour. But in terms of period of time of exposure, he found that generally longer was better: people seemed to get better faster, the longer they had the stone on them. But, since people couldn't keep the stone on them twenty-four hours a day, Jay started making mud packs that were easy to keep on the body during the course of the day, as well as easy to put under the sheet in the bed so the exposure could continue throughout the night. The other advantage of the mud packs is that they are easy for Jay to adjust to any energy level needed. It was with the packs that Jay started his experimentation to see what dosage gave the best response to the greatest number of people. He started the packs at 0.15 mRems/hr. But some people were not getting a fast enough response at that dosage, so he increased it to 0.5 mRems/hr.

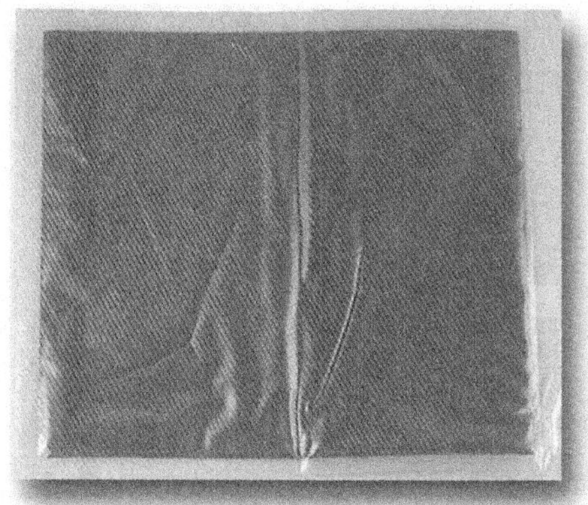

The Mud Pack.

Knowing that his products were at a dosage that was still considerably under anything that could be harmful, he kept increasing the dosage until he saw responses that were immediate, but not overwhelming. At one point, he went as high as 0.6 mRems/hr. But people who had had no previous exposure to low-level radiation would sometimes become overwhelmed. The packs have been kept at 0.4mRems/hr for many years now, and the responses have been consistent and effective. Unlike the green stone, the packs do not have to be warm or hot to make them effective. Temperature will not vary the energy level.

Jay's instructions are to put a thin cotton material between the skin and the pack, and place the pack over the effected area for at least eight hours a day (more is better). Sleeping with it is an excellent way to get uninterrupted usage. If the packaging breaks or leaks, it is not dangerous to have skin contact. In fact, one woman decided that she wanted to use the mud in her pack as a face mask, and deliberately punctured the plastic wrapping. She claims that her face appreciated the daily mud mask she gave it, and that all her friends thought she had had a face lift.

THE WATER STONE

The water stone puts out between 6 and 10 mRems/hr. The stone is placed in a jug of water and left to sit overnight. After this period of time, the water will have absorbed the radiation and reached a saturation point. Whether the stone sits in the water another hour or another year, the water will maintain the same constant level of radioactive hotness. The water will absorb the radiation and in turn will put out about 0.06 mRems/hr as it flows through the body. The water retains its charge for approximately three hours after the stone has been removed.

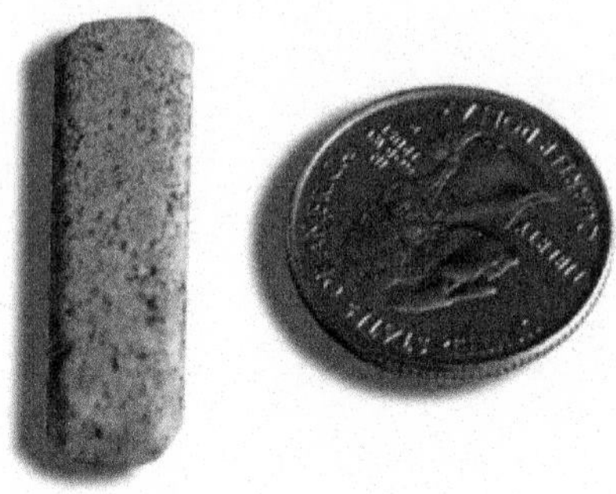

The Water Stone.

Any water can be used (though filtered is best), and there is no change in its effectiveness refrigerated or not. Jay suggests that when beginning the practice of drinking radioactive water, drink one to two glasses a day until the body has adjusted.

When you start, it is not uncommon for an aggravation period on the area of affliction of between two and thirty days. Other detoxification symptoms can also be expected for the first one to four days such as nausea, headaches, slight fever, dizziness, etc. This is a sign of the healing reaction that your own body is orchestrating. Other effects usually include good sleep and increased energy. After this initial period, any amount of water can be drunk.

THE PENDANT

Except for the cancer stone, the stone in the pendant is the strongest stone Jay creates—2-4 mRems/hr. (though it is often the smallest—size and "hotness" are unrelated). The pendant is the stone to wear to radiate energy on the chest area. Jay has had great success with the pendant stone in treating breast cancer, lung cancer, thyroid problems, and other problems that arise from this part of the body. But one needn't have an affliction to derive benefit from this stone. The necklace is very beneficial for anyone to wear.

THE GRAY STONE

This stone, used specifically in most cancer cases, measures from 8 to 12 mRem/hr. When necessary, when time is of the essence because of an encroaching disease, Jay will make the stone as strong as 30 mRem/hr. For instance, if someone has a month or less to live, Jay makes the stone as "hot" as he feels the patient can tolerate without stimulating an acute radiation reaction. Unlike the other stones, which operate on a more systemic level, the gray stone is used directly on the site of the tumor, enhancing its ability to resolve the immediate life-threatening problem on a local level.

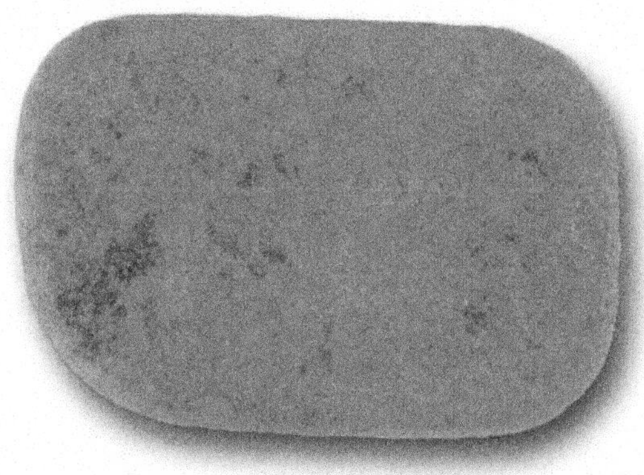

The Gray Stone.

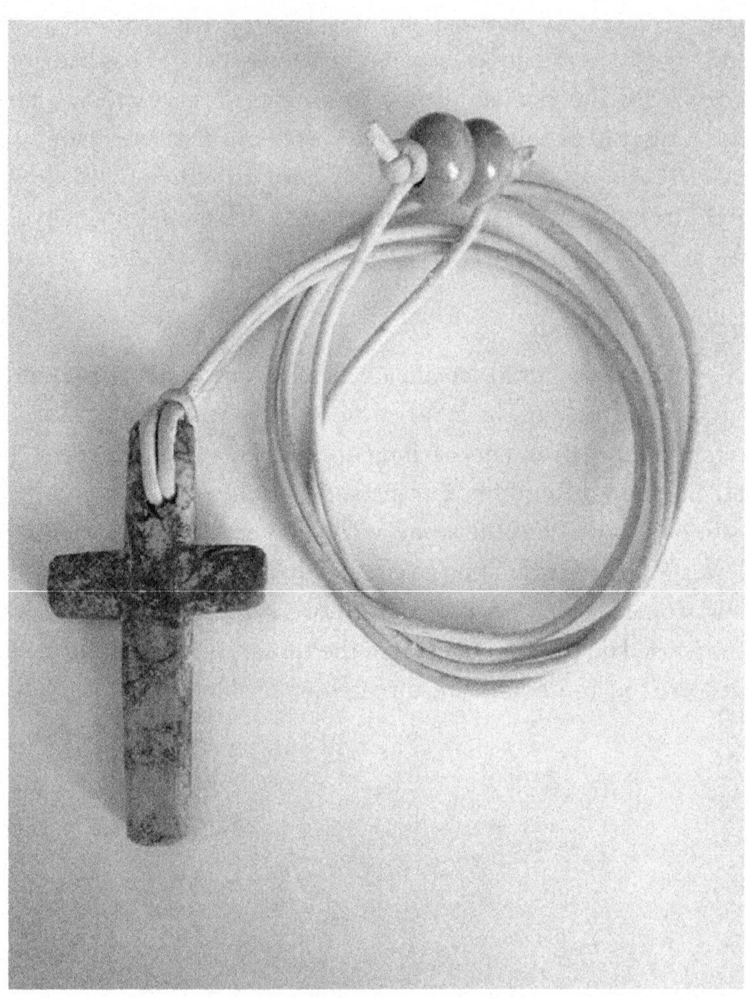

The Green Stone Cross Pendant.

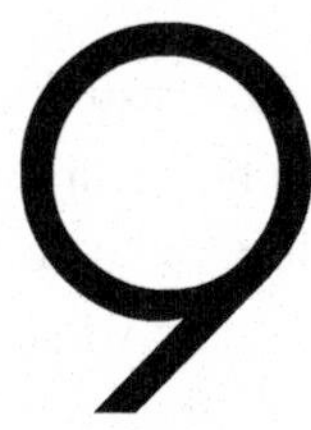

WHO'S DYING? AND WHO'S NOT?

Not only do the current models of radiation carcinogenesis disagree with modern oncology, but most important they have contributed to a number of misconceptions about radiation risks. What concerns me most is whether the radiological doctrines have sometimes caused greater health and environmental problems than those we seek to avoid. — Prof. Gunnar Walinder, former Chair, Swedish Radiobiology Society, *Has Radiation Protection Become a Health Hazard?*

AMERICANS ARE DYING. WE'RE DYING at a faster rate than any other industrialized country and we're all spending too much money to do it.

Our present need for the technology of the application of low-level radiation is desperate—both for health reasons as well as financial concerns. In 1901, the cancer rate in our country was at 7 percent. It is now hovering at 47 percent, and still climbing. One statistician has postulated that in twenty years, if the rate continues to climb at its present rate, we will have 100 percent of the population being afflicted with cancer.

We spend 50 percent more of our economy on health care than any nation on earth. Each American pays $7,600 a year per person for healthcare—16 percent of the GDP. Yet, our health care produces remarkably poor results. We actually rank *last* out of nineteen countries for unnecessary deaths, despite the vastly increased use of a wide variety of "wonder drugs" and vaccines.

Premature deaths caused by inappropriate, and overpriced interventions are increasing at an exponential rate. Fatalities now account for 23 percent of all reported adverse effects of prescription drugs. Overall reports of side effects from drugs increased a whopping 38 percent in the first quarter of 2008, compared to the previous four quarters.

The reason the U.S. ranks so poorly is because our system focuses on disease mongering and sickness care, whereas the health care systems in most other countries rely more heavily on prevention. As a result, the people in those countries live longer, healthier lives.

Just fifty years ago, according to IMS Health (a company that tracks the pharmaceutical industry), the two biggest sellers were over-the-counter drugs Bufferin and Geritol. At that time the prescription drug business was microscopic. In 1954, Johnson and Johnson had $204 million in revenue. By 2004 it had grown to about $36 billion.

Merck's drug sales in 1954 were a minuscule $1.5 million; by 2002, that figure was $52 billion. Last year, 3.8 billion prescriptions were filled. That's a 72 percent increase in prescriptions in just ten years, from 1997 to 2007. In that same period, the average number of prescriptions filled by each person in the U.S. increased from about nine a year in 1997, to almost eleven in 2006, and thirteen in 2007. The current average annual prescription rate for seniors is twenty-eight prescriptions per person.

However, there are signs that the tides are turning for America's dependence on drugs, and U.S. consumers' willingness to find alternatives for health care. For the first time in a decade, U.S. consumers are trying to get by on fewer prescription drugs. As people around the country respond to financial hard times, drugs are sometimes having to wait.

The drug giant Pfizer, which makes Lipitor, the world's top-selling prescription medicine, said U.S. sales of that drug were down 13 percent in the third quarter of 2008. And although the overall decline in total prescriptions was less than 1 percent, it represents the first downturn after more than a decade of steady increases in prescriptions.

The nation's top accountant, the Comptroller General of the United States, David Walker, has totaled up our government's income, liabilities, and future obligations and concluded that our current standard of living is unsustainable unless some drastic action is taken. Walker thinks the biggest economic peril facing the nation is being ignored: it's not the falling prices of real estate; it's not the failure of banks; it's not our lack of savings; it's not our nation's debt. It's the health crisis upon us.

As Walker points out, we have the largest uninsured population of any major industrialized nation. We have above average infant mortality, below average life expectancy, and much higher than average medical error rates for an industrialized nation. He continues:

> I would argue that the most serious threat to the United States is not someone hiding in a cave in Afghanistan or Pakistan but our own fiscal irresponsibility.

He warns us that without dramatically and fundamentally reforming our health care system in installments over the next twenty years, the result could easily be the bankruptcy of America.

Joseph Mercola insists that there is no doubt that a vast majority of the population is severely overmedicated with expensive and nearly always unnecessary drugs, considering the multitude of natural therapeutic options. He points out that the

> only way to turn this devastating situation around is to remind the public of the basic truths that nearly all their ancestors knew: Health has nothing to do with pills, and everything to do with sensible lifestyles that include a healthy diet, stress relief, and exercise.

Who's dying? Most of us will die prematurely. Scientists tell us that we're genetically programmed to live at least 120 years. Health enthusiasts Norman Walker and Bernard Jensen died at 117 and 92 respectively. Neither of these men paid a dime for medicines or drugs or even doctors' visits (except when Jensen was in a car accident at the age of eighty-four). They both died peacefully in their sleep. To an overwhelming extent, the people who die prematurely are the ones who don't take care of the essential ingredients that go into sustaining a long and healthy life.

With cancer specifically, Jay says that he spends more time cleaning people out from chemotherapy than he does from treating their cancers. He finds that if the body can be enabled to produce white blood cells, then there is an immune system that can become activated, and the person can fight and survive the cancer. In low-level radiation, the energy from the rays is transferred to the molecules in whatever living material the rays reach. This energy creates transient reactive chemicals that slightly damage the DNA, causing defects in the genetic instructions. Unless it can repair this damage, the living organism will die when it grows and tries to duplicate itself. This is the process of the death for the fungus and other pathogenic cells. But, when the organism does succeed in repairing itself, the strength and health of that organism is even better than it was before the damage.

However, the stones are only a place for people to begin their journey into health. The power of the stones is infinitely magnified when their use is coupled with following sound and proven principles of health.

10

THERAPEUTIC SOUL SISTERS

> It is time to scientifically challenge the old tenet that cancer risk is always proportional to dose, no matter how small . . . It is time to update our thinking and policies. — Marvin Goldman, past HPS President, *Science* 271, Mar 1996

THIRTY YEARS AGO, HOLISTIC PRACTITIONERS could change a patient's diet, give them some tips on how to do more effective detoxification, and the patient would get better. But, our world has become so polluted in the last twenty years that we live in a virtual sea of toxins. Nearly every person in the U.S. has at least 125 toxic chemicals in their blood.

Recent studies have found rocket fuel in 100 percent of breast milk samples taken from women across eighteen states. One study identified 287 industrial chemicals in babies' umbilical-cord blood, including 180 known to cause cancer and 217 that are toxic to the brain and nervous system.

Additionally, we have become so deficient in essential life-sustaining substances, that modification of diet alone, even when combined with standard detoxification procedures, is often insufficient for health restoration and maintenance.

The holistic health movement has grown exponentially in

response to the need, and other therapies now augment the basic principles of the importance of nourishment and detoxification.

DIET: THE TROJAN HORSE

If it's a food, it's not considered poisonous. Yet, food carries other organisms that are poisonous. In terms of fungi, it appears that our food is the pathway for the delivery of these poisons to our bodies. The toxicogenic fungi and their mycotoxins, which are characteristically present in stored and fermented foods, are using our food chain as a Trojan horse.

It has been documented that over half of German adults have ochratoxin in their blood, that leukemic children have aflatoxin in their blood, that patients with urinary tract cancers have ochratoxin in their blood, that patients with Crohn's Disease have aflatoxin in their blood, and finally, 18 to 90 percent of nursing mothers have mycotoxins in their breast milk.

We know that there is an abundance of mycotoxic growth in peanuts, corn, cashews, and all dried and stored foods. Corn is an especially serious problem as many different fungi have been found on virtually all corn, including even organic corn. The fungus fumonisin contaminates corn with the greatest frequency and is present in corn in particularly high concentrations. (An additional problem is that corn oil is contaminated with mercury because of the way it is processed.) It is suspected that the use of corn as a major staple in their diets of Hispanics, and the over-use of hi fructose corn syrup in packaged foods, may be a prime reason for the epidemic of diabetes that we are now witnessing. It is estimated that 50 percent of Latin-American Hispanics, by the time they reach 45 years of age, will have diabetes. The health situation, caused by the fungal infestation of corn and corn byproducts, seems no less than dire.

Animals fed fungal colonized-mycotoxic feed are not only at risk for developing mycotoxicoses, but their meat and their fat constitute another vehicle for human exposure to excessive mycotoxin intake. Animal fat is increasingly being documented to be a major risk factor for a number of human cancers and atherosclerosis. Humans who eat these foods are ingesting both the toxicogenic fungi and their mycotoxins. These fungi are capable of surviving in the intestinal stream where they may continue to produce their toxins.

DETOXIFICATION

All spiritual traditions, ancient and modern, have periods of time allotted to systematic cleansing. Native Americans would periodically purify themselves through their sweat lodges. Communally, they would subject themselves to intense heat, thus eliminating accumulated bodily toxins. Similarly, the Ayurvedic tradition recommends Panchakarma cleansing three times a year, at the change of the seasons, in order to maintain well-being in healthy individuals or to restore balance in those who are ill. Panchakarma consists of a series of therapies, including colon cleansing, designed to remove deep-rooted biological toxins.

The yogic tradition, too, has developed techniques for purification that lead to rejuvenation. In Sivinanda Yoga, these techniques are called *kriyas*, a word that means sacrifice. Yogis spend many years mastering elaborate techniques of muscular control in order to cleanse even deep internal organs. The Jewish tradition devotes one day a week—the *Shabbos*—to eating lightly and resting; Jews fast all day on Yom Kippur, allowing their bodies to detoxify as they turn their mental and spiritual attention to atonement, release from guilt and from negative thinking. Catholicism embraces the concept of abstinence in its celebration of Lent, also known as The Big Fast, a period of forty days in which participants cleanse themselves of desire.

These beliefs in abstinence, cleansing and rest are not frivolous notions. They are based on sound understandings of the nature of health. Ancient peoples understood that without setting aside specific times for periodic purification, vitality and regeneration were not possible. They understood as well, the notion that the occasional denial of pleasure and desire leads to the greater benefit of consciousness and healing. This notion is the essence of detoxification.

WHAT GOES IN MUST COME OUT

It is unfortunate that American doctors have contended for decades that the number of bowel movements an individual has is unrelated to health. They have convinced most of us that they are correct. Many of us think that we are not constipated if we are having one bowel movement a day. Yet, we eat three meals a day. Where are the other two meals going if they're not being eliminated through the colon? The answer actually is somewhat frightening. The rest of the food that is not absorbed by the body as nutrients stays around the body in unlikely places—against the colon walls, in tissues and organs, in arteries—any place at all in the body can serve as a receptacle for un-eliminated waste. Humans are the only animals who have such insufficient bowel functioning. Breast-fed babies, indigenous peoples, birds and animals all evacuate their bowels shortly after each meal.

Dr. John Harvey Kellogg, of the famed Battle Creek Sanitarium, maintained that 90 percent of modern diseases are the result of improper functioning of the colon. British physician, Sir Arbuthnut Lane concurred after performing hundreds of bowel resections where diseased portions of the bowel were removed. He noticed that during the time that the patient was recovering from the surgery that other diseases, seemingly unrelated to the colon problem, were cured.

Sir Lane came to understand that a large part of the problem in many diseases was the body's inability to adequately carry out its normal waste disposal functions. He calculated that a healthy intestine requires emptying every six hours. Yet, more commonly, it is sluggish in its performance and is emptied every twenty-four hours.

There is scientific research, as well, showing the relationship between bowel functioning and health. British and South African scientists have shown a lot of interest in this issue and have conducted elaborate experiments involving the clocking and weighing of feces of human volunteers. It has been confirmed that too few bowel movements and too little bulk in the stool is related to a variety of disorders, including heart and gallbladder diseases, diverticulitis, varicose veins, hiatal hernia and cancer of the large intestine.

There is also a study of over 1,000 women with histories of constipation. Fluid was extracted from the breasts of the women. This fluid showed abnormal cells which are the same abnormal cells found in women with breast cancer. These cellular abnormalities occurred five times as often in women who moved their bowels fewer than three times a week than in women who did so more than once a day.

Normal bowel functioning means there is waste for everything that goes in except distilled water. We need to find those other, lost meals.

Many holistic centers, including La Casa Day Spa, have colon therapists who specialize in helping people to know how to take care of their bowels. They also perform colonics, which is an intensive cleansing of the entire colon tract.

WHY WATER?

Water has always been a part of any spiritual detoxification. The Mineral Palace and La Casa Day Spa, as well as all of the hot springs spas around the world, use heated water as the delivery system for low-level radiation. The therapeutic use of water is a time-honored tradition. Ancient cultures used water to utterly transform the body.

In yogic tradition, for instance, you never say you're going to take a bath or a shower—you say you're going to perform *Ishnaan*. There's a reverence, a grace to the concept of immersing your body in water and allowing the water to work a magical transformation and healing on you.

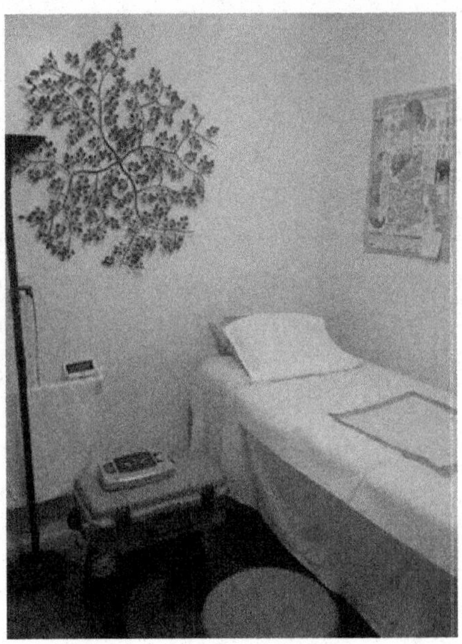

La Casa Day Spa, New York City.

It is, in a way, unfortunate that modern plumbing brings water to us so easily. It has gotten us to be too indifferent to the magic and possibility of transformation through the therapeutic use of water. In ancient times, hydrotherapy required 500 men to fill the huge tub. The tub had to be placed forty feet above the ground in order to create enough water pressure to get the desired effect.

The science of hydrotherapy is extremely precise and it is in the ancient yogic tradition that its laws were first discovered. Water therapy forces the capillaries to open and when they close again, the blood returns back to the organs. Each organ has its own blood supply so in doing this you have just given each organ a nice flushing out of old blood and replenishing of revitalized blood. When the organs get a flushing, the glands have to change their secretions. When the glands change, according to yogic tradition, youth returns. If the glandular system is revitalized, it secretes chemicals that are young chemicals, thus returning the body to youthfulness and health.

Perhaps what makes hot water therapy so effective—almost magical in its effectiveness—is that it represents our origins. Life itself arose out of the primordial soup that was warm and moist.

Hot water has the effect of increasing the overall temperature of the body. The heart rate and respiration also increase, as does the rate at which the body uses oxygen and excretes waste material. Perspiration eliminates metabolic waste products, and this cleansing augments the sensation of calmness and relaxation.

Relaxing muscles has an effect on both the skeletal system and the nerves. Nerves run through muscle tissue and constantly constricted muscles can pinch these nerves. Because muscles are attached to bones through tendons, tightness in a muscle can exert pressure on the bones to which they are attached. Each of these conditions can be quite painful. But when muscles are enabled to let go of their tightness, nerves are soothed, pressure on bones is alleviated and pain is relieved.

YOU ARE A SHINING, VIBRATING BEING OF ENERGY

Until relatively recently, scientists believed that life was mostly a biochemical process. The idea that magnetic fields could significantly influence living systems seemed far-fetched. Perspectives have shifted rapidly, however, and many scientists now believe that as much as being a mix of chemicals, we are, too, fundamentally electromagnetic creatures.

Einstein is actually the one who paved the way for a scientific understanding of what shamans, yogis and healers had known for over 5,000 years. The understanding of this formula is so absolutely simple. All Einstein meant was: energy and matter are dual expressions of the same universal substance. That universal substance is energy. Energy is vibration.

Since Einstein, research has confirmed his theory. The modern science of superstring theory teaches that fundamentally the universe is pure vibration. Quantum physics has similarly shown us that at the particle level, all matter is really energy.

Vibrational-energy medicine (the use of frequencies in healing) has become established as a cutting-edge approach to health and vitality. This paradigm shift takes us away from the Newtonian-Cartesian worldview focused on the world of matter, things and nouns and has propelled us into the world of energy, processes and verbs.

As beings of energy, we can be affected by energy. Not only can we convert matter into energy, we can also convert energy into matter. Energy can be imparted to us from an external source—materials of the cosmos, a person, even a machine; we can give others energy; we can transform our own energetic states. The universe itself is a healer; everyone is a potential energetic healer to everyone else, and we are all healers to ourselves.

Everything living vibrates at certain frequencies—and this is true not only for electrons, atoms, molecules, cells, tissues and organs, but also for parasites, bacteria, and viruses. And, it is true for humans, and for all parts of our bodies. We humans, like the universe in which we reside, are beings of energy. We are actually a series of interacting, multidimensional energy systems that are manifested on the physical, emotional, mental and spiritual planes. Each part of the body—even the smallest constituent—is a part of this bioenergetic communication network, continuously generating a stream of vibratory information. We are so much more than mere flesh and bones, cells and proteins; we are shining, electrical, magnetic (and perhaps other forms of energy not yet discovered) beings. And we exist in dynamic interaction and equilibrium with a universe of energy that is, similarly, shining, electrical and magnetic.

We know that the human body, awake, averages a frequency of 62-72 Hz. Disease sets in when the frequency drops. Flu occurs when the electrical frequency drops to 58 hz.; candida occurs at 55 hz.; Epstein-Barr occurs at 52 hz.; cancer occurs at 42 hz. The frequency of the body also drops when the body comes into contact with substances that have lower frequencies: junk food, canned or otherwise denatured food, drugs, even synthetic vitamins. Research has shown that merely holding a cup of coffee in your hand can drop your frequency (probably through the aroma which has a more powerful effect on us than any of us would imagine).

Vibrational-energy medicine is one of the most widely studied fields of medicine today. It is based on the intersecting aspects of the sciences of biology, physiology, chemistry and physics, and looks at the subtleties of human structure and patterns of energy in interaction. Significant bioenergetic principles as well as treatment modalities have emerged, and there is now global interest and research in the clinical application of vibrational medicine. Homeopathy is one part of vibrational medicine, and has been used by various systems of medicine throughout history. Advancements in modern technology have made it possible for the previously unseen and subtle to be now seen. Subtle energy systems, invisible to the naked eye, and their influence on the physiologic behavior of cellular systems, have been confirmed.

For the past fifty years, physicists and other researchers following Einstein's quantum model have been working on ways to detect, measure and manipulate the subtle energy systems of the human body. The discoveries made through this research have made it possible for today's health care practitioners to work with subtler forms of energy, both in the diagnosis and treatment of illness. Thus, it is now possible to view and measure the body's subtle energy fields, as well as changes in these fields after vibrational medicine modalities have been applied. Vibrational medicine stimulates the body's restorative systems without the side-effects associated with the use of pharmacological substances.

MAGNETIC PULSE THERAPY

Magnetic Pulse Therapy (MPT) is a well-established form of energy medicine. Extensive research has been conducted on it and pulsed magnetic machines have FDA approval as a medical device. As a treatment for healing bone and joint fractures, it is used routinely in both the U.S. and throughout Europe, in over forty countries world-wide. But its usefulness has been shown in clinical usage to be much more systemic to all functions of the body. The treatment works by addressing the underlying cause of all disease: stagnation at the cellular level. MPT improves cellular metabolism through encouraging a flow and release of cellular sluggishness. Bodily traffic jams are restored to an even flow of orderly transport of oxygen and nutrients to the whole system. Thus, MPT both detoxifies as well as promotes better absorption of nutrients. Exposing the cells to pulsed magnetic energy from a MPT will increase the cell's energy, thus optimizing all its functions. Unlike both electric and electromagnetic fields, pure magnetic fields penetrate freely everywhere in the body.

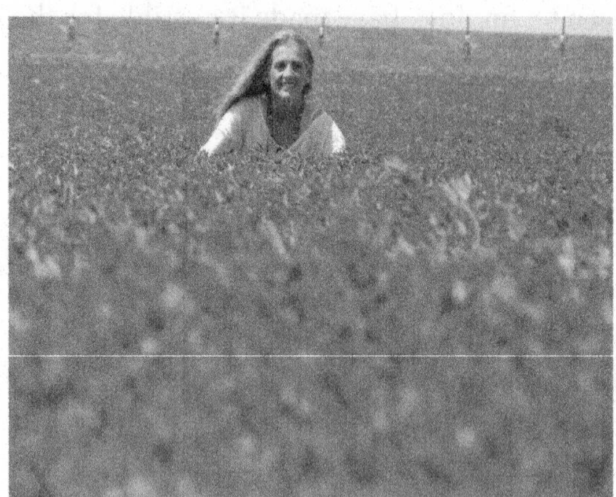

Faye in an abundant and healthy field of alfalfa, grown using radiation hormesis-treated water.

One of the more interesting magnetic theories about our current state of pervasive illness postulates something called "Magnetic Field Deficiency Syndrome." It is offered as an explanation of biomagnetic effects by Dr. Kyochi Nakagawa of Japan. The Earth's magnetic field is not fixed in position or strength. In the last hundred years, it has weakened on the average by about 6 percent. In the last thousand years, it has fallen nearly 30 percent. Dr. Nakagawa argues that since humans evolved in a magnetic field, it is necessary for proper health. A falling magnetic field puts us at risk and magnetic therapy makes up the deficit (just as a therapeutic dosage of low-level radiation makes up a deficiency in radiation).

11

IF YOU CAN DO IT IN JACHYMOV, YOU CAN DO IT AT HOME

If all electric and heat energy in the United Kingdom were produced in nuclear power plants, the radioactive waste generated in those plants could be accommodated within one football field. — Professor Fukasz Turski, National Academy of Sciences Center for Theoretical Physics and College for Sciences in Warsaw.

MANY OF THE THERAPIES AND healing techniques that are done at the Mineral Palace and at La Casa Day Spa, and at all of the radon spas around the world (including several in Jachymov, the Czech Republic) can be, and should be done at home.

CREATING A RADON STEAM USING YOUR STOVE

Put the green stone and the water stone in a pot of boiling water. Place a towel over your head, and breathe in the steam that is being generated from the radioactive boiling water. This is the most efficient and effective way of getting the radiation to enter your lungs directly, and then into your bloodstream. This is particularly recommended for all respiratory ailments, including asthma, bronchial conditions, and lung cancer.

CREATING A RADON BATH IN YOUR BATHTUB

You will need to go to a pool or spa store and get a plastic cover that fits over your bathtub. Run the water as hot as it will get. Place the stones in the water. Put the plastic sheet over the water to help the water retain the heat. After three hours, the water will be sufficiently radiated. Hop in and enjoy.

THE UN-FUNGAL HOME DIET PLAN

You can easily reduce the intake of fungal toxins which are present in stored grains, nuts, seeds, meats, grain-fed animal products (meat, animal fats, butter, milk) and fermented foods such as beer, bread, cheese and wine. As well, an increased fungal growth/toxin production is caused by diets high in sugar, fruit, grains, and some fats. On the other hand, a decreased fungal growth/toxin production is due to the anti-fungal action of high fiber foods, all vegetables, fish, fish oils, garlic, onion, herbs and spices. While fruit is a source of fiber, the high sugar fructose content of fruit stimulates fungal growth: fructose increases blood cholesterol and uric acid levels which are associated with increased risk of hypertension and atherosclerosis.

Here is a five point anti-fungal dietary-cleansing plan:

1) Starve the fungus: This is a low carbohydrate dietary program that dramatically cuts back on sugar that feeds fungi. Although carbohydrates are known to be fuel for the body, this is true only in a non-toxic individual. In a fungally-toxic individual, carbohydrates actually suppress energy. This program is also very low in mold/fungi infected foods and high in vegetables, which are known to

carry out mycotoxins and inhibit their toxicity.

2) Move your bowels: As fungus is killed inside your body, it is imperative that you move it out, and quickly. The next section outlines procedures for bowel cleansing.
3) Repair the damage: Repairing the oxidative damage is crucial. Use powerful free radical scavenger such as: Pycnogenol, Grape Seed Extract, Vitamin C.
4) Kill the fungus: Physicians will prescribe drugs like Nystatin, Lamisil, Nizoral, Diflucan, or Sporanax to kill the fungus. However, you can do just a good of a job with natural remedies: olive leaf extract, oregano oil, capryillic acid, pau d'arco, apple cider vinegar (malic acid), garlic.
5) Replace the good bacteria: This can be done with lactobacillus acidophilus and a high quality propionic.

Eating properly, and keeping your fungal load down, is also dependent on maintaining the proper acid/alkaline balance in your body. To get an electrical charge, you need to have both a positive and a negative pole. So too with the body; we need an acid/alkaline balance, which is, in effect, the electrical charge of the body. The fact that we have an acid/alkaline ratio means that we are not just a conglomeration of chemicals, but are also an entire system of highly organized electrical reactions.

There is an extremely small parameter of this delicate balance in which good health is maintained. We each have an alkaline reserve and every time we eat foods that create too much of an acid condition in our bodies, then our alkaline reserve leaps into action in order to neutralize the acids. But this reserve is limited. It's just a back-up if you abuse yourself with too much acid-producing food.

You can maintain the proper acid/alkaline balance by choosing foods in the ratio that your body needs. This ratio should be 20/80, in the alkaline favor.

Acid foods: meats and fish; dairy products, including

butter, cheese, whey and eggs; sugar and honey; potatoes and yams; grains; most nuts, including brazil, filberts, pecans, pine and walnuts; most oils, including olive and vegetable oils; most beans, including kidney, lima, navy, split peas, chick-peas and pinto; most legumes, including cashews.

Alkaline foods include most fresh vegetables and most fruits, both fresh and dried (dried prunes are acid). When citrus fruits are ripe, they are alkaline; when picked before they are ripe, they change to an indigestible acid. The fresher and sweeter the food tastes, the more alkaline it is.

Injuries, either physical or psychological, produce an acid condition.

Pathogens in the form of viruses, fungi or bacteria can survive only in an acid environment. The acid/alkaline balance is effected by exercise. The better your nutritional program becomes, the more alkaline your body will become. If you become too alkaline, your bowels will not work well. Every time you exercise, you produce lactic acid which will restore the balance.

DETOXIFICATION THROUGH COLON CLEANSING

Colon cleansing can be approached from, so to speak, either the top end or the bottom end—the mouth or the rectum.

The simplest way of beginning colon cleansing is to add bulk to the diet. Fiber is present in all fresh, raw vegetables. Cooking softens the fiber and renders it ineffective. Dietary fiber in food is indigestible. But when present in the intestinal tract, it supports a multiplying population of intestinal bacteria, and this can be an aid in both digestion and elimination. The detoxifying powers of fiber were demonstrated in a study where rats were fed poison, and simultaneously put on a high fiber diet. These rats survived without harm, while other animals fed the same poison, but without the fiber, became ill and died.

Enemas are effective in reaching the low part of the colon, but have the disadvantage of not reaching the entire organ. Adding ingredients to the water in an enema can, however, greatly enhance its detoxifying power. Coffee enemas stimulate the liver; flaxseed tea enemas relieve the colon of inflammation; bentonite, or clay water, greatly increases the absorption of toxins from the colon walls.

The colema board was developed more than thirty years ago by V.E. Irons. It is a home unit that combines the ease of the enema with the thoroughness of the colonic. It is a gentle bowel cleansing, following the body's own natural rhythm for retention and expulsion of water. The water enters the intestinal tract, and it is the colon's own spontaneous contractions that pushes water out. Thus, the colema works like an exercise program. The water trains the colon to begin to correct its atrophied condition. Because the muscles in the colon are stimulated, the colon sends messages to the rest of the body to release stored toxins and to bring them down through the normal eliminative channels. Pockets of putrefied material embedded within the colon walls can be dislodged through the colema. We encourage the use of the colema board because the advantage of being able to do it yourself at home makes it economical and convenient, as well as effective.

To improve bowel functioning:

1) Eat flaxseed cereal: grind up two tablespoonfuls of flaxseed. Add to goat yogurt.
2) Eat prunes stewed in hot water.
3) Do an enema, colema or colonic. Each has a specific effect. Choose the one that best suits your needs at that time.
4) Drink an aloe smoothie: blend one inch portion of fresh aloe leaf (with green skin on) with juice of a whole lemon, honey to taste (you'll need lots to combat the bitter taste of the aloe skin, but the skin is the part of the leaf that has the purgative effect).
5) Herbal laxatives may be taken. Whole leaf aloe capsules are a good choice. There are many special formulations on the

market. Laxatives with either senna or cascara sagrada may cause peristaltic cramping as they are both herbs that work through irritating the intestines.

OXYGEN: THE BREATH OF LIFE

Ninety percent of the body's energy is created by oxygen. Every single activity of the body is regulated by oxygen. It is a life-giving, life-sustaining element. We can live without food for months and without water for weeks; without oxygen, we can live for only a few minutes.

The more oxygen we have in our system, the more energy we are able to produce. In fact, a good definition of vitality is the body's ability to assimilate oxygen.

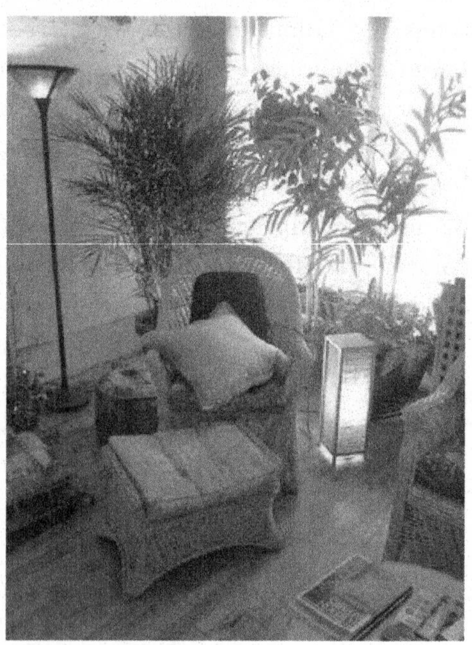

La Casa Day Spa, New York City.

Recently scientists were stunned to discover that the air bubbles in fossilized amber contained oxygen levels of 38 percent. Today, the average oxygen content of air is only 19-21 percent. In larger cities, where the pollution is greater, the oxygen content often dips as low as 12-15 percent.

This stunning finding suggests that there was a time on earth when the oxygen content of the air was more than 50 percent higher than it is today. We might well wonder whether or not our bodies have made the evolutionary changes that would be required to maintain good health with so much less oxygen than we are used to. We think not. In fact, when the oxygen content drops down to 7 percent, human life cannot be supported. Large, polluted cities are getting dangerously close to that level. In Japan, we now see the use of oxygen booths on the streets.

The link between oxygen and disease has been firmly established. The result of an insufficient oxygen supply can be anything from mild fatigue to life-threatening disease. Otto Warburg's words describe the core causation of cancer: "Cancer has only one prime cause. The prime cause of cancer is the replacement of normal oxygen respiration of body cells by an anaerobic (oxygen-deficient) cell respiration." Cancer cells simply cannot survive in an oxygen-rich environment. Renowned molecular biologist and geneticist, Stephen Levine, has concluded that the lack of oxygen in human cells and tissues is the underlying root cause of not just cancer, but of all chronic degenerative disease.

Oxidation, the process of burning, is the method through which the body is supplied with oxygen. Oxidation contributes to metabolic function, circulation, assimilation, digestion and elimination. The link between oxidation and toxicity is particularly strong; in the absence of normal oxidation, cells are incapable of burning cell waste. These wastes then accumulate throughout the body, causing all kinds of disease, including but not limited to cancer.

The key to cellular oxidation is electricity. Electricity involves the exchange of electrons. Of all the elements, oxygen is the greatest giver and receiver of electrons. We cannot have a healthy nervous system without sufficient oxygen.

Because it is always best to do things naturally, we can increase our oxygen load by learning, simply, how to breathe. Breathing well is actually not as easy as one might think. Unfortunately, we have lost much of our knowledge about this automatic process and we have to relearn it. We come into this world with the excellent talent for knowing how to do diaphragmatic breathing. Infants all breathe deeply from their diaphragms. As we get older, however, we forget this talent and we breathe primarily from our upper chest. This means that only the upper portion of our lungs has air moving in and out; the lower regions contain stale air. But since gravity pulls most of the blood supply to the lower lungs, our bloodstream never gets the benefit of the fresh, oxygen-rich air. This shallow breathing can cause a plethora of problems. The oxygen level of the entire body and brain is lowered. Physical and mental problems can ensue: respiratory disease, low energy, sluggishness, senility, heart disease, loss of memory.

> *Deep breathing:*
> Place a hand below your navel point. Push out against your hand, expanding the diaphragm as you inhale. The lungs will then naturally expand. Push in with your hand, contracting the diaphragm. Exhalation will follow naturally and the chest will decline. Continue this method of breathing; take long, slow and deep breaths with one continuous flow.

THE BEST HOME EXERCISE: JUMP FOR JOY

Rebounding is performed on a mini-trampoline. All sporting goods stores carry them, usually for less than $100. Rebounding is unique as an aerobic exercise because it stimulates, strengthens and cleanses every cell in the body. This is because it uses vertical motion rather than the horizontal motion that is used in all other forms of exercise.

Simply explained, when you bounce up and down, your entire body goes through repetitive vertical acceleration and deceleration, working against gravity. At the bottom of every bounce, your entire body stops for a split second. At this moment, the force of gravity shoves down on every cell in your body. This is the deceleration working with gravity. Then your body shoots back upward, again stopping for just a split instant. This is your moment in space. The movement upward has exerted pressure on your body from the opposite direction of the downward movement. This is the acceleration working against gravity. Because of the repetitive pushing and pulling on all your cells, the tissues and fibers and muscles in your body all grow stronger. This includes your heart fibers and the muscle layers within the arterial walls, even if you don't dramatically get your heart rate up.

Also, rebounding cleanses and purifies every cell. Your cells depend on the diffusion of fluid through the permeable membranes in order to carry oxygen, nutrients, hormones and enzymes into the cell, and to flush out metabolic waste. This process is increased by a factor of 300 percent by rebounding. This is because at the top of every bounce, your body actually becomes weightless for a fraction of a second. The cells therefore oscillate between increased G-force and no G-force, providing a constant compression/decompression factor. This on-going compression/decompression of the cell membranes significantly boosts the diffusion of fluid into and out of the cells, carrying fresh oxygen and nutrients, and flushing out the toxins. There is literally no other form of exercise that has this same capacity for total cellular cleansing.

The lymph system, specifically, cleans the body of debris. Lymph fluid surrounds every cell in your body. The human body contains three times more lymph fluid than it does blood. The pressure that is exerted on the lymphatic system in rebounding activates the valves in the lymph channels to their maximum capacity, increasing lymph flow by as much as thirty times normal. In fact, the entire lymph system can be cleansed in the span of a single, short session on the trampoline. Clogged lymph nodes are cleared; tonsils and adenoids are cleansed, as are the larger organs of the appendix and spleen.

Jumping can also substantially boost the immune system by increasing the activity of lymphocytes within the bloodstream. Any form of exercise can, of course, do this. But research shows that when the body is exposed to higher than normal gravitational pressure, such as that produced in rebounding, that the lymphocyte activity is increased to the greatest extent. With more lymphocyte activity, infectious organisms are more quickly zeroed in on, attacked and neutralized by the lymphocytes, and infection is much less likely to settle in.

For all these reasons, NASA has embraced rebounding, and has shown that it is 68 percent more effective as a fitness conditioner than running or any other form of aerobic exercise.

EWOT - EXERCISE WITH OXYGEN THERAPY

EWOT (pronounced ee-watt) stands for Exercise with Oxygen Therapy. This method of prolonging your life is so simple that it's hard to believe it could work, but it does. All you need is an oxygen concentrator, which you should be able to pick up used on the internet for about $300, and a nasal canula (costs about $3). And your trusty trampoline.

One of the main reasons for aging is the failure of enzymatic systems that are responsible for your body's uptake and utilization of oxygen. When your cells don't get enough oxygen, they degenerate and die and so you degenerate and die. It's as simple as that.

Human beings can take a lot of punishment, mentally and physically, so these frequent drops in your ability to utilize oxygen efficiently are not going to kill you immediately. You would have died a long time ago if that were true. But each oxygen deprivation can take its toll, and if a few cells die here and there due to constant external (or internal) stress, it begins to add up. The end result is premature aging.

So if a simple system can be used that constantly provides the body with additional oxygen, these stress factors can be, to a certain extent, neutralized. EWOT does just that.

Exercising (rebounding), while breathing oxygen, dramatically increases the amount of oxygen in the blood plasma, i.e., the portion of the blood outside the red and white cells. This can be easily determined by testing the blood oxygen level in the arteries or veins. Doctors will say that you can't increase the oxygen in your blood by breathing oxygen. But what they mean is that you can't increase the amount of oxygen in your red blood cells, which are responsible for transporting oxygen to the tissues. The reason the amount of oxygen in the red cells cannot be increased is because, under most circumstances, they are already 97 percent saturated with oxygen. Doctors say, rightly so, that a 3 percent increase will make little difference and the red cells won't accept the extra oxygen, anyway.

While this statement is true, it ignores the role of oxygen in the plasma, the "juice" within which the red cells flow. The oxygen content of plasma can be dramatically increased and thus oxygen will be "pushed" into the body's cells. This mechanism is called the Law of Mass Action. If you build up the concentration of a certain component in a chemical mixture high enough, chemical combining will take place with other elements of the mixture that ordinarily wouldn't happen.

Most of the oxygen in the plasma under these high-saturation circumstances will be "wasted" in that it will not be absorbed by the cells which expect to be "fed" oxygen by the red cells. But if only one-tenth of 1 percent of the oxygen gets through, and you offer your cells this extra "meal" every day, there will be an extensive increase in your total tissue oxygen level. The objective is to keep the oxygen level of your blood as close to optimum (100 points) as long as possible; ideally, for your entire life.

After 15 minutes of EWOT, there is a dramatic "pinking up" of the person's skin. If this can be seen so easily by simple observation, then it is obvious that the tiny capillaries, vessels tinier than a strand of hair, are carrying extra oxygen to cells of the body. Every organ (your brain, kidneys, heart, eyes, and even the tips of your toes) is being bathed in extra amounts of life-sustaining oxygen.

You don't get the same effect if you exercise vigorously, such as a long jog. You don't similarly increase the oxygenation of the blood and hence your tissues. You can run ten miles and you will not increase the oxygen content of your blood. You will, in fact, temporarily decrease your blood oxygen as the body bums oxygen to cover the work load.

Moderate exercise, as in walking, has been confirmed as the best exercise. It is well-known that during exercise, blood is sent to the muscles to provide oxygen where it is immediately needed. And the blood is not "oxygen-enriched"—the longer you exercise, the less oxygen the blood contains. That's why you feel fatigued after heavy exercise.

EWOT is not strenuous exercise. It is moderate exercise for a limited period of time, fifteen minutes of jumping, in the presence of extra oxygen. This will give you "oxygen-rich blood."

WHAT'S ESSENTIAL

If you do some research into the Royal English Archives, you'll come across an interesting little tidbit. It's a recipe for "thieves' oils." So the story goes: in the 17th century, when all of Europe was in the thrust of the Black Plague, a small band of marauding thieves seemed immune to the disease. They would enter the homes of Black Plague victims and have no fear of touching the bodies as they searched for jewelry and money. The King demanded to know their secret.

Their secret had to do with the oils they rubbed on their bodies. Because their family was from a long lineage of apothecaries, they had knowledge about how to use oils medicinally and prophylactically against disease. The King got the exact formulation they were using against Black Plague and this saved his

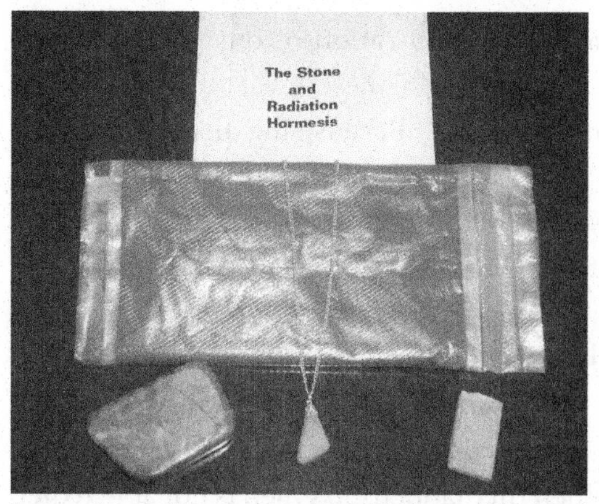

Jay's radiation hormesis product known as "The Kit," which includes several stones, a pendant necklace, and a mud pack.

entire family from the disease.

Today we think of essential oils as mere pleasant additions to a relaxing massage. But in olden days, some cultures valued oils even more than gold because their powerful healing properties were known.

Essential oils have the same function in the plant as blood has to the human. When you cut yourself, blood comes out of the cut. The blood cleanses the wound and kills bacteria so that regeneration of the tissue can begin. Similarly, when you cut a plant, resin, or the oil of the plant is released.

Blood is a transporter. It carries nutrients to the cells. Oxygen is the constituent of blood that delivers the blood through the cell walls. When oxygen is taken out of the blood, the cells mutate and give off a toxic gas. This, then, creates a host condition that will breed disease. So, too, with plants. Oils serve as the defense system in plants. These oils oxygenate the plant and carry nutrients, vital elements and chemical constituents to every cell in the plant. They contain each of the plant's healing nutrients including trace minerals, vitamins, hormones, amino acid precursors and other components. They give the plant the ability to destroy infections, stave off infestations, initiate and maintain growth and repair structural damage. The essential oil of the plant is literally the life force of the plant.

When essential oils are applied to human skin, they carry the same healing force as they do to the plant. Because they themselves carry such a high concentration of oxygen, they also produce in the human system the highest level of oxygenating molecules of any substance on earth. Because the oils are so highly concentrated, they are at least fifty times more therapeutically potent than the plant itself or herbs made from the plant.

Essential oils detoxify the body. Oxygen pushes unwanted chemicals out of the cell. Normal cell function and balance is established only when there is sufficient oxygen.

The absorbability of essential oils into the human system is unsurpassed. If you are deficient in oxygen, your cell membranes will begin to thicken. When this happens, oxygen is not able to get its nutrients through this thick wall. You may have been eating all the nutritional food in the world, but if the blood can't get the nutrients into the cell, you may have well-nourished blood but you won't have well-nourished cells. Essential oils are soluble with the lipids in the cell membrane and thus go through the cellular wall.

As well, essential oils have the capacity to change the electrical frequency of the body. As well as our bodies being electrical, so is everything around us, including our television, our lights and our microwave. The difference between us and our electrical appliances is that we have a harmonic, coherent frequency whereas appliances operate at incoherent, chaotic frequencies. Our appliances have the ability to fracture the frequency that we operate at.

The electrical frequency of essential oils ranges between 52 and 320 Hz. They have the highest frequency of any substance known to man. Because they are living substances, their frequency is harmonic with the human frequency. When essential oils come into contact with our bodies, the frequency of our bodies becomes raised to a degree that we become inhospitable hosts to pathogenic organisms.

Essential oils are also valuable because they carry a unique capacity for retarding mold growth. Researchers have found that wrapping baked goods, such as bread, with cinnamon-laced wax paper protects it from molding. Even with bread already tainted with mold, you can wrap it in a paper containing 6 percent cinnamon oil, and it will inhibit the mold's growth by 96 percent.

Essential oils can be applied directly to the skin. Within twenty-one minutes of being placed anywhere on the human body, essential oils will penetrate every cell within the body. We rub our bodies with oils as specific medicines.

Merely breathing in the fragrance of essential oils is a powerful healer. The healing begins in the brain. There are 800 million nerve endings in the nose which detect odors. The nerve from the olfactory bulb extends back toward the mid-brain and then on to the pituitary and pineal glands and finally to the amygdala. Anyone can grow their own plants from which to make essential oils. Mint, lemongrass or lemon leaves can be crushed in your hands and you can just breathe in the aroma. You will be breathing in the fragrance of the essential oil as it oozes from the plant, just as blood oozes from our skin when we are cut.

Essential oils can also be diffused in the air. Research has shown that oils can kill most air-born microorganisms. A French study colonized 210 various microbes; within thirty minutes of misting the air with a mixture of oils only four colonies remained alive. You can mist your air with the fragrance of an essential oil by simply placing a few drops of oil—ten to fifteen—in a regular plant water mister diluted with some water.

As well, the therapeutic effect of food supplements and herbs is greatly enhanced when essential oils are part of the formula. When herbs and food supplements are prepared for sale, they are dehydrated. This dehydration releases 90 percent of the essential oil of the plant. Without the oil, most of the life force of the plant has been evaporated out. This is one reason why herbs used today are less effective than when our ancestors used to just go to the fields and pick what they needed. When the essential oil is reintroduced into the supplement, you are guaranteed that the nutrients will reach the cellular level in your body.

YOU CAN'T FIGHT GRAVITY—BUT WHEN YOU CAN'T FIGHT 'EM, JOIN 'EM

Because we live day-in and day-out with the force of gravity, we don't often think about how much energy we exert fighting it. Yet, when we feel tired, we are sensitive to the effects of gravity and feel compelled to lie down to ameliorate some of gravity's inexorable pull. When we go to the zoo and look at the animals on all fours, we develop a great appreciation for our up-rightness. However, we don't often think about how much stress our being erect puts on our bodies. When we walk or run, we're putting all of the gravitational pressure of our entire body on one small spot, creating thousands of pounds of pressure per square inch. Merely standing creates tremendous gravitational force against the feet and the spine.

Wherever there are weaknesses in our bodily structure—in the knee and hip joints, the lower back, the neck and abdomen—there will be more frequent injuries. In fact, the single largest health problem in the United States is back pain, an effect from our perpetual struggle against gravity. As well, gravity affects us on a cellular level. Many biologists now feel that gravity plays a significant role in the cell's loss of ability to replicate itself, thus contributing directly to aging and death. Bernard Jensen has said that there is not a single disease in which gravity does not play a part.

However, our bodies have evolved in a way that they normally work, not too badly, with the law of gravity. For instance if we look at the construction of the intestinal tract, we see that through most of the journey, food follows a downward slope. When the food reaches the beginning of the colon, it is now mostly liquid, and thus responds easily to peristaltic movement. In the ascending colon, the appendix lies below, and this organ, usually thought of as useless, actually acts as an irritant to force the food material uphill. By the time the material reaches the descending colon, gravity is able to exert its force to pull the waste downward.

To find an occasional reprieve from gravity, the logical question is: since gravity is the force that keeps pulling everything down, why not change the direction of our bodies so that what was going down in us now goes up, and what was going up now goes down? In other words, since we can't change gravity, we have to change ourselves. We can turn ourselves upside down. In this way, we are using the force of gravity for healing.

Yogic science discovered the importance of upside-down thousands of years ago. They invented the shoulder stand and the head stand. The slant board is, you might say, the short-cut version of these yoga postures.

When you are standing up, the pull of gravity, and thus the pull on the flow of blood and all other fluids in your body is five or six feet. When you lie on the slant board, with your head lower than your feet, the pull of blood to the upper part of your body is about eighteen inches. It's not a lot, but plenty enough to accomplish a considerable task.

Brain anemia may not be a medically recognized disease entity, but anyone suffering from chronic fatigue has it. If muscle tone or circulation is not good enough, then the blood can't travel uphill to the brain sufficiently to feed the brain. Without sufficient blood to the brain, virtually all of our functions will be weakened. The cerebellum, the back part of your brain, is where every physical organ is regenerated. You cannot breathe, you cannot hear, see or taste, you cannot think properly, nor move any part of your body without your back brain getting enough blood flow. This is, as well, the first part of the brain to be adversely affected by gravity.

Animals instinctively feed their brains the blood that is needed by how they sleep. An animal is always in a prone position during sleep, and its head falls lower than the rest of its body. In fact, if you hold an animal up by his front feet for long enough (for a dog, it's four hours, for a rabbit, it's three quarters of an hour), the animal will die because its heart and arteries cannot pump enough blood into its brain to keep it alive.

One of the conditions that we find the most responsive to the slant board is prolapsus of the internal organs. Any of us who have been on a traditional western diet, with refined foods, for any extended period of time, will have a prolapsed bowel. The transverse colon, which crosses over the abdomen, will dip in the middle, thus forcing the waste products in the colon to actually have to go upward, against gravity. This almost always proves too difficult, and a prolapsed colon then becomes a clogged colon. Bladder and prostate difficulties generally arise because the organs have fought against gravity for too many years, and the bladder is no longer in its proper place. Uterine fibroid tumors can be caused by the organs above bearing down, causing pressure on the uterus. The uterus, then, becomes mal-positioned, thus rendering the uterus less capable of throwing off toxic material.

Lying on the slant board repositions all of the internal organs. Gravity pulls the organs upwards, thus creating space between the organs so that the oxygen can reach the organs more easily.

Simply lying on the slant board with your arms stretched out above your head is wonderful. You may have noticed that between 3 and 5 p.m., it gets harder to keep your energy level up. This is because at this time, the sun and moon change their configuration in relation to each other. The fluids in our bodies make a concomitant change in response. It's best to find time to do the slant board around this time and you will find that you have renewed vigor for the rest of the day. In fact, fifteen to twenty minutes on the slant board renews your body the same as an hour of sleep.

THREE MINUTE DETOXIFICATION: DRY SKIN BRUSHING

Bernard Jensen tells the story of Samson, "the Saxon Giant," as an illustration of the health benefits of detoxifying through skin brushing. Samson was a weight lifter and wrestler brought to the

United States from Europe by Florenz Zeigfeld. Samson was one of the features in the Zeigfeld Follies in the 1920s. Besides his strength, Samson was also known for his baby-soft skin, an attribute which Samson attributed to his daily regimen of skin brushing.

Then one year, Samson lost the world's championship heavyweight weight-lifting contest by just ten ounces. Jensen was able to examine Samson's diaries, and found a stunning theory. Samson attributed his loss of the contest to the fact that he had neglected to dry-brush his skin for three weeks prior to the contest.

Jensen decided to do a little experiment to see why Samson would have reached such a conclusion. He bought a skin brush and stood on brown wrapping paper while he brushed. After he had collected enough debris that had fallen from his body from the brushing, he sent the material to a lab. The lab found a lot of dead skin, which would, of course, be expected; but the lab also found dried catarrh, urea, sodium chloride, sebum and metabolic acid wastes. Jensen came to understand that when these substances are not removed from the skin by skin brushing, they can become backed up in the muscle structure and cause a loss of vitality.

Jensen himself is testimony to his own theory. At a cancer conference, before his death at ninety-two, he told his story of recovering from cancer at the age of eighty-five (he was eighty-eight as he told the story with great vigor). He showed those of us attending the conference the skin on his arms and legs; there was not a single wrinkle, line or blemish anywhere on this man's body. He attributed the beauty of his skin, its tautness and elasticity, to his daily regimen of skin brushing.

WORKING WITH CONSCIOUSNESS

Meditation and psychoanalysis both work with the processes of the mind. They are both radar and sonar—sight as well as sound. They both have the power to project into the infinite consciousness and then bounce back to us. When we quiet our brain chatter, we are able, then, to break through all the interfering voices that arise out of mental speculation and that prevent us from hearing our own true voice. Meditation and psychoanalysis erase self-defense and self-justification. It is said that prayer is talking to the divine and that meditation and psychoanalysis are tools of listening.

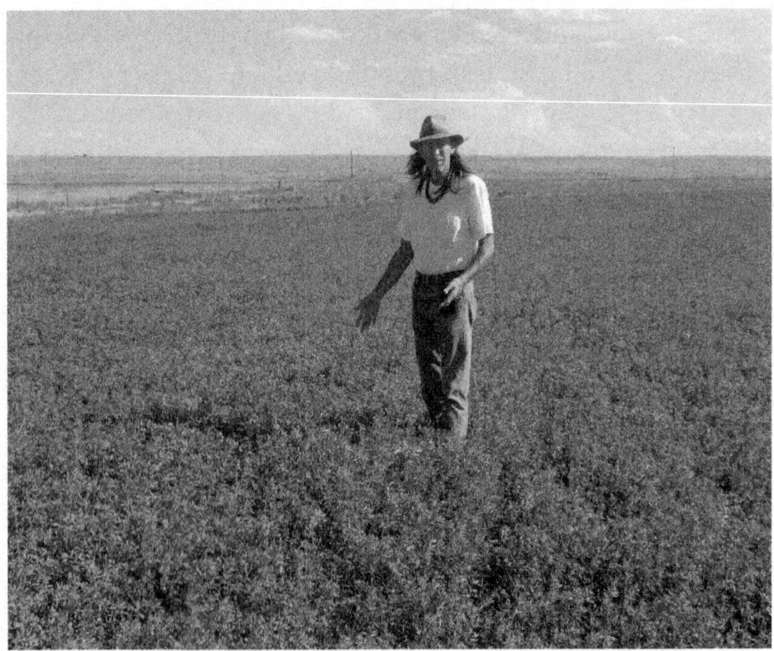

Jay Gutierrez standing in a crop field that has been nurtured with radiation hormesis-treated water. In comparison to non-treated plants, Jay's crops are notable for their vibrancy, growth, color, and yield.

APPENDICES

APPENDIX A

Testimonials

FROM JAY'S PATIENTS USING RADIATION HORMESIS

☛ Wednesday, April 05, 2006
Subject: the rock

Another cool one. I worked on a lady that had back surgery 5 weeks ago. She was in so much pain that she could hardly stand to be on the table. I put a rock on her back and did some energy work and light massage and guess what happened next.

Yes you are right no pain. Took all of 15 minutes to get her completely out of pain. She had been suffering so that she was completely amazed. Once more hear it for the rock.
Doc BJ

☛ Monday, November 06, 2006
Subject: RE: Healing Stones
Hello Jay,

October 2005 I was already schedule for a knee replacements surgery. Beginning that month I postponed for January 2006. Besides strong pain I really did not like the idea of the surgery plus the situation that I'm a golfer and I had to suspend for 6 months at least. During November 2005 I learned about Hormesis from a Japanese professor who does this in his country, is a senior person and very wise.

I did Radon inhalations for 20 days (3 a day) and also drink water with radon for 3 months. After a month, no more pain and I recovered all my faculties to do a normal life. Today I believe that no surgery is necessary and I play at least 3 times a week. As a matter of fact I play Saturday, Sunday and today (holyday) and I feel great and full of energy at the moment I'm writing this message to you. Last month I did again a 20 day therapy as it was recommended.

In a few words, that's what happened to me and I'm convinced about the benefits of underexposed.
Jorge Gutierrez

☛ May 8, 2007
Subject: skin cancer, from naturopathic doc
Hi Jay,

Here's an update on my skin cancer lady. Got back her AMAS test results from Oncolabs on the on the 27th of April. She's clear. Florence is the 84 year-old lady up in Stockton, Massachusetts that you sent the small stones and the special small mud packs. She was diagnosed with Merkel Cell Carcinoma in late December after a skin specialist botched an attempt to remove what he thought was a small tumor from her cheek. It turned out to be a lot more than he imagined. Tissue samples were sent to the lab. The doctors told Florence that Merkel Cell is a rare form of skin cancer that has a poor cure rate. They proposed putting a port in her body so that they could administer chemo to try to "maintain" her for the rest of her life. She was appalled at the idea and called me for a nutritional protocol.

Well this one sure went very fast. Florence started her protocol around the 7th of March. The test was performed on the 23rd of April. That is barely seven weeks. She has been a delight to work with. She says that the protocol reminds her of the way she ate when she was growing up on the small family farm: All fresh food. We fashioned a sling that she could fit over her head so that the small stone could be secured right up against the mass on her cheek. She slept with it that way. Sometimes she would sleep with her cheek up against the small mud pack.

I am happy to say that the numbers on the test are all in the right place. I called Oncolabs just to be sure. We still have a little swelling to work on, but the malignancy is gone. I suspect that the swelling is scar tissue from the surgery. Will keep you posted if there are any new developments. I will send Florence back for another AMAS test in about eight months.

Here's hoping this letter puts a smile on your face.

Blessings,
Maxine Murray, ND, CNHP, CNC

☛ August 20, 2007
Subject: breast cancer
Dear Jay,

These are just a few lines to bring you up to date on the breast cancer case I told you about last month. Remember when I was considering using escharotics but feared that it would be too traumatic? As you know, I'm out here in the middle of Pennsylvania Dutch country where there are many Menonite and Amish villages. I am writing about the Menonite lady who took to her bed after an unfortunate fall that dislocated her hip. As I understand, her doctor refused to do anything for her. After he advised her earlier this year that she had breast cancer, she refused chemo, radiation, and surgery. They quarreled over her decision, so he told her that she might as well go home and call hospice.

Her family called me the first week in July about a nutritional protocol. What I walked in on was not a pretty sight. Her right breast was just a hard movable mass about three inches square. There were approximately half a dozen oozing sores which she said had been there since February. Nothing the doctor had given her had helped. She tried to keep it clean as best she could, but it was always oozing a very smelly discharge. You could pick up this odor when you walked in the front door long before you got to the bedroom. When I called you about her case, we talked about the connection of fungus to cancer, and decided that a "hot" rock would probably kill the fungus and allow the breast to start healing. You sent the rock out; I got it over to the family around the 29th of July. I advised that the rock be kept on the breast 24/7. This has not been the easiest family to work with, for they don't always understand the importance of keeping in touch. Finally, after three weeks of silence, I heard from them on Sunday. It was the lady herself, calling me, glad to report that not only had the sores gone away "almost overnight," but that the actual mass was softening and felt as if it might be shrinking. She said that, after putting on the rock, the oozing had stopped almost overnight and that every single one of the sores had started scabbing over in about two or three days. She was delighted to finally see new pink skin where the open sores had been. She said that she did not experience any discomfort. Having seen some success, she is ready to get serious with her nutrition.

You know, I think this case is pretty remarkable, in that this woman is doing little or no supplements, plus she is osteoporotic. Her body has been very acidic for a long period of time and she has trouble remaining compliant to her nutritional protocol. Yet the breast is well on the way to healing. It just goes to prove one more time that we are dealing with fungus. The low-dose radiation killed the fungus, and the breast started healing. I am so grateful that you were there to help me with this one. Thank you very much.
Maxine Murray

☛ Sunday, August 26, 2007
Subject: smelly oozing cancer sores closed up
Hi Jay,

Oh joy! Just wanted to let you know that I finally heard from Mary Bowerman, the lady with the bad breast. She called to tell me that the breast is completely and totally healed. Every single one of the oozing smelly sores has closed up and healed. The hard lump inside has softened and is almost gone, and there is no more pain. She said that once she got to where she could have the stone on the area 24 hours a day, it was completely healed in about two weeks. I told her that I would like for her to keep the stone on

for a little longer just to be sure we get it all. Her doctor (the one who told her to call Hospice) came over to visit her on Wednesday night and could not believe his eyes. He expected to find someone near death. What a surprise to find her looking very well, indeed. With this success behind her, Mary is ready to do whatever I ask her to do to get completely well and out of that bed. Oh happy days.
Blessings
Maxine Murray

☛ Wednesday, September 05, 2007
Subject: stones plus surgery for breast cancer
Hi Jay,

Here are the details of my path so far . . . In May 07, I felt a small lump in the right breast that felt hard and was shaped like a pea. It was different than the fibro-cystic masses that I was familiar with. After an ultra-sound and biopsy, they said in 1 of the 5 tissue samples there were some low grade abnormal cells that needed to be dealt with. By this time, it was the end of June. The surgeon was willing to give me the month of July to pursue the alternative methods that I was getting info on. One of these was radiation hormesis and the products that you have. I purchased the green healing stone, a water stone, the mud pack and you also made me a necklace from a water stone. I began to use these each day.

The green stone was pulling things out and sometimes it ached after many hours. You said that this was a sign it was doing its work. The necklace stone began to have black spots all over it, again doing its job. After the month of July, I had a MRI. The lump had grown a minute amount which you said sometimes happens as its healing. It still showed some low grade cells in the lump but no other area was affected and the lymph nodes were clear. I was getting pressure from the surgeon to remove it and after checking with intuitive medical people and other alternative people I work with, I decided to remove it. I felt it was necessary to remove the old energy to make way for the new energy to come in.

The surgery was quick and easy. The recovery has been smooth and the test results could not have been any better. The area was clean, the lymph nodes were negative and the lump was half the size it was in the biopsy, ultra sound, and MRI. It had grade 1, slow growing cells in it. I will continue to use the stones and mud pack to ensure continued health. I do not feel regular radiation would be beneficial. Thank you so much for you research, help, continuing support and encouragement!!
Many blessings
Gael Holderman

☛ Sunday, October 28, 2007 12:07 PM
Subject: brain cancer treated with stones and chemo
Hello Jay,

I was originally diagnosed with adult onset brainstem gliomas in December. On Dec 30th they implanted radioactive seeds into the tumor. I received your stones sometime in January I believe. I have to be totally honest here I was really skeptical, but my Mom believes in this and the healing powers of "Jay's Rocks." I had used the stones haphazardly at best. I had faith in western medicine—the Doctor said that the seeds would eradicate the tumors so I figured six weeks would go by and I would be fine.

Well, six weeks went by and the tumor (actually it is a group of small tumors) were only reduced by about 30 percent, so the Doctor said more seeds and chemo. I have to be honest I turned to the stones not because I thought they would "cure" the cancer so to speak but more because I finally put two and two together and realized that they had really helped with the pain. So I started sleeping with them and clipping them to my head with a hair clip during the day for pain relief. I really didn't want to do chemo, so I went one time, and then skipped one time, then I skipped the next time. The Doctor was a little peeved and did another CATSCAN to see where we were and low and behold ... the unexplainable happened, I only have two small tumors left. So the Doctor wants to finish chemo, I agreed to one more round of chemo and then another CATSCAN so we will see what that bring.

I have to tell you Jay I am a believer now! I used to call my Mom the VOODOO doctor because I just couldn't get my brain around the healing power that she possesses. I am so in awe of her and the way she works with people. I truly believe that it is her love for people that makes her so special. At any rate, there is the latest update of where I am.

Words can't possibly describe the gratitude I feel in my heart for you, thank you so much for the stones, I think they may have saved my life, I am certain that they saved me from a great deal of unbearable pain.

I will keep you updated.

Jodi

☛ Sunday, October 28, 2007

Subject: prostate, written to Madeleen Herreshoff, Director of CANHELP

Dear Madeleen Herreshoff,

I am glad to offer my experiences to the healing power of Jay's stones. I need to give a brief medical history to help you understand my medical history. In the spring of 2001 I visited my urologist and I had an enlarged prostate. I put off seeing him again till after a family trip to Europe. On the long flight back, I did not do much walking in the airplane. I was obese and 80 lbs. overweight. On the flight back, an aneurism broke in vessel behind my stomach. I was not aware of this action till 6 months later, most of it in the hospital. It took that long to locate the source of my internal bleeding. I got out of the hospital in 2002. I was confined mostly to the house the rest of the year. I lost 80 lbs in the hospital.

In 2003, I was strong enough to revisit my urologist. He

did a biopsy and it turned out positive. The biopsy score was much lower than the lab score of the removed prostate. He operated and removed my prostate. The 20 pints of blood that I had received in the hospital from my leaking aneurism drained down on my pancreas and on to my prostate. I am a brittle diabetic because of the damage to my pancreas by the draining blood. It took the doctor almost 2 hours to remove the enlarged organ. The outer layer of the organ was hardened and looked like a walnut shell. In the removal process, the doc knew that he had spread cancer cells all over the area where the prostate was because of the difficulty in the removal process. He had the removed prostate examined in a lab and the cancer growth was past the time to have removed the organ.

The cancer level was very high. I went back to urologist after 3 months to review the PSA score. It came out to a minus 0. 03something. I went back in 3 more months and the PSA was a positive 0.02. It was during that time that I had the pleasure of working with Jay. He gave me a stone and I started to use it every night. I placed it in my crotch area and slept with it there. I always use the raw stones against my skin. I use the stones to relieve many other pains in my body all of the time. I currently sleep with 4 stones. Two in my crotch and 2 large stones on other areas of my body that are hurting or the help maintain my pancreas and keep a low PSA score.

I went back for another PSA test 3 months later. This test came out with the same score of 0.02. I have continued to use the stone ever since Jay introduced it to me. I am convinced the Jay's stones do offer pain relief and have healing power in many other medical conditions. My last PSA test was August of 2006. My score then was still 0.02. The doctor is very happy and so are we. I did drink some green tea for a while, but I can not verify that the tea was any real help.

Regards,
Ray Bonella

☛ Sunday, October 28, 2007
Subject: doubting Thomas
Dear Jay,

Let me preface this letter with the fact that I was the Ultimate "Doubting Thomas." In early 1990, I was at the peak of my game. I was the assistant to the VP of the world's largest animal health products, running my own tax preparation company, and composing music. On June 30, my life came to a screeching halt. I was struck down with a rare form of spinal meningitis that not only attacked my spine and brain, it attacked my body. The doctors told me I contracted it from birds. I never kept birds as pets so it was very confusing to me how I could have picked up this awful debilitating disease. I have remembered tending to a sick bird in my yard. My IQ dropped from 145 to 93. I began showing signs of chronic fatigue syndrome, immune deficiency, sensory loss, memory loss, skin disorders, bladder disorder, COPD, seizures, fibromyalgia, chronic headaches and spine pain, and on and on.

I was given morphine to control pain and many medications to control all my disorders. I went into severe clinical depression and just couldn't cope with all the major changes in my life. For many years I have suffered (as stoically as I could) through one health crisis after another. My doctors tried every way possible to help me. I even spent 3 years at a rehab hospital desperately trying to overcome my difficulties. I managed to get out of a wheelchair after a year but I still have trouble falling down and walking into things. I can't tell you how many well-meaning people would bring me all the latest "cures." For a while I tried them and became broken-hearted when nothing worked. I sought out the best specialist in the country. Absolutely nothing seemed to help me. I had to accept the fact that I wasn't going to get any better. So, I just lived life the best way I could without complaining and bearing a lot of terrible pain.

It has been 17 years of extreme difficulty. Then a miracle did happen. A friend of the family came home on vacation from

Singapore and dropped by to visit. She brought me a stone called "The Stone." She had gotten this stone from a friend who had several. Her friend lived here in Phoenix and swore this stone would heal anything. Well, my "Doubting Thomas" nature kicked on and I set it down on the kitchen table with my myriad of med's. A few days later, I had one of my infamous headaches, my chest was hurting unbearably, my stomach was in pain and an oxygen tank had fallen on me and broke my left wrist.

Early in the morning, out of sheer desperation, I saw the stone there on the table and began rubbing my wrist. It took the pain away immediately. As well as the bruise. So I rubbed it on my head, neck, chest and stomach. When I was finished, I was shocked to see my stone had gone from a light clay white to a very dark brown with large areas of round black spots. I used it for several days on my joints and other painful areas and the outcome was the same—No pain after use! I was beyond shocked!

Today, July 1, 2007, I was watching the concert for Princess Diana when Tom Jones came on a strange pattern was spinning on the screen behind him. It sent me into a grand mal seizure. My friend was helping me and she grabbed the stone and began rubbing my head with it. The seizure actually stopped after a few seconds and I didn't have the awful lethargic stupor afterwards! There really is no other explanation for all this pain relief and what happened today—except The Stone.

Now, I will take any oath or swear on anything sacred that this is all true. My health condition is slowly improving (even though my spelling might be off!) and I want everyone I know to use this stone. I am getting my pain under control and spending more and more time out of bed—up and doing things!

I will give you permission to requisition medical records from any of my doctors if you wish to show just how sick I have been. Please realize I am not yet cured, but I'm moving in that direction day by day! For the first time in 17 years I have had days when I don't feel the horrible pain.

Thank you! Thank you! Thank you! I cannot express how much gratitude I feel for your efforts and for my friend bringing me this miracle! If you have any questions for me, please don't hesitate to contact me.

With my best regards and loving gratitude,
Cindy Pelletier

☛ Monday, November 12, 2007
Subject: breast cancer

In June of 2001, I was diagnosed with breast cancer. It was classified as stage 2 and the lump was removed as well as lymph nodes. The treatment I chose at the time was IPT (insulin potentiated therapy) with a Dr. in Denver who was using alternative treatments along with some traditional. I chose not to do traditional chemo and radiation that was recommended to me at the Cancer Treatment Center of America in Tulsa. It just didn't feel right for me. My body and spirit was in conflict when I considered that form of treatment. I also did my due diligence in study of what I could find during the 6 weeks from surgery to treatment time. So I did not come to this decision without a lot of prayer, study, and consideration of all the effects on my body and life.

Now time has passed since 2001 and during this time, I have made a conscience effort to live a healthy life. I am not a purist so my lifestyle was that of what I figured to be an 80/20 of eating the right foods and nutritional supplements, balance of physical activity, spiritual life, emotional and mental. All my tests were clear and life was good.

In the summer of 2006, I seemed to be having some back muscle problems. I went to a massage therapist (a couple of different ones over time) and a couple of different Chiropractors—I would get some relief but it never seemed to hold and by Oct it was getting worse. For me, something else was happening that I still cannot say that I really comprehend. I had strange thoughts about missing my husband—for no apparent reason—and at times feel like I was going to have to be alone—now the reason I bring this up is that I believe this caused distress or stress at a very base level that I wasn't recognizing. I just pretty much dismissed these feelings as strange and disturbing but so not real in my world. By late Oct, my massage therapist told me that my right rib that was causing me considerable discomfort and sometimes outright pain, just didn't feel right and that I needed to get that checked out. I intended to do so but had a lot of things going on and figured I'd do it a little later.

My husband Dick in the meantime was having a few strange things happen to him. He would have indigestion type pain once in awhile but it didn't seem connected to anytime or any activity or meal. At 69 he looked maybe 55 and had the energy and strength of many younger than that as well as me at 57. He hiked the mountain behind us at least 2 times a week sometimes more. Also he started building our timber-framed home at age 65—an incredible accomplishment when you consider that he had never built anything in his life. He worked on the house every day, unless we were off and running, visiting family and friends. We did a lot of travel in between finishing the house. So in Oct he went to the VA here in Alamosa to get a physical. All was well—he was healthy and all his tests looked great. But they wanted to rule out that this pain could be a heart problem, so they scheduled a stress test in Denver at the VA hospital where they had the equipment.

On Nov 20, 2006 we made our way there to meet the appt at 12:30. We enjoyed our drive up and talked and laughed as we usually did. We exchanged our smiles and love as he walked down the hall to do the test. That was the last I saw him alive. He was on the treadmill for 4 min, heart rate at 110, EKG fine, and then he said "I feel lightheaded"—and never took a breath after that. They worked on him for 30 min and could not bring him back. It was unreal to me. The love of my life, my strength, my joy, my best friend—gone. Now in the arms of Jesus—not mine.

Now the pain really took over—in every way. And when all of this happened, I also lost over half of my income. I was now not able to financially take care of myself as well. The fog, the depth of darkness, the fear of what was ahead of me—even at times the questions of did I really want to go forward with my life—not in a suicidal thought—but in wanting to live –and for what purpose. Yes, I had my children, my grandchildren, my parents and aunts and uncles, my church family, my close friends—all surrounding me with love and support. God has so blessed me and surrounded me with love—but was it enough?—that is so hard—because my life was with Dick—we were one as much as any two could be—a part of me was gone forever and now my body was so open to the cancer to just take over.

Finally in March, I got to a Chiropractor that saw how bad I was and knew it was more than the grief and just muscle problems. He insisted I get x-rays—and that was when it was diagnosed that I had metastatic cancer—it was in my lungs, my rib, and on my spine. I went back to the Dr I had gone to in 2001, he alarmed me. He said I had no time and that alternative wasn't going to help me that I needed to do radiation on my spine before I got a fracture and was crippled and full dose chemo to attack the rest. He also told me that there was no hope of any type of cure and that the best that could happen was to maybe get it under "control" for awhile. But God had other plans.

Just the week before I had a chance encounter with a friend whom I normally would not have had contact with for a long time. She gave me the name of Dr. [Raphael] d'Angelo and said I might like him and he might be able to help me. So always wanting more information before I make a choice—I wanted a second opinion. Dr. d'Angelo was so kind, encouraging and gave me hope. He told me that at this time standard medicine really had no answer to cancer, and alternative although better, didn't have any strong answers either. But, he said—he had recently met a man by the name of Jay Gutierrez who had introduced him to Radiation

Hormesis which already he had 2 other cancer patients on it and they were doing very well. He took his time and did a little drawing and explained a lot to me. He also encouraged me to get in contact with Jay as well as check out more information on the web in regards to the Radiation Hormesis.

I did these things, as well as get a pack and a rock that day. Jay was so full of hope and encouragement that I felt for the first time that maybe I was to stay here and survive and have a new purpose in my life. In a few days, I went out to his "rock shop" and met him. I knew then, this was of God and He had so graced me with this gift of His creation—and the gift of friendship with Jay.

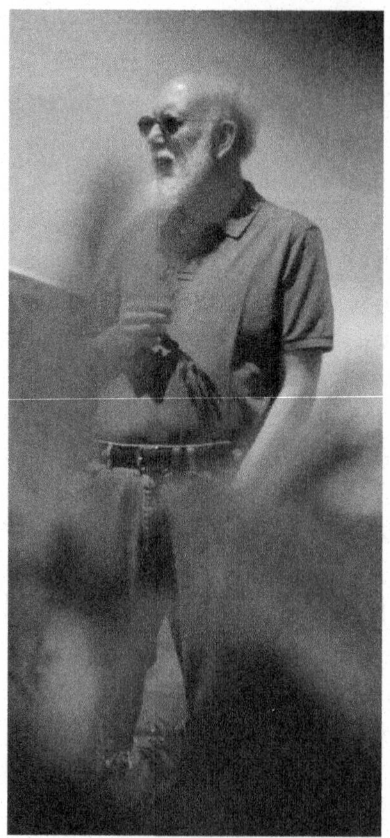

Dr. Raphael d'Angelo.

I diligently slept on the pack—then moved to 2 packs—as well as devised methods on which to wear the stones on specific areas on my person during the day. Jay made me some half packs as the full packs were too heavy to wear. So from March through July, that's what I did. I also went back to a stricter healthier diet, took some specific nutritionals for cancer fighting, and continued to work on my mental, emotional, and spiritual being. I have always believed that cancer or any other disease in a whole person problem.

In July we went for the tests. I was concerned and yet ok

at the same time. Jay couldn't wait to hear the results—of course he by now had seen so much that he was sure we had gotten a hold of it. And he was right—all the areas that we knew of the cancer had stopped!! It was such great news. How can it be cancer anymore if it isn't growing?? My understanding is that—that is what cancer is—out of control mutant cells that kill and take over the good cells. Also at that time, my upper leg had been really giving me problems, so we did an MRI on the femur. Sure enough—there was an area there that had cancer as well.

I then came up with a way to keep a stone on that area too now. My leg continued to bother me and when I had come back from being with family for a month—Jay got me a stronger rock—we had also upped the level radiation packs in the meantime. Now time to wait again. Another 4 months had passed. After one conversation with Jay about how my leg was still in a lot of pain—he just said—it can't be the cancer—it just can't. So last week I met with Dr. d'Angelo and we talked and then did an x-ray. Sure enough—that cancer had stopped too. There had been no change, the bone looked normal although you could see the dark area where the cancer was, and my joint was healthy. What was going on was muscle atrophy—I had been not using my leg like I should because weight bearing made it hurt—so now had created the problem from limited use. He was right—the cancer could not continue to grow in the radiation field. Radiation Hormesis works. All the other things I have been doing and continue are good for the overall health of my body but the final component that stopped the cancer was the Radiation Hormesis—of that I am sure. I believe in time my body will rid itself of the bad cells and the damage they have caused. Now that they aren't perpetuating themselves, my body will be able to heal itself. And I will always sleep on my pack for the rest of my days.

Whatever life brings our way—we need hope. God gives us that hope through many different ways. Through radiation hormesis (which He created)—He gives us hope in cancer (and

maybe many other challenges) that our lives here are not yet done –we have more to do—I believe He will draw those to us who know about this to share this gift of healing. Again—thank you Jay for being so willing to speak the truth in a world that doesn't always want to hear it. And for others willing to seek and share what we have been given—thank you too. God's Blessings.
Helen Carlson

☛ Thursday, November 29, 2007
Subject: menstrual cramps
Hi Jay

I am writing to let you know of another fascinating healing story using your necklace. I wear mine all the time and last night, at dinner with dear friends, 15 year old Jennifer was in serious pain with menstrual cramps. She could barely keep her head up, was nauseated by the smell of food, looked bleary-eyed and had very low energy. After about a half hour together, I took off my necklace and handed her the stone, explaining briefly about the healing qualities. She was skeptical at first.

Almost immediately, upon holding it in her left hand, she began to perk up. She noted that the stone felt warm in her palm, and that she was experiencing a tingling feeling. Within minutes, she was full of life again. Her pain had subsided and she was eating! She handed the stone to her friend Olinda, but almost immediately asked for it back—she could feel that she needed it. For the rest of our dinner, she held the stone and was high spirits, energetic, laughing, talking, eating. I had never seen the stone work so immediately—and this was the small necklace stone!
Rhonda Ruretzky

☛ Wednesday, December 26, 2007
Subject: arthritis
Just wanted you to know the stones have helped my arthritis in my knees a whole bunch. I can go up and down my stairs very well

now. Something I haven't been able to do for 2 years. Scotty has had to carry my laundry down stairs and then back up when I am done. I used to have to hold on and pull myself up one stair at a time. Now I can go up and down with the laundry with no problem. Wonderful stuff Huh???? I tell everybody about them. A lot of people look at me like I am talking Voo Doo Ha Ha!! That's ok . . . I am undeterred with their opinions.
Melba Scott

☛ January 12, 2008
Subject: pancreatic cancer
Hi Jay,
Admission date to the Hospital Emergency center: 7/20/2007
Hospital Diagnosis: Pancreatic Mass (about 1 inch in diameter)
Acute Renal Failure
Diabetes Mellitus Type 2
Hypertension
Hyponatremia
Depressive Disorder
Smoker
Cardiomyopathy

Brief Summary of Hospital Course/Complications: 71 year-old male with a history of diabetes and HTN, who presents with acute on chronic renal failure, jaundice, weight loss and a pancreatic head mass found on ultrasound. CT-guided brush biopsies of mass were obtained and pericutaneous biliary drain inserted on 7/20/2007. Brush biopsy cytology was inconclusive. CT scan for staging which showed no pulmonary or hepatic metastases but did show peripancreatic nodes. Percutaneous biliary drain became problematic for patient with pain. Following oncology consult patient and family have agreed to not pursue further treatment of biopsies (because of high risk with a needle biopsy), and focus on home hospice care. We then placed a permanent metal stint to allow for physiologic biliary drainage and removal of external drain prior to patient discharge to home.

Patient has been home and has home hospice services since discharge: 8/1/07

Since September, 2007, Bill has been doing low radiation stones therapy with Jay Gutierrez. He is drinking radiated water (with water stone), has placed (taped) radiation stones, 1 green and 1 higher radiation, over his pancreas on his stomach. Has worn the stones constantly except when showering. He also has a radiated mud pack that was originally a lower radiation dose, and now wears a mud pack of more intensity. He also is taking dietary supplements of Limu and Colostrum.

On: 12/18/07 Bill had another ultrasound test. The results showed "something" on the pancreas that was about 1 inch in diameter. There was no change showing at all. Since the diagnosis when we left the hospital was that we could expect him to die within a range of 2 weeks to 6 weeks and to have unbelievable pain (he has not had the first twinge), we tend to think what Jay thinks. The tumor is gone and has left a mark, or scar tissue, and of course it is Jan. 12, 2008 and Bill is still walking around.

This week (1/13/08) our doctor has consulted with a radiologist who will be calling Bill to do another kind of scan in the near future. Dr. T. has also requested 7 fasting blood sugar readings be sent to him, and he then will decide if Bill will go back to an insulin regimen.
Sue M.

☛ January 12, 2008
Subject: cure of Lyme's disease
Dear Night Hawk,

I am a patient of Opus Arts Holistic Health and have been struggling with chronic and late stage Lyme disease, fibromyalgia, disautonomia, low thyroid, rapid heart beat, high blood pressure, numerous cancer surgeries and chronic fatigue syndrome. Needless to say I have been severely lacking in energy. So severe that I couldn't stand up and walk across the room. If I did anything, I became extremely dizzy and felt as though I was blacking out. My joint pain was so severe that I could not walk and had to use wheelchairs to do my shopping. This is how severe my illnesses were back in 2005.

I began seeing John and Laurie on October 23, 2007. They immediately recommended the Green Stone, the Stone for my water and the mud pack. So I started with this treatment right away. I will bathe with the Green Stone or rub it on specific painful areas. And I sleep with the mud pack as well as drinking lots of the stone water daily. I experienced only a mild nausea on the first day which John and Laurie explained might happen.

Since then I have seen tremendous gains in my energy levels. I no longer have to stay in bed most of the day or nap. I am able to focus my attention better and my short term memory loss has improved too. My pain level is much better. I never have to take pain medication anymore. Even on days when the weather has become cold or wet. I have now stopped using a wheelchair and walking stick.

Unfortunately, since my type of Lyme disease is so difficult to cure I sometimes suffer relapses. My last relapse was about 3 weeks ago and since then I've changed the way I use the Green Stone treatments. I've been instructed to use hot water with the water stone and then cool it down for drinking. I use hot water before rubbing the Green Stone on specific painful areas, i.e., joint pain and lymph node pain.

I think that anyone in my condition could benefit from using this treatment.

Thanks to you, Night Hawk and to Opus Arts!!

Sincerely, Diane Black

☛ Thursday, January 17, 2008

Subject: A Doctor with MS finds pain relief using the Stone

Dear Jay,

I want to give you some feedback on my experience with the use of the regimen of "the stone." First, some background on me. I am currently 55 years old. I was diagnosed with relapsing-remitting multiple sclerosis at age 35—20 years ago. At that time I was a professor of anesthesiology. I developed a vertigo, loss of proprioception (ability to tell where my body parts were located in space), visual difficulties, and very low stamina. I had to stop working for two years. I optimized my diet, took reasonable supplements, and practiced yoga to maintain my body's flexibility. I was able to return to graduate school, and I earned a PhD in behavioral medicine, with a focus on neuroscience and neuropsychology. From my anesthesiology training I was well-versed in pharmacology. My last job was as a professor of advanced pathophysiology and pharmacology at Georgetown University.

From 1995-2000, I was prescribed various forms of beta interferon. This drug produced a side-effect that never went away. It created pain in all of my muscles and joints that was debilitating. I switched from interferon to copaxone. While this drug did not cause the muscular pain, the pain from the interferon treatment never went away. I also continued to have extreme fatigue. The problem with copaxone is that it caused severe injection site reactions—pain, redness, and swelling, reactions which took weeks to subside.

Even while taking interferon and copaxone, I would have exacerbations of my MS symptoms about every 6 weeks, and I would have to spend about a week sleeping 16 hours per day and wasn't able to maintain my yoga routine or take care of household chores. It would take me about 10 days to start feeling better.

Four months ago stopped taking copaxone, and I began using the combination of the green eliat stone and the mud pack and the thorium stone in water. I spend at least eight hours per day with the pack against the skin of my lower and upper back. I rub the green stone over aching joints and muscles, which provides me with relief of my pain (a decrease from a 7 on a 1-10 scale to about a 3.) My greatest improvement has been in my stamina and in my coordination of my ocular muscles, and in my proprioception, which I attribute to drinking the water. I drink about a gallon of the water per day. My productivity has increased considerable, since I am able to read longer without fatigue, I can move about with less pain, and my overall energy has improved significantly. I have not had any exacerbations of my symptoms in four months, and overall I am feeling better than I have in years. My mood seems more stable, and it is easier for me to perform my light exercise with low weight dumb bells and a more physically demanding yoga sessions.

I plan to continue on this regimen. In my experience, it provides better disease management than any of the ABC drugs that are currently the mainstay of multiple sclerosis treatment. As a student of pathophysiology, I have thoroughly reviewed the literature on radiation hormesis. It makes sense to me that steady exposure to low doses of ionizing radiation would be beneficial in any condition where stability of the immune system is crucial to disease management. I will continue to keep you updated on my condition. Thank you, Jay, for finding me an answer.

Sincerely,
John M. Evans, CRNA, MPH, Ph.D.

☛ Friday, February 22, 2008
Subject: liver and pancreatic cancer

Hi Jay—thought I would share some good news with you. I have the liver and pancreatic cancer, and you had sent me a liver stone. I went in for a CT scan and blood work after four months of wearing the stone for 10 hours per day (at night usually). My doctor told me that that cancer had not grown – it is slow growing and rare. One noticeable test showed my chromogranin A lowered from 7974 to 515. Normal is 0 – 32, but this is a substantial drop. It is a protein tied with the pancreas and used as a marker in the blood which is used in pancreatic and prostate cancers. This was good news to me and my mom.

I tape the stone over the liver and then change to closer over the pancreas. Hope this is the right way. I do believe that the Lord puts things on this earth to help where others fail. I count this as a blessing. I thank you for your help. If you have any other suggestions, please let me know.

Thank you again –
Willi Moore

☛ Monday, March 17, 2008
Subject: Miracle Mineral Dog
Hi Jay,

Perhaps it was just circumstance, (or maybe not!) but the very day that we received our Water Stone, our dog became violently ill with a diagnosed case of parasitic infection from drinking contaminated water in our backyard. By that evening, he was not even able to lift up his head from his pillow. Around midnight, I taped the Water Stone to his abdomen. By next morning at sunrise he was up and ready to go. I took him for a two hour walk and he left me panting for breath. Thanks again Jay! I'm sure that we would have lost him had it not been for the Stone.

Jim Dooley

☛ Friday, May 02, 2008
Subject: My Mother
Jay,

Sorry for the delay in the email—I wanted to get the accurate numbers for the CA 125 test. Today was a spectacular day for my mom and my family. First I wanted to briefly go over where we have been in this cancer journey. My Mom was diagnosed with stage three ovarian cancer in July 2006. In August she had an emergency surgery: they performed a hysterectomy and removed several tumors one the size of a grapefruit. One month later she was started on Chemo—carboplatinum based—6 cycles. After six months she was off the Chemo and her CA125 had dropped back to around 40. Within one month she experienced pain in her side and stomach—her CA125 level started to shoot up as it was obvious she was carboplatinum resistant. We opted at that time to enroll her in a Phase 2 study at the University of Arizona which was an antibody treatment using Genentechs, Tarceva and Avastin.

She started to have good results for about 5 months—the problem was that the drug caused massive skin irritation to her face and various parts of her body. Initially in the study she had a drop in her CA 125 down below 100. Unfortunately the CA 125 started to shoot back up in October-November 2007. She was taken off the study and we were running out of options.

My mom opted to take a brief break from the medical treatment to give her body and soul a chance re coup. She took a pilgrimage with my sister to Lourdes France in search of some divine intervention in January (Lourdes being a Catholic pilgrimage destination for healing). Her CA 125 level was up to 500 in December, 1500 in January, 2,500 in February—and then at the end of March it went all the way to 8,700. Basically 8,700 is off the charts. She was holding off starting the next leg of CHEMO hoping that some of the natural path things she was doing would take hold (high doses of Vitamin C). She was started on Gemzar at the end of March (2 rounds of Chemo once a week for two weeks and then one week off).

I had flown to Phoenix to be with her prior to the second round of her first cycle. She also began to develop Ascites as her stomach began to fill with cancer cells. We had her stomach drained of about 2.5 liters of fluid as the bloating became very very uncomfortable. On the next day after the Chemo it became apparent to me that she was at an extremely critical juncture—to be truthful I could sense that the Ascites was already filling up again (which was extremely negative) and that she was basically was losing the battle. I had realization that the Chemo was being applied to late and was frankly not working.

My sister had recommend your webpage two months before and I simply mentally filed it in the "whacko" category of more cancer cure nonsense. It was then that I had begun to do research on your web page and the internet. Suddenly with death seeming far more evident I began to search information on the historical studies as well as the information on your web page. I appreciated you directness and sincerity when I spoke to you and really started to believe that this was a real possibility for my mother. So I ordered two kits one for my mom and one for myself as I wanted to do things with her to see how it effected me (I liked the idea of better sleep as well). So to give you a brief overview of the CA 125 tests: CA125 started at 8700 in late March. After using the Rock therapy for two weeks it dropped to 4,500. After three more weeks CA 125 dropped to 850 (as of last Tuesday). The fact is that the cancer was far more advanced then it should have been when we started the Chemo. This level of reversal has been extremely dramatic and the Doctors are very very happy with the progress. I did not inform the Doctors of the rock therapy as I knew what their response would be.

The fact is that most of the scientific community would say that the drop was a result of the Chemo—I can only reflect what I believe in my heart of hearts—the reason I started my mom on this therapy was that I believed the CHEMO was not working and she was dying. I anticipate taking her off CHEMO in the next four weeks due to the physical toll. I believe with my rational mind and emotional heart that the radiation Hormesis saved her life. The CA 125 empirical data supports the drastic drop. Chemo advocates will believe the CHEMO is working—what I know is that the radiation hormesis therapy is what's killing the cancer and saving my mom's life. Thank you—thank you—thank you for all your kindness, help, and dedication.

Michael Treon

☛ Tuesday, May 20, 2008
Subject: No Mass & No Tumors
Aloha Jay:

While visiting my doctor today, I had a chest x-ray. My doctor called me into her office to review the results. She was concerned about water in the lungs or water surrounding the heart as I was retaining water and had some swelling. None of that showed up. I looked at the x-ray and asked my doctor where the mass or tumors, which was diagnosed as stage IV lung cancer in January was and she replied "I don't see any." I said "Thank you Lord." I knew at that moment that I had received a miracle. I cannot thank Our Lord enough for putting Jay Guiterrez in my life because according to the pulmonary surgeon I visited in January, I should be dead by now. I never had any radiation or chemotherapy. The only radiation I used was radiation hormesis from the stones Jay sent me. Please believe anything is possible through Our Lord and never stop thanking Jay for his help, patience and dedication while working with all the people who call upon him for his hope and support when none was offered by the medical field.

Heartfelt Thank You Jay and God bless you.
Kay Noto

☛ June 9th, 2008
Subject: Woman's son gets bitten by a brown recluse spider.

This is our story . . . My son and his fiancé moved into a duplex last fall. When the weather started to warm up this spring, they noticed spiders moving into their house. They realized that the spiders were brown recluse spiders and that his home was infested with them. One morning he woke up to realize that he had been bitten on his ear with the recluse spider still lying next to his pillow. He immediately went to a clinic near his home and the Doctor told him there was nothing he could do for it and that Tyler would most likely have to have reconstructive surgery on his ear.

I had an aunt who was bitten by a recluse spider on her hand when she was a child. I know the severity of a brown recluse bite and did not want that for my son. My fiancé looked on the internet for about 6 hours trying to find something that could help Tyler. We decided to try Pascalite/Bentonite Clay because it said that it was the only known cure for Recluse Spider Bites.

I happened to email my very close friend that day to tell her what had happened to Tyler. She told me about the stones you use and how effective they are. More importantly, she was driving to Kansas City that weekend where my son lives. Talk about perfect timing! She met Tyler and gave him the stone to use. Tyler used the stone as directed to him and within just a few days the ear was completely healed. When I say completely healed, I mean no scabbing or scarring. I believe that things happen for a reason. Because you are a friend of my friend and because she just happened to be driving to Kansas City from Colorado that weekend was not simply coincidence. "Thank you" doesn't seem good enough but I don't know how else to let you know grateful we are that you were there for us at that moment.

God Bless,
Connie

☛ Tuesday, June 10, 2008
Subject: Knee

Jay, I wanted to make sure of the results before I wrote you. I have used the pack and rock on my knee. It works, the pain is gone. The radiation did something to repair, restore or heal the damaged Mencius in my knee.

Gene Moore

☛ Wednesday, July 23, 2008
Subject: Just had to share

Well, this is great. Today is the 21st day since I received my stones. I'm feeling so good today. I have been able to do a few things, even prepared my own breakfast and lunch without a lot of trouble. I can walk through the house, all the way through the house. That's compared to dragging across a room and having to rest for an hour the day before and for the last 3 weeks. I am so happy. Now I can't wait until tomorrow to see how much better I'm going to be. I have a feeling this is going to be a wonderful weekend, I can hardly wait. I'm almost giddy with excitement. I knew this day was coming but it just seemed to be taking so long. Now that it's here all I can think of is how wonderful the rest of life is going to be.

Thanks so much Jay for what you do. I'll keep you posted on how the rest of my recovery is coming. I can't wait to go to the lung doctor and see the improvement in my lungs. Like I said, I'm almost giddy I'm so excited. Oh, while I'm bubbling over with so much joy I should tell you about the great things the stones have been doing besides working on my lungs. I burned my thumb back when I first received the stones. It was a painful burn but I remembered the necklace and rubbed the stone between my thumb and my index finger and in less that one minute the pain was completely gone. There was no redness or spot from the burn. I didn't even have a twinge from that moment on.

Also, I got some really nasty organic shampoo in my eye. Anything that hurts that bad can't be good for us. Anyway, I didn't think about the stone for a couple of hours. The eye was raw and red. It wouldn't quit hurting and burning even though I'd washed it out thoroughly. Then suddenly I remembered how well the necklace stone had worked on my thumb. I took the necklace off and began rubbing the stone over the eyelid. In just three or four minutes the pain was gone. The redness was gone and my eye was like new. These stones are wonderful.

Also, I've had an arthritic shoulder for a couple of years. The joint was frozen in place and attempting to move my arm was excruciatingly painful. I began putting the green stone on my shoulder the day I got it. In three days I was able to lift my arm over my head to the front. I could also lift it as high as my shoulder up from my side. It is working great now. It's still a bit tender in certain positions but I am certain that will ease up shortly. After all it wouldn't move at all for months. So I'm amazed with the results.

My husband had golf elbow (or tennis elbow) in both arms. He put the green stone on each elbow and left it for a couple of hours and hasn't had any pain in his elbows since then.

OK, that's all the wonderful things I can think of for the moment. But I just love these stones. They are great for absolutely everything.
Joann Kyce

☛ Wednesday, July 23, 2008
Subject: Fw: So much for cancer
Jay,

Remember the PSA was 85. Now it is—are you sitting down? .9. That's right and yes you can holler. I did, and my a1c which is for diabetic less than 7 is ok and mine was 35 is now 12 praise God and You for following his works. I am going to do the test again in 30 days to see where I am and will let you know, I have started using the stones on the upper part of my body and now those glands are kicking up so here we go again. Heather also drew for fungus can't wait to see the results on that but that will take 2 to 3 days. I couldn't wait to tell you the news.
Mark had a PSA of 85! Now it's 0.9. Incredible!
Mark Morrison

☛ Monday, July 28, 2008
Subject: spinal disc
Hi again Jay,

Hope you had a great weekend!

This is such a wonderful Monday morning. I received a call from my daughter just a few minutes ago. She was on her way home from her doctors appointment. They did an x-ray. So you know who she is. I am Joann (Jody) Kyce. My daughter is Sybil Goff. She had a back injury and had 4 discs removed and bone grafts put in their place two years ago. About 3 or 4 months ago another disc exploded and they were planning on doing another surgery as soon as she was physically able to have it. This time they were going to put a rod in her spine to strengthen it because so much of her lower spine is gone. She also has lupus.

She received her package on July 7th and began using everything right away. She immediately became ill with diarrhea, headaches, nausea and symptoms of the flu. So she had to cut back on the water and the amount of hours she was using the stones and mud pack. She only slowed down but didn't stop using them.

This morning when she removed her body cast to have the ex-ray, her doctor asked what was inside her brace. It was her mud pack. She only told him it's something she'd been using to help with her back. When he did the ex-rays he was astonished. He was only checking to see how much the inflammation in her spine was going down so he could estimate when the surgery could possibly take place. But to his astonishment the soft tissue around the disc has started to heal. He told her that from what he was seeing she may not need surgery, after all. Given the condition of her spine he had not expected this tissue to begin healing. He sent her to see the therapist this morning to schedule therapy to extend her range of motion. Of course it is good to know that he thinks she is strong enough to begin stretching exercises.

Jay, this is what we have prayed for. The mud pack is working just like you told me it would. I am so thankful to you for sharing these wonderful stones. I am seeing more and more evidence everyday that they work. I am definitely on cloud nine and so is my daughter. Neither one of us can jump up and down and dance a jig to show our excitement but because of the stones we will be able to in the very near future. Thanks again Jay, I certainly appreciate you much more than words can convey.

Maybe someday I can come to your stone store and meet you so I can shake your hand.
God Bless,
Joann (Jody) Kyce

☛ Friday, August 15, 2008
Subject: Jack's Lung Cancer
Jay,

We purchased stones from you about two months ago and Jack had his first CT scan since he started wearing the necklace, using the mud packs, etc. All of the tumors are at least half the size they were in the last scan and at least one doesn't show up at all any more. I will keep you informed as we go forward—but I wanted to let you know our progress to date and to thank you for your help. I may just have to order a few more necklaces for the family.
Sincerely,
Polly Case

☛ Saturday, August 23, 2008
Subject: bye bye diabetes
Dear Jay,

Just wanted to update you on my progress. I'm still getting much better. I have tons more energy and the swelling in my body is going down and I'm losing weight which I haven't been able to do for years, no matter how little I ate. My doctors took me off my diabetic medications and have been trying to figure out what happened I told them what I was doing with the rocks, and the foot baths, she said she didn't recommend it, but then again she couldn't argue with success, and my blood work had been amazing. I'm still on my blood pressure meds. But the skin sores I've had for around 7 years that the regular doctors haven't been able to figure out are healing and almost gone. I have had two very small set backs though one was when I went back to Cheyenne.

I wasn't following my program well because I was under a

lot of stress and very busy but if you remember I was pretty much bed ridden four months ago, so that was probably a lot for my muscles. I had been that way for many years and for several days now I've had itchy welts on my arms and legs but by morning they seem to disappear and my skin is looser which I've been telling doctors for years that it feels like my skin tightens up and folds into itself. It feels like it's unfolding now. I know that sounds crazy but that's what it seems like to me. Also as it unfolds, it seems like hair like long fibers come out.

Anyway I'm still wondering about how we could use this in making something like a natural pool that I could have my whole body in because the only other thing that has ever helped me was soaking in a hot tub or spending lots of time in a pool and that never helped to this degree. But I think it could have kept me from dying. I used to pray a lot for how to heal myself and it seemed to me that God always had me soaking in water. I knew at that time he was telling me something about energy but I didn't really understand however he always prompted me to go and pray on this hill.

I wanted to pray for the town and I kept feeling like I was supposed to go there so I just did it. Some people from the church that I was going to kept telling me that that was crazy—God wouldn't say that because he answers prayer from anywhere. I know that, but on the other hand, God hasn't ever lied to me yet. So even when it seems not to make sense to me at the time, I've always found out later there are always reasons. Now I believe that maybe there were some of those rocks there and it was a maintenance program of sorts. Ha ha. God's a multi-tasker. Anyway, I've prayed about this and I really believe something that combines these two things like I said would be worth figuring.
Teresa Rhodes

☛ Date: Dec 1, 2008
Subject: Cancer free

Hi Jay,

Just thought I would let you know how things are going for me at this time. If you recall I came to you in June 2008 and here is my story: I am a 56 year old woman that had been told in April 2007 by my gynecologist during a routine pap smear exam that there was a lump about 5 mm in size in my rectum that should be checked by my physician. January 10, 2008 I finally had a colonoscopy that showed the lump had increased in size to 8 mm. The biopsy showed adenocarcinoma colorectal cancer. The tumor was 1 cm from top of dentate line which meant I was not considered a candidate for surgery with resection due to the close proximity to the sphincter muscles and the required margin needed to completely remove any possibilities of recurrence. So a permanent colostomy was what the doctors told me is how it would be. It was recommended strong chemotherapy and radiation for 5 to 6 weeks with 6 weeks to heal then the colostomy surgery and after all that there still would be no guarantee that there would be no recurrence of cancer.

My reaction was NO WAY, I did not want chemo or radiation and the permanent colostomy was not something I was willing to accept. I had a PetScan February 28, 2008 the results were not very promising. My husband and I searched the web for anything that would get me back to health. There is a lot out there but you are a guinea pig and with all cancers time is of the essence. My first alternative was to go to Tijuana, Mexico for 21 days of treatment to build the immune system. I got back to Colorado the 1st of April, and started having acupuncture treatments and taking supplements continuing to support my immune system. On the 21st of May, I had my second PetScan. The news was even worse.

The size of the tumor had increased to 1.6mm with increased metabolic activity identified (cancer activity) from 4.1 to 9.7 and now the lymph nodes were involved. What was I to do? I went to a Dr. that was a specialist in only colon surgery to get another answer and of course I did not get another answer, just more of a maybe on the colostomy if the chemo and radiation shrunk the tumor so the margin needed was enough for resection and was told I wouldn't know if I would have a colostomy until I came out of surgery.

Mid-June I spoke to a friend that my husband and I met while in Mexico, she told me about Night Hawk Minerals, Jay Gutierrez and that the stones were helping people live. What did I have to lose? I called Jay, it was late Saturday afternoon and told him my story. He explained about the stones and he would send them to me on Monday, I said I would come to his house and pick them up on Monday. My husband and I went to Jay's home and out to his rock shop. Jay told us that I would be fine in 4 to 41/2 months—not to worry. He said the tumor would probably have some scar tissue remaining that may show up on my next scan but that would be all.

Two months went by I was worried the stones weren't working so I called Jay in a panic, asking if he was sure the stones were working. Jay calmly replied that yes indeed, the stones were working as long as I was using them as he'd said and that he would email me some testimonials and that I wasn't to worry, I would be fine. I received the testimonials and I did calm down and felt I was truly on the right path.

November 13, 2008, 4 ½ months later my PetScan showed marked decrease in size of the tumor with no cancer activity and complete resolution of the metastatic presacral lymph node as well. *I was cancer free.*

Jay—Thank you, Thank you, Thank you! Words cannot express my gratitude. May God Bless you for all your work, to give those who ask, a second chance at life.
Sandra Mayer

☛ December 12, 2008
Subject: Diagnosed with Breast Cancer

I was diagnosed with Stage III Invasive Ductal Carcinoma

Breast Cancer on April 3, 2008. I was incredibly shocked. I wasn't sure what I was going to do but I had a good idea it would not be the western protocol of surgery, chemotherapy and radiation. After the biopsy, my doctor wanted me to have a MRI of my breast so I did. In doing the MRI they found another lump. I knew a holistic doctor and pharmacist in Kansas City and I called them immediately. They suggested that I come up to Kansas City and start nutritional IV's so that is what I did. I had an I.V. every day that week, started applying Black Salve directly on the tumor and also started an oral nutritional protocol geared for oncology. I went home with the plan to have the pharmacy overnight the IV's and have them administered in my home town but that did not work out so I had to look for another plan. I heard about a nutritionist in Colorado, so I contacted him to see if he could help me. We had a long talk and my husband and I drove to Colorado to see him. He had healed himself of cancer several years ago so I felt that he would be able to guide me to health also. He started me on Essiac tea and a fermented soy powder that had a history of successfully treating breast cancer.

Meanwhile my youngest son and his wife were planning on me coming to help them with a new baby. I didn't want to disappoint them and everyone thought it would be good for me so I went. I was there two weeks and kept applying the black salve and following the oral nutritional oncology protocol. I arrived home on May 5th.

I had to stop taking the fermented soy powder because of side effects and that was disappointing and discouraging. For the next two weeks I went back and forth trying to determine what would work best for me and I considered going forward with the typical Western protocol because I felt like I needed something more than what I was currently doing. But I dragged my feet on this because it just didn't feel right.

On Monday, May 19th Mark (the nutritionist in Colorado) called me and said a lady had just left his office that had had breast cancer but he had not been able to detect cancer in her body. She told Mark that she had been using healing stones which acted as radiation hormesis and gave Mark the name of the man to contact for more information. That man's name was Jay Gutierrez. Mark called Jay and talked to him a long time finding out about this process. Then he called me. I immediately called Jay and he answered the phone. I told him what I was dealing with and he said "Breast cancer is a piece of cake, can't you get something harder?" I laughed and said, "Well, I really didn't want to!" We made plans for my husband and me to meet him at his home on Wednesday, May 21st. In the meantime I went to his website and read and researched all I could find about radiation hormesis.

We arrived at Jay's home and he took us to his rock shop. He went over everything very carefully and two hours later we left armed with everything I needed to heal my body from breast cancer using radiation hormesis. It all seemed so easy and I felt very happy and grateful to have found out about this. Jay was so kind and said to call him anytime. And I did. I am ever grateful to both Jay and Mark for their unending support. Jay never failed to answer my call or call me back and always put my fears to rest. Mark did the same; I couldn't have stayed the course without their support. I might add that I had been eating a raw food diet for almost two years, and this is one reason I was so surprised that I had cancer. I continued with this way of eating but I believe the radiation hormesis would have healed my body if I had not been eating raw.

I had some tests done in September and they all came back negative. I am thankful for Jay and the work he has done with radiation hormesis. Jay, thank you from the bottom of my heart for being true to God's calling for you. I am one grateful woman.
Janie A.

☛ February 20, 2009
Subject: from old lady stoop back to youthful vigor

My severe back pain started upon the death of my mother

in September 3, 2004. One morning I just couldn't get out of bed without excruciating pain. At 6am the following morning I went to Walgreen. When I went to the cashier to ask where the Aleve was the cashier offered to leave the cash register to get it for me. Being a health food junkie Aleve was a last resort. I knew I was in trouble since I was walking like an old lady without a cane: hobbling and holding on to walls, rails, bent over and moaning every once in a while when I moved the wrong way.

For 2 years I was afraid to do things. My life consisted of ICE, walk to work, ICE, did my job, walk home, ICE again, take Aleve, receive acupressure treatments once a week. During the early stages of my acupressure treatments (2004) we placed an entire chair on top of the massage table to decrease pain because my back was so inflamed.

In the spring of 2006 I became adventurous and went to the gym finally to workout. Since the late 1990s I had a Fitness Center Membership but during the time of back pain I was afraid to use it.

May of 2006 I was given a large green stone by someone who knew of my past history with Quartz crystals and Marcel Vogel. Actually I was trained as one of his teachers. My instruction with the green stone was to take it home and sleep with it to decrease pain and build my immune system. I did as instructed.

To my surprise and delight I *did* feel pain relief and more importantly my body felt better all over. This meant a lot to me because that May of 2006 I was going to the pyramids in Egypt as a single traveler for an astrologically-inspired solar return trip for my birthday. There was much fear in me but I really wanted to go. This was to be the fulfillment of a lifelong dream, even if I couldn't climb down into the pyramids. My fear was that I could go down easily, but then I wouldn't have the strength to climb back out.

Much to my surprise again I not only eventually went into a pyramid and climbed out, I felt better and stronger each and everyday! (except for a brief bout of diarrhea). Faithfully each night I slept with my green stone.

That was the beginning of a new life for me. So amazed at my results of how this stone was healing my physical body that two things occurred:

1. I asked Jay in September 2006 if I could be a distributor.
2. I encouraged a longtime client also suffering of back pain to try the green stone which he did. Eventually he taught all of us to wear the mud pack in our pants during the day.

Fast forward in time to January, 2008. I was in Ministerial School and running my business when Jay called to ask if I would help promote him across the U.S. I answered, "absolutely!"

Around the same time I started drinking radiation hormesis water and using a mud pack which we didn't have until around September, 2007 along with the green stone.

With the use of Jay's entire radiation hormesis system throughout 2008, I saw my left knee return to its normal size and pain in my neck release while range of motion in my neck returned to normal. Those who meet me now never guess that I had been so debilitated.

How grateful I am to have met Jay Gutierrez and have him in my life as my mentor, friend, coach.
Sincerely, Carol Thomas, Phoenix, Az.

☛ Feb 21, 2009
Subject: Hampton the cat and his many disappearing tumors

Early March, 2008 while in ministerial school and extremely busy in my business I realized my cat, Hampton, was being ignored. In an attempt to give him attention while petting his belly I discovered 8 tumors.

Hampton is a male cat who likes to be an alpha male so he has territorial fights with other males.

About 8 months previous to my finding his tumors he was scratched on the chest in one of those territorial fights. The wound was nasty so I lanced it. Whatever I used after that to heal it wasn't working - herbs, silver nitrate, homeopathics. I even tried taping stones to the wounded area, but he removed them within an hour. The wound would close for a while then it opened on and off for those 8 months.

My guess is that Hampton's wound allowed fungus to grow within his system that then developed into tumors. I couldn't possibly have discovered them at a worse time since I was extremely busy organizing my first lecture in Phoenix for Jay on top of everything else.

Jay said to feed the body with irradiated Stone water to heal funguses. When I heard Jay's voice in my head I put a water Stone in each of Hampton's water bowls. From then until now he has only drunk Stone water.

After 10 days of Hampton's drinking that water his tumors disappeared. Unfortunately then I found a much larger tumor at the base of his sternum. So, I trusted.

He kept drinking the water, and the tumor was shrinking by the time Jay gave his first free lecture in Phoenix. Now I was checking his body everyday for "irregularities." He got pretty tired of that.

By our last lecture time in Phoenix, Sunday April 20, I announced to the group that Hampton's large tumor was ½ gone. That night, as usual, I checked his sternum again to discover—Hampton was clear, *no tumor* - yeah!!

Hampton's tumors have never returned and his fur has returned to it's normal sheen. As any healthy male cat - he is rubbing me all the time. I *love* that cat!
Sincerely, Carol Thomas

☛ 2009
Subject: Eye Blisters.

When I first met Jay, I started working in the accounting office of a helicopter company. I was immediately amazed when I found out that he was working with these beautiful stones and what he was doing with them. He would constantly show me letters and emails of people that had been helped with some pretty serious diseases. Mainly cancer. Myself, I was having issues with my sinuses. I asked Jay if his stones could help me.

He gave me two small green stones and a mud pack to put on my eyes. Within a very short time, these huge nasty like pimples started forming on my eyelids. I was in a panic.

I went to the doctor and he was astonished. He said he hadn't seen anything like this. He said they would have to drain them and that they would probably scar pretty bad.

Jay told me to stay with using the stones, that it was drawing toxins out that could be detrimental to my health later on.

The gunk that they drained out of my eyelids was green and brown. As for scars, I used the stones to help heal the eyelids after the operation and you can't even tell they were operated on.

Jay says that the toxins that my body pushed out were a precursor to a much more serious health problem that we could now avoid.

I was so impressed, I quit working my job when Jay did, and started working with Jay fulltime. We keep getting stories in every day that are nothing short of miracles. I am now the General Manger of The Mineral Palace, along with traveling with Jay to educate others on the benefits of Radiation Hormesis. I am on a journey now to save lives and let God use me as he feels.

I would like to thank Jay with all my heart for changing my life and the lives of countless others for the better. God Bless.
Faye Cox*

*[Note from the publisher: Faye is now Jay's wife, as well as lecture coordinator of Night Hawk Minerals, LLC.]

APPENDIX B

What's So & What's Not On Radiation & Nuclear Power

BY THEODORE ROCKWELL, SC.D., MARCH 2003

Myth: Man created radiation. It's unnatural, little-understood, an unprecedented threat to the earth.
Facts: Radiation has been with us since the dawn of time. Life evolved in a sea of radiation. Our soil, our water and our bodies are naturally radioactive. Radioactive processes light the sun and the stars, keep the earth's core molten and our environment livably warm. Radiation is better understood than most environmental challenges. Tests show it is probably essential to life.

Myth: We're fouling our nest and degrading the gene pool by continually adding to the earth's radioactivity.
Facts: Fission changes long-lived uranium into shorter-lived fission products, ultimately *decreasing* earth's radioactivity. All the radioactivity we produce is less than the natural decay that continually decreases earth's total radioactivity each year.

Myth: The quantity of nuclear waste is so great! What can we do with it?
Facts: Nuclear plants produce less than a millionth of the volume of waste from an equivalent coal-fired plant, so it can be put into sealed drums and controlled, rather than dumped into the environment. The 50,000 tons of radwaste destined for Yucca Mtn was produced by all 103 U.S. nuclear plants over the past 40 years. This is less than *2 pounds per person served* for the whole 40 years.

This is small compared to wastes produced by most other industries, or even our homes. The waste volumes associated with construction and operation of solar, wind, and other renewables are larger, on a per-kilowatt-hour basis, than nuclear wastes.

Myth: Radwaste stays toxic for thousands of years. Humanity has never faced such a long-term hazard.
Facts: Radioactive wastes continually decrease in toxicity, whereas other toxic wastes like mercury, lead, arsenic, selenium, cadmium, chromium, etc. retain full toxicity forever. After 500 years, you could eat a pound of it. We bury it 2000 feet underground. The top 2000 feet of U.S. soil contain millions of times more lethal doses of natural poisons than all the nuclear power waste together. We make *10,000 times more lethal doses of chlorine each year*, and put it in our drinking water to kill germs.

Myth: Shipping these "Mobile Chernobyls" (*spent fuel casks*) past schools and homes is a terrible risk.
Facts: These casks pose no significant risk. They are nearly indestructible, being tested by collision, explosives and fire. They contain no liquids and can't "go critical" like a reactor. In tests, armor-piercing missiles blew a hole in one side, but the small amount of radioactivity released was not harmful.

Myth: Nuclear power is an especially unforgiving technology. A momentary slipup and it's catastrophe.
Facts: Just the opposite. *Nuclear plants are uniquely robust*. They can resist earthquakes, hurricanes, power loss, sabotage and operator errors. Even if the core were to melt, even with containment breached, analyses and tests show that few, if any, persons would be seriously injured or killed. Hundreds of nuclear plants worldwide, operating for decades, have confirmed this.

Myth: But Chernobyl killed thousands of people and disabled millions.

Facts: Not true. Thirty workers and firefighters at the plant were killed. But a 16-year investigation by the UN and WHO concluded that there were no public radiation deaths or injuries. No significant increase in any illness resulted except for 2000 cases of childhood thyroid cancer, a highly treatable disease from which there have been few if any deaths. But *fear of radiation* led to unnecessary evacuation of large population groups, causing unemployment, depression, alcoholism and suicides. In the year after the accident, there were 100,000 additional abortions downwind of the accident, presumably in unwarranted fear of bearing a "nuclear mutant." Deformed "Chernobyl victims" used to raise money for relief were later found to be a scam—unrelated to the accident. Some were from far away, others were deformed before the accident.

POINT PAPER ON NUCLEAR "PROBLEMS" BY THEODORE ROCKWELL

Many people hold contradictory beliefs about nuclear energy. For example:

1. The UK applies a carbon tax to fossil fuels, to encourage power sources that do not generate global warming gases. When asked if this tax would be applied to nuclear plants that generate no such gases, the Energy Minister replied, "Of course! Otherwise nuclear would have an unfair advantage over coal."

2. Many patients at the Taipei Municipal Hospital are given a diagnostic "radioactive cocktail," assured that it will not hurt them. After some hours, some of the cocktail is excreted in the urine, which is collected in a tank to allow the 8-hour half-life to decay before disposal. On Jan 14, 2003, some of this urine was spilled,

creating a "radioactive contamination emergency." The treatment center and the intensive care unit were shut down and sealed off, the press reported the "public health scare," and a formal incident investigation was performed.

Note that this radioactivity was deemed not harmful when all of it, fresh, was inside a person's body, but was a full-blown public health emergency when a small portion of it, decayed for many hours, was spilled.

3. The European Community has been struggling with the fact that many substances are naturally radioactive, some in excess of regulations for nuclear facilities. Current regulations address this by requiring that materials released from nuclear facilities be less than 1% as radioactive as materials with "natural" radioactivity, even when the radioactivity is from the same radioisotopes.

4. Soil over most of the earth contains uranium, some in quite high amounts. Careful studies show that this has not harmed the health of inhabitants. When this uranium is processed for use for in nuclear power, most of the radioactivity, is removed, leaving "depleted uranium." This depleted uranium is thereafter falsely characterized as a special health hazard.

5. In many diverse cultures world-wide, natural radon spas have been used for centuries to treat a variety of illnesses. Patients are often sent there by physicians, with the treatment paid for by the national health insurance. The evidence for benefit is impressive. Yet, while spas boast of their high radon, elsewhere "radon police" warn people that radon in their homes, although much lower than at the spas, is a health hazard.

6. Nuclear power plants are forced to go to great extremes to reduce any potential environmental pollution to far below natural levels. Yet when it is suggested that coal miners should stop

pushing the tops of mountains into pristine streams, it is objected that this would make coal plants uneconomical.

7. Europeans are particularly concerned about the safety of their food. Luxembourg prohibits the import of any irradiated food and inspects it at the borders. But the only sure test that food has not been irradiated is the presence of pathogens. So they test to be sure there are pathogens.

8. An intensive program during the 1970s and 80s, in which the federal government participated, measured the release of radioactivity from molten reactor fuel and monitored its dispersion in the air. It was found that nearly all the radioactivity stayed bound in the fuel, or dissolved in the water, or plated out on adjacent structure. Very little escaped into the air, and that which did did not remain long in respirable form. This confirmed results of the Three Mile Island and Chernobyl accidents, where few if any fatalities occurred among the public. Yet government-sponsored "studies" are repeatedly released, claiming tens of thousands of deaths would result from such accidents, even hundreds of miles away.

9. The only way one can "predict" large numbers of deaths from a nuclear accident is to *multiply the expected trivial individual radiation doses by very large populations* assumed to be exposed. This practice has been called scientifically indefensible, even by the organizations who recommend it as a "prudent course." Yet emergency plans are all based on such "predictions."

10. "ALARA," the practice of requiring that cumulative radiation dose be kept As Low As Reasonably Achievable, restrains workers from performing needed inspections (e.g., for leakage and corrosion) and preventive maintenance in radiation zones, decreasing assurance of plant safety in the name of "prudence."

APPENDIX C

Excerpt From the Unpublished Memoir of Stafford Warren, M.D.

"The atomic bomb was dropped on Hiroshima on August 6, 1945 and on Nagasaki on August 9, 1945. General Groves ordered me to proceed to those cities as soon as surrender was accomplished. Lt. Col Hymer Friedel and I, with a small team of doctors and laboratory men were to assure the radiological safety of the U.S. troops that would later occupy these areas. We were to record the amount of radioactivity on the ground, estimate the casualties, and report the amount of blast and other damage.

"Under War Department orders, we flew to Hiroshima on September 8, 1945, and later flew to Nagasaki. The Japanese emperor, in his surrender broadcast, had ordered his people to cooperate with the Americans, and they did. During the survey no awkward incidents occurred, although we were there before this area of Japan was occupied by our troops.

"Our survey with portable Geiger counters with earphones showed that in these two cities there was only a small amount of residual radioactivity, most of which resulted from neutron-induced reactions with objects on the ground beneath the high bomb detonation. The amount of induced radioactivity was of such a small amount that no biological damage was produced on any Japanese individuals entering any of the slightly contaminated areas any time after the catastrophe. The areas were declared safe for our troops as well as for the population. These conditions were a result of the predetermined height of the explosion (1800 ft) and the intensity of the subsequent updraft of hot gases which carried the radioactive materials high into the air, to be dispersed by jet streams over a wide area of the globe in almost undetectable amounts.

"The Geiger counter batteries of our survey team lasted well enough (3-4 weeks) to permit an extensive survey of the destroyed areas, including the torpedo works and other industrial plants in both Hiroshima and Nagasaki. The survey was hampered in the former city by lack of roads in the downwind areas. However, ground contamination with radioactive materials was found then and later to be below both the acute and long-time hazardous levels. In fact, it was not much above ground-background levels in most areas. There were no surprises in any of the predicted findings, except for the immensity of destruction and mortality."

APPENDIX D

On the Life-span of Nuclear Physicists, Researchers & Engineers

The first radiation standards were set up in 1928. Prior to that, researchers were casual about exposure. Radiation exposure of radiologists was high until a lot of them developed skin burns. Then they began wearing radiation detection films and controlling exposure. The cancer data on radiation researchers reflects this casualness. Prior to 1925, the cancer rate was higher than average. After that, it became, and stayed, below "expected," i.e., below the rate for the unirradiated—the "radiation virgins."

◆ MARIE CURIE (1867-1934): died at 67
Dr. Curie was concentrating radioactive ores in a huge caldron that was so potent that she could literally read at night by the radioactive glow. (Think what she was inhaling.) During WW I, she worked on the wounded brought in freshly from the battlefield, holding the film with her bare hands as x-rays were taken. She got *lots* of radiation—it wasn't even measured until detection instruments were invented, developed and deployed. Yet, she still out-lived the normal life-span for that time period.

◆ CORNELIUS A. TOBIAS (1918-2000): died at 82
President of the Radiation Biophysics Committee, International Union of Pure and Applied Physics; from 1955 onward, Dr. Tobias was a professor of Medical Physics at the Donner Laboratory of the University of California at Berkeley. From 1960 to 1967, he was the vice chairman in charge of Medical Physics for the Department of Physics. From 1967 to 1971, he chaired the Division of Medical Physics; from 1969 to 1973, he chaired the graduate group in Biophysics and Medical Physics. In 1965 he became a professor of Electrical Engineering and, from 1977 onward, he was a professor of Radiology at the University of California,

San Francisco.

♦ GLEN SEABORG (1912-1999): died at 87
Nobel Laureate, discoverer of plutonium. Until close to his death, still maintained an active schedule of committees and speaking.

♦ THEODORE "TED" ROCKWELL (1923-2013): died at 90
Ted worked in nuclear technology for 66 years. In 1943 he was in the war-time atomic bomb project at Oak Ridge, Tennessee. After the war he transferred to the Oak Ridge National Laboratory and became Head of the Radiation Shield Engineering Group. He received distinguished Service Medals from both the Navy and the Atomic Energy Commission. He was Technical Director of Admiral Hyman Rickover's program to build the nuclear Navy and the world's first commercial atomic power station. He was awarded the first "Lifetime Contribution Award," henceforth known as the "Rockwell Award," by the American Nuclear Society. Aside from a few joint pains, Ted was in perfect health until his death.

♦ DON LUCKEY (1919-2014): died at 94
Nutrition consultant for NASA's Apollo moon missions. Dr. Luckey wrote a number of works on radiation hormesis.

♦ LAURISTON TAYLOR (1902-2004): died at 102
Taylor was Chief of the Biophysics Branch in the Division of Biology and Medicine of the Atomic Energy Division and one of two members of the Commission on Radiation Units and Measurements (ICRU). He was the first Chairman of the National Council on Radiation Protection and Measurements (NCRP). In an interview in 1995, Taylor related how, in 1929, he was accidentally exposed to a large amount of whole-body radiation from an x-ray machine at NBS. That exposure in addition to medical radiation treatment for bursitis and other benign conditions and from radiation experiments resulted in an estimated whole-body dose-equivalent in excess of a thousand rem. He experienced no discernible adverse effect. He related that experience to juries with great effectiveness while testifying in cases of alleged radiation injury involving small radiation exposures.

APPENDIX E

Places To Go For Radon Therapy

☆ LA CASA DAY SPA
41 E 20th St., New York City, New York 10003, USA
Tel: 212-673-2272 (CASA)
Email: lacasa@lacasaspa.com
www.LaCasaSpa.com
www.youtube.com/lacasadayspa
www.facebook.com/LaCasaDaySpaNY

☆ GASTEINER HEILSTOLLEN
Bad Gastein, Austria
Heilstollenstraße 19
5645 Bad Gastein, Austria
Tel: +43 6434 37530

☆ CURIE SANATORIUM
Agricolovo nám. 1036
CZ-362 51 Jáchymov, Czech republic
Tel: + 420 353 832 111 (reception)
Fax: + 420 353 831 683
Tel: + 420 353 836 666 (reservation)
Fax: + 420 353 832 777
Email: curie@laznejachymov.cz

☆ FURSTENZECHE BERGWERK
Lam, Germany
Tel: +48 12 278 73 75
Fax: +48 12 278 73 80
Email: sekretariat@kopalnia.pl
Email: fueze@degnet.org

✯ KURBAD SCHLEMA
Schlema, Germany
Pension “Haus Siegmar”
Sylvana und Swen Gerber
Gleesbergstr. 26
08301 Schlema
Tel: +49 (0) 37 72 / 2 83 86
Fax: +49 (0) 37 72 / 38 24 68
Email: swengerber@asz-online.de

✯ KURMITTELHAUS SIBYLLENBAD
Neualbenreuth, Germany
Drucken
Tel: +49 (0) 96 38 - 9 33-0 | Fax: +49 (0) 96 38 - 9 33-1 90
Email: info@sibyllenbad.de

✯ BEHOUNEK'S SANATORIUM
Jachymov, Czech Republic
Akademik Behounek
Lidická 1015
CZ-362 51 Jáchymov, Czech republic
Tel: + 420 353 834 111 (reception)
Fax: + 420 353 831 283
Tel: + 420 353 834 444 (reservation)
Fax: + 420 353 834 777
Email: behounek@laznejachymov.cz

✯ RADIUM PALACE
Jachymov, Czech Republic
Tel: +420 353 833 333

✯ GUARAPARI, BRAZIL
Atlantic coasts of Brazil are covered with sand that originated from nearby naturally radioactive monazite and zirconite hillsides.

MEET JANE G. GOLDBERG

JANE G. GOLDBERG, PH.D. is a psychoanalyst, blogger for *Huffington Post* and *Musings from 20th Street*, and the author of seven books, including the acclaimed, *The Dark Side of Love*. She is the owner of La Casa Day Spa in New York City, now celebrating its 21st year anniversary.

In her specialization of working with cancer patients, Dr. Goldberg has integrated her psychoanalytic work with the field of holistic health. She has worked with many cancer patients who, through commitment to sound principles of health as well as an interest in the exploration of their mental, emotional and psychic states, have defied the statistical odds and consider themselves fully healed.

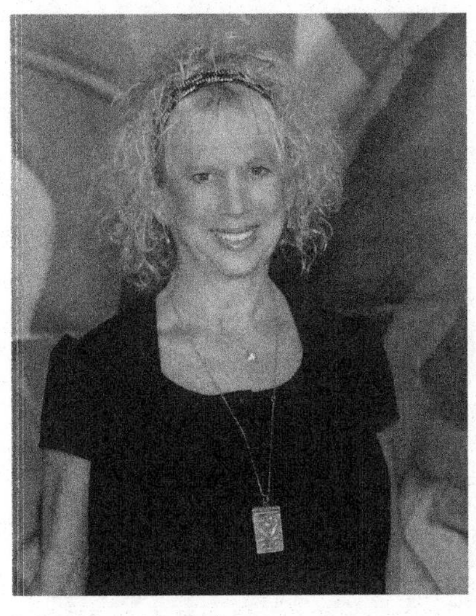

Dr. Goldberg is also the Founder and Director of Brainercize, a system of interactive integrative brain exercise classes designed to maximize brain functioning. She is also the Founder and Director of RRRPM (Restorative, Regenerative, Rebalancing Post-Mastectomy).

INFORMATION

Website: drjanegoldberg.com
Brainercize Website: brainercize.org
Facebook: facebook.com/jane.goldberg.399?fref=ts
Twitter: twitter.com/JaneGoldbergNY
Publisher's Website: SeaRavenPress.com

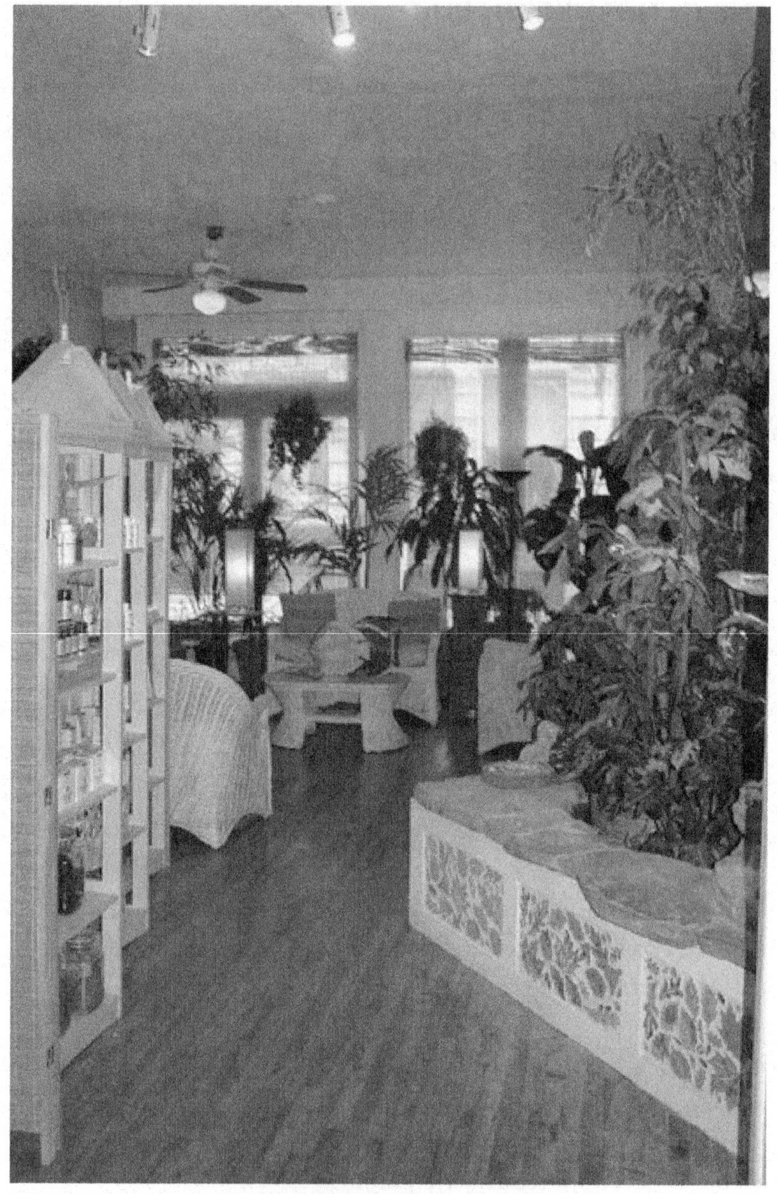

La Casa Day Spa, New York, NY.

ABOUT LA CASA DAY SPA

LA CASA DAY SPA offers a healing experience that has its origins in the wisdom of the ancient world. Throughout the ages, the experience of healers and sages is that life is not linear and fixed but rather a world of gradations and of phases of subtlety. Underlying the apparent phenomenal world is a more refined realm of energy and creation; this is the realm of the 5 elements: *Earth, Water, Fire, Air and Sky*. It is the principles of the 5 elements and their healing energies upon which La Casa bases all of its treatments.

La Casa offers the following therapies: colon cleansing (colonic irrigation, alkalizing colonic, and intensive colonic), foot detoxification, salt sauna, massage, facials, magnetic pulse therapy, oxidative exercise, super-enriched oxygen steam baths, floatation, vibrational re-balancing and radiation hormesis. As well, La Casa sponsors its *Medical Series Lectures and Seminars* in conjunction with the Concordia Foundation and New Realities.

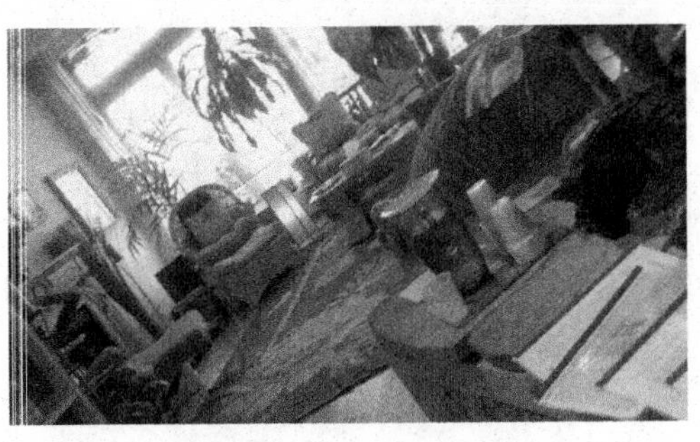

Dr. Jane G. Goldberg is the Founder and Director of La Casa Day Spa. Radiant Float (radon bath), Vibrational Therapies (Guardian, Scenar, North Field Magnetic Oscillator), Magnetic Massage Magnetic Pulse Therapy, Massage, Colon Cleansing, Reflexology, Ion Foot Baths, Ozone Detoxification Baths, EWOT (exercise with oxygen therapy), Raindrop Therapy (essential oil application), and Psychoanalysis.

INFORMATION

Address: 41 East 20th Street, New York, NY 10003 USA
Office telephone: 212-673-2272
Email: lacasa@lacasaspa.com
Website: lascasaspa.com
Facebook: facebook.com/LaCasaDaySpaNY
YouTube: youtube.com/lacasadayspa

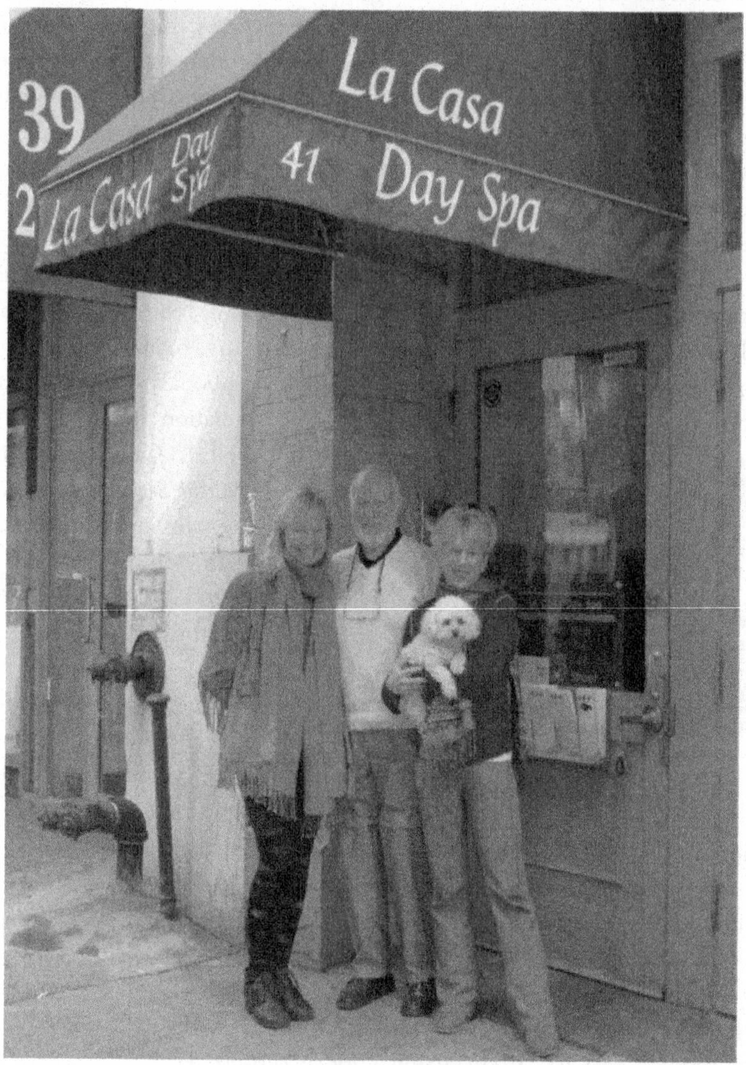

Entrance to La Casa Day Spa, New York City. Left to right: Paula Gloria Tsakona, Gregg Lalley (manager of La Casa Day Spa), the renowned Lilly, and Jane G. Goldberg.

MEET JAY GUTIERREZ

JAY GUTIERREZ spent 20 years in the Air Force and Army as an F-16 jet engine mechanic and a helicopter engine and airframe mechanic. He has received many awards and has numerous helicopter mission stories.

One day while flying on a mission he discovered some blue and green stone on the ground and made some jewelry out of it and gave it to some friends. Later he found out the stones were mildly radioactive. He attempted to buy the jewelry back, thinking he may have injured those people he cared about.

Remarkably, instead of their being sick, they remained unusually healthy and attributed that health in large part to wearing those stones. Ever since, Jay has made it his main mission in life to help others become aware of the healing energies associated with low-radiation stones.

Today Jay is considered an expert in the field of natural radiation hormesis. After traveling several times around the country and working with clients, doctors, healers, and scientists, he and his wife Faye are now successfully fighting serious degenerative diseases such as cancer. Night Hawk Minerals, their company, is the only U.S. company they are aware of that actively promotes the use of natural radiation hormesis.

As a byproduct of helping health challenged individuals, Jay has discovered additional ways to use these energies in other important areas affecting all mankind—modalities that he will present in an upcoming book to be published by Sea Raven Press.

INFORMATION

Address: PO Box 146, Pritchett, CO 81064 USA
Email: jay@nighthawkminerals.com
Publisher's Website: SeaRavenPress.com

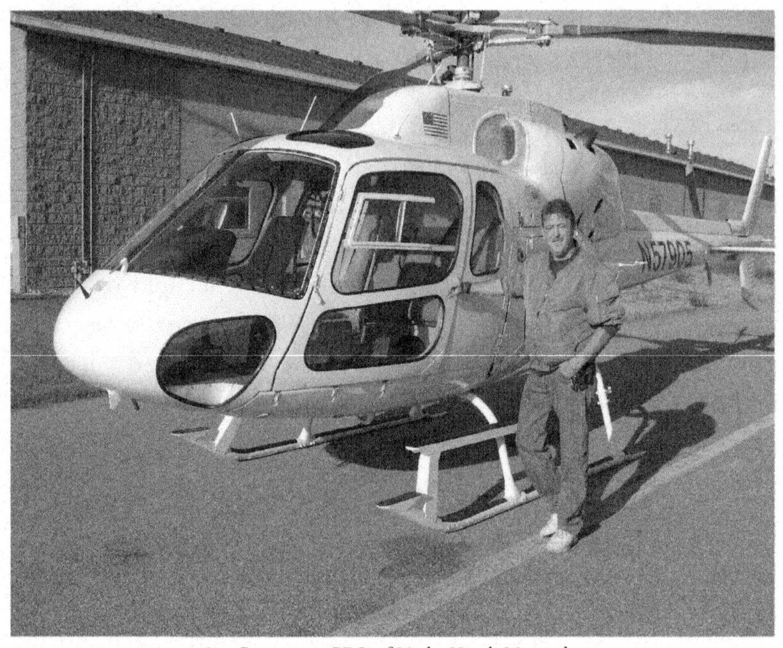

Jay Gutierrez, CEO of Night Hawk Minerals.

ABOUT NIGHT HAWK MINERALS

NIGHT HAWK MINERALS offers information and products concerning radiation hormesis, and is headed by founder Jay Gutierrez and his wife Faye Cox-Gutierrez.

The Night Hawk Minerals Webstore includes: a full selection of radiation hormesis stones, research material on radiation hormesis, instructions on how to use the stones, articles, PDF files, radio interviews with Jay, FAQ, Jay's video blog, health benefits, information on treating cancer, diabetes, candida, heart problems, general pain issues, autoimmune diseases, and a host of other illnesses, recommended Websites and books, monthly specials, evidence for radiation hormesis, natural living news, testimonials, a history of the company, and Wellness Instructors.

The Hormesis Effect: The Miraculous Healing Power of Radioactive Stones, is also available on the Night Hawk Minerals Webstore.

INFORMATION

Address: PO Box 98, Pritchett, CO 81064 USA
Office telephone: 1-888-563-8389
Email: info@nighthawkminerals.com
Website: NightHawkMinerals.com
Facebook: facebook.com/Nighthawkminerals
Twitter: twitter.com/healingrocks

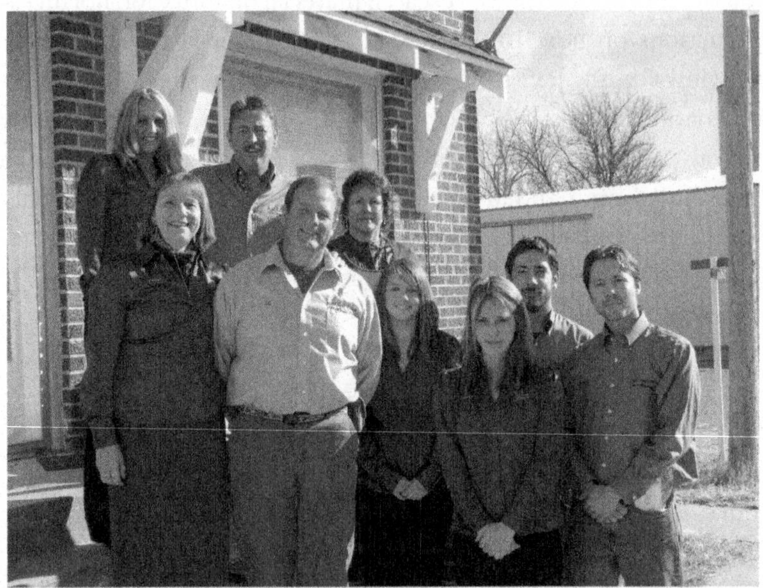

The "We Team"staff at what was once known as the Mineral Palace. From upper left: Faye (General Manager); Jay (Director, Owner). First row from left to right: Carol (Workshop Director); J. C. (Speaker); Theresa (Chef); Tanna (Patient Information); Amy (Patient Coordinator); Cisco (IT); Adam (Rock Shop Manager)

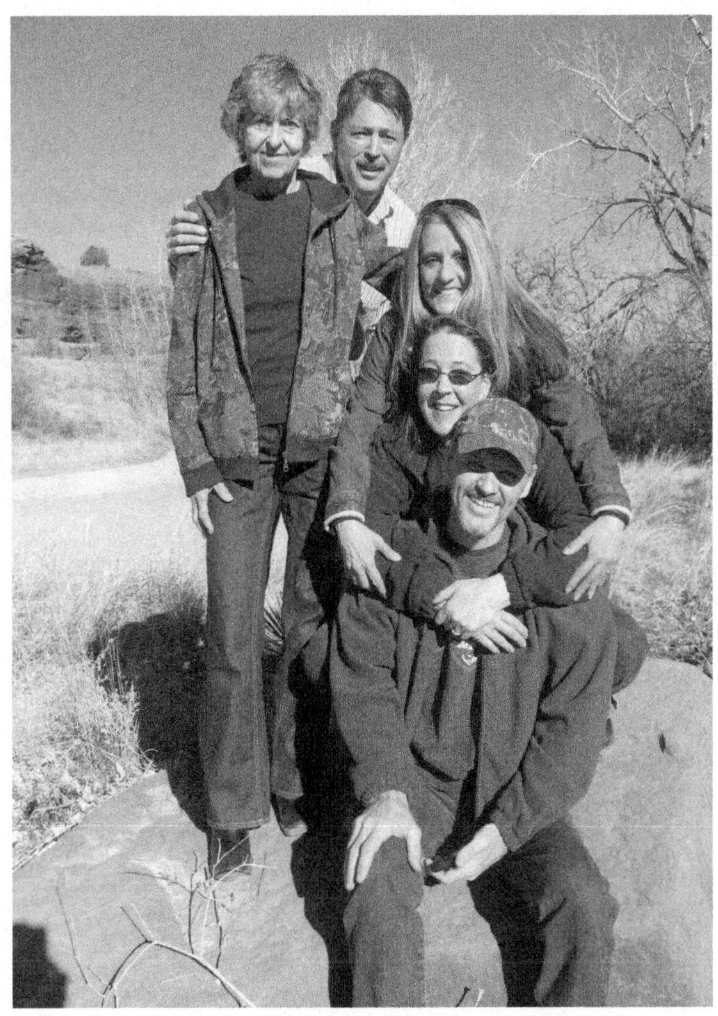

Jay (top right) and Faye (below Jay) with friends at Pritchett, Colorado.

MEET RAPHAEL D'ANGELO

DR. RAPHAEL D'ANGELO is an integrative family physician semi-retired from a 35 year medical practice in 2011. He spent his earliest years as an Air Force medical technologist, serving a tour in Vietnam before exiting the service to become a doctor.

After graduating from the University of Oklahoma College of Medicine in 1976, he reentered the Air Force for seven additional years, during which time he completed a residency in family medicine. After departure from the military he practiced in Oklahoma as well as in Colorado, which is now his home.

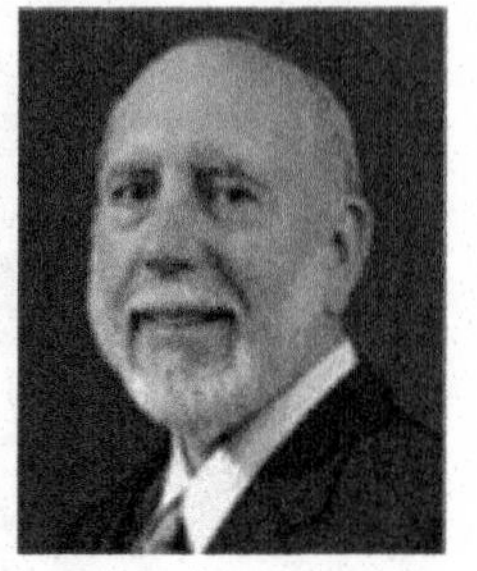

Board certified in family medicine and integrative/holistic medicine, Dr. d'Angelo provides comprehensive consultations in the diagnosis and natural treatment of parasitic problems through the ParaWellness Research Program. As a medical advisor to Night Hawk Minerals, the doctor is frequently in close contact with Jay Gutierrez and various people from his program.

INFORMATION

Address: Center for Holistic and Integrative Medicine, 18121 E. Hampden Ave., Unit C #123, Aurora, CO 80013 USA
Office telephone: 303-680-2288
Email: info@ParaWellnessResearch.com
Website: ParaWellnessResearch.com
LinkedIn: linkedin.com/pub/r-d-angelo/10/a40/b6b

THE WISDOM

- ✦ We believe in arming people with knowledge.
- ✦ We believe that knowledge leads to intuition and that intuition leads to wisdom.
- ✦ We believe that wisdom leads us to make the best choices for ourselves.

Jane G. Goldberg and Jay Gutierrez have been initiated as Stone-Carriers Medicine-Woman and Medicine-Man of the Nemenhah Band and Native American Traditional Organization. As such, they believe that the modern world would benefit by returning back to the age of the stone.

True to the vision and wisdom of the Nemehah American Indian tribe, both the Mineral Palace and La Casa Day Spa embrace the concept of using the 5 basic elements of life—*Earth, Water, Fire, Air and Sky*. Using the radiation-hormesis stones in our daily lives not only re-balances the body (as has been proven in countless medical studies), but, as well, gives a profound sense of awareness of and trust in this earth we share with all its other living beings.

There are only two ways to live your life. One is as though there are no miracles. The other is as though everything is a miracle.

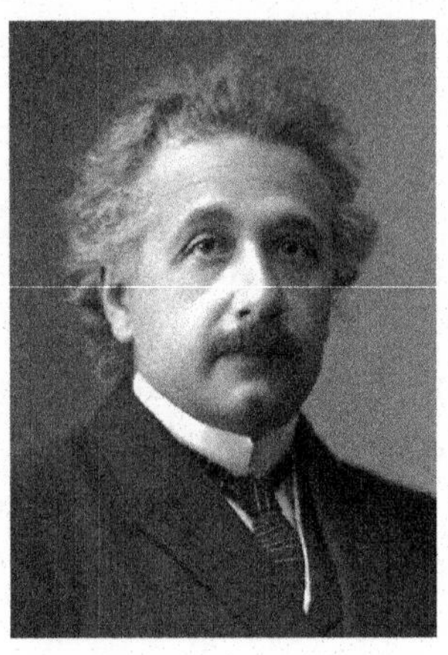

Albert Einstein

BIBLIOGRAPHIC REFERENCES

Abbatt, J.D., Hamilton, T.R., and Weeks, J.L. "Epidemiological studies in three corporations covering the Canadian nuclear fuel cycle." *Biological Effects of Low-Level Radiation.* Vienna, Austria: International Atomic Energy Agency; 1983:351–361.

Aldridge, D. "Unconventional medicine in Europe." *Advances: The Journal of Mind/Body Health* 10:1, 1994.

Amsel, J., Waterbor, J.W., Oler, J., et al. "Relationship of site-specific cancer mortality rates to altitude." *Carcinogenesis.* 3:461–465, 1982.

Auxier, J.A. "Reactions to BRC." *Health Physics Society Newsletter*, 16, 5, 1988.

Azzam, E.I., de Toledo, S.M., Raaphorst, G.P., et al. "Low dose ionizing radiation decreases the frequency of neoplastic transformation to a level below the spontaneous rate in C3h 10T1/2 cells." *Radiation Research*, Vol. 146, No.4, pp. 369-73, 1996.

Bailey, S. "True reports on the underground cure for arthritis." *True Magazine,* 16-20 and 28-29, Dec 1955.

Becker, K. "Health effects of high radon environments in Central Europe: another test for the LNT hypothesis." *Nonlinearity in Biology, Toxicology, and Medicine* 1(1):3, 2003.

——. "Is radon dangerous for our health?" *Proceedings of the 7th International Conference on Nuclear Engineering Special Symposium*, Tokyo, 1999.

Beir IV, Committee on the Biological Effects of Ionizing Radiation. U.S. National Research Council. National Academy Press, Washington, D.C., 1988.

Berrington, A., Darby, S.C., Weiss, H.A., and Doll, R. "100 years of observation on British radiologists: mortality from cancer and other causes 1897–1997." *Br. J. Radiol* 74(882): 507-519, 2001.

Bettelheim, Bruno. *The Uses of Enchantment: The Meaning and Importance of Fairy Tales*. New York: Random House, 2010.

Bhattarcharjee, D. "Role of radioadaptation on radiation-induced thymic lymphoma in mice." *Mutation Research,* 358, 231-235, 1996.

Blot, W.J., et al. "Indoor radon and lung cancer in China." *Journal of the National Cancer Institute*, 82, 1025, 1990.

Bogen, K.T. "A cytodynamic two stage model that predicts radon hormesis (decreased, then increased lung-cancer risk vs. exposure)." Lawrence Livermore National Laboratory, Univ of California, Preprint UCRL-TC-123219. Based on data of Cohen B.L. "Test of the linear-no threshold theory of radiation carcinogenesis for inhaled radon decay products." *Health Physics*; 68: 157-174, 1997.

——. "Mechanistic model predicts a U-shaped relation of radon exposure to lung cancer risk reflected in combined occupational and U.S. residential data." *Human & Experimental Toxicology*, 17:691, 1998.

Bogoljubov, W.M. "Clinical aspects of radon therapy in the U.S.S.R." *Z. Phys. Med. Balneol. Med. Klimatol.* 17, 59-61, 1988.

Boltwood, B. "The ultimate disintegration products of the radio-active elements. Part II. The disintegration products of uranium." *American Journal of Science* series 4, volume 23, 77-88, 1907.

Bross, I.D.J. "Hazards to persons exposed to ionizing radiation (and to their children) from dosages currently permitted by the Nuclear Regulatory Commission." NRC Public Meeting, 4-7-78 (7590-01), 1978.

Brucer, M. "Radiation hormesis after 85 years." *Health Physics Society Newsletter*, 1987.

——. *A Chronology of Nuclear Medicine.* St. Louis: Heritage Publications, 1990.

——. Letter to *Time* magazine, from the files of Peter Beckman.

Calabrese, E.J. *Biological Effects of Low Level Exposures to Chemicals and Radiation*. Boca Raton, FL: Lewis Publishers, 1994.

——. "Hormesis: changing view of the dose-response, a personal account of the history and current status." *Mutat Res*, 511(3):181-9, July 2002.

——. "Historical blunders: how toxicology got the dose-response relationship half right." *Cellular and Molecular Biology,* 51: 643-654, 2005.

Calabrese, E.J. and Baldwin, L.A. "Radiation hormesis: origins, history, scientific foundations." *Human & Exp Tox* 19(1):2, 2000.

——. "Radiation hormesis: its historical foundations as a biological hypothesis." *Hum Exp Toxicol*,19(1):41-75, Jan 2000.

——. "Tales of two similar hypotheses: the rise and fall of chemical and radiation hormesis." *Human Exp Toxicol*, 19(1):85-97, Jan 2000.

——. "Defining hormesis." *Hum Exp Toxicol*, 21(2):91-7, Feb 2002.

——. *Nature*, 421,691, 2003.

Cameron, J.R. "Radiation increases the longevity of British radiologists." *Br J Radiol,* 75:637-638, 2002.

Cameron, J.R. and Moulder, J.E. "Proposition: radiation hormesis should be elevated to a position of scientific respectability." *Med Phys*, 25:1407–1410, 1998.

"Cancer postponement with radon." *Access to Energy*, 24, 1-3, Feb. 1997.

Clarke, R.H. "Progress towards new recommendations from the international commission radiological protection." *J Brit Nucl En Soc, Nuclear Energy* 40(1):37. 2001.

Cohen, B.L. "Test of the linear-no threshold theory of radiation carcinogenesis." ICSE Conference, Paris, 1993.

——. "Relationship between exposure to radon and various types of cancer." *Health Physics*, Vol. 65, No. 5, pp. 529, 1993.

——. "Test of the linear-no threshold theory of radiation carcinogenesis for inhaled radon products." *Health Phys.*, 68:157–174, 1995.

——. "Test of the linear no-threshold theory of radiation induced cancer." Presented at the annual congress of the south African radiation protection association, Kruger National Park, South Africa, 1998.

Congdon, C.C. "A review of certain low-level ionizing radiation studies in mice and guinea pigs." *Health Phys.*, 52:593–597, 1987.

Constantini, A. V., Wieland, H., and Qvick, L.I. *Prevention of Breast Cancer: Hope at Last* ("Fungalbionics Series"). Freiburg, Germany: Johann Friedrich Oberlin Verlag, 1998.

Cuttler, J.M. "What becomes of nuclear risk assessment in light of radiation hormesis." *Proc of 25th Ann Conf Can Nucl Soc.*, Toronto, June 6-9, 2004.

——. "Health Effects of Low Level Radiation. When will we acknowledge the reality?" *Proceedings of 27th Annual Conference of the Canadian Nuclear Society,* Toronto, June 11-14, 2006.

Cuttler, J.M. and Pollycove, M. "Can cancer be treated with low doses of radiation?" *J Am Phys Surg* 8(4):108, 2003.

Darby, S.C., Kendall, G.M., Fell, T.P. et al. "A summary of mortality and incidence of cancer in men from the United Kingdom who participated in the United Kingdom atmospheric weapons tests and experimental programs." *Br. Med. J.* 296, 332-340, 1988.

Day, T. "Complex mutagenesis dose-response relationships after exposure of pKZ1 mice to DNA damaging agents." *Hormesis: implications for toxicology, medicine and risk assessment,* June 6-8, 2005.

Low Dose Irradiation and Biological Defense Mechanisms. Amsterdam, Excerpta Medica, 1992.

"Discarding the truth." *Access to Energy*, 17; 5:3-5, Jan 2000.

Delpha, M. "Fear of nuclear power could be met with data from Hiroshima." *Nuclear Europe*, 42, 3, 1989.

DiSantis, D.J. and DiSantis, D.M. "Wrong turns on radiology's road of progress." *Radiographics*, 11:1121–1138, 1991.

Duke, R.C., Ojcius, D.M., and Young, J.D. "Cell suicide in health and disease." *Sci Am.*; 275:80–87, 1996.

"Effect of X-Rays on the Skin." *Electrical World*, Dec. 1896.

Eisenberg, D., Kessler, C., Foster, F., et al. "Unconventional medicine in the United States: prevalence, costs, and patterns of use." *New Engl J Med* 328(4):246, 1993.

Eisenberg, D., Davis, R., Ettner, S., et al. "Trends in alternative medicine use in the United States, 1990-1997." *JAMA* 280 (18):1569, 1998.

EPA. *Radon: the Health Threat with a Simple Solution. A Physician's Guide.* Publication 401-K-93-008, Washington, D.C., 1993.

"Epidemiological study group of nuclear workers (Japan), first analysis of mortality of nuclear industry workers in Japan, 1986-1992." *Journal of Health Physics*, Vol. 32, pp. 173-184, 1997.

Eskenazi, S. "This week's 'terrorist attack' is only a drill." *Seattle Times*, 11; B1, B7, May 2003.

"Experiments with x-rays upon germs." *The Electrical Engineer*, August 19, Vol. XXII. No. 433, 176-7, August 19, 1896.

Falkenbach, A. "Combined radon and heat exposure for treatment of rheumatic diseases: a clinical approach." *Thermotherapy for Neoplasia, Inflammation, and Pain*, Tokyo: Springer-Verlag, 2001.

Feinendegen, L.E. "The role of adaptive responses following exposure to ionizing radiation." *Hum Exper Toxicol.*, 18:426–432, 1999.

——. "Evidence for beneficial low level radiation effects and radiation hormesis." *Br J Radiol*, 78 (925):3-7, Jan 2005.

Feinendegen, L.E., Muhlensiepen, H., Bond, V.P., et al. "Intracellular stimulation of biochemical control mechanisms by low-dose, low-LET irradiation." *Health Phys.*, 52:663–669, 1987.

Franke, A., et al. "Long-term efficacy of radon spa therapy in rheumatoid arthritis—a randomized, sham-controlled study and follow-up." *Rheumatology* 39: 894, 2000.

Freire-Maya, A., and Kreiger, H. "Human genetic studies in areas of high natural radiation." *Health Physics*, 4, 61, 1978.

French Academy of Sciences—French National Academy of Medicine. "Dose-effect relationships and estimation of the carcinogenic effects of low doses of ionizing radiation." March 30, 2005.

Frigerio, N.A., Eckerman, K.F., and Stowe, R.S. *Carcinogenic hazard from low-level, low-rate radiation, Part I.* Rep. ANL/ES-26, Argonne Nat. Lab., 1973.

Frigerio, N.A. and Stowe, R.S. *Carcinogenic and genetic hazard from background radiation, Biological and environmental effects of low-level radiation.* IAEA, Vienna, Vol. II, 385-393, 1976.

Gager, C.S. "Effects of the rays of radium on plants." *Mem. N.Y. Bot. Garden,* IV, 1908.

Gerber M. *On the Homefront.* 1992.

Gilbert, E.S., Fry, S.A., Wiggs, L.D. et al. "Analysis of combined mortality data on workers at the Hanfort Site, Oak Ridge National Laboratory, and Rocky Flats Nuclear Weapons Plant." *Radiat. Res.* 120, 19, 1989.

"Global Liars." *Access to Energy.* 25; 4: 1-4, Dec 1997.

Gribbin, M.A., Weeks, J.L., and Howe, G.R. "Cancer mortality (1956-1985) among male employees of Atomic Energy Limited with respect to occupational exposure to low-linear-energy-transfert ionizing radiation." *Radiat Res* 3, 375, 1993.

Hanley, C.J. "U.S. and Russia measure threat from 'dirty bombs.'" *Seattle Post-Intelligencer,* page A6. From Associated Press, March 15 2003.

Hashimoto, S., Shirato, H., Hosokawa, M., et al. "The suppression of metastases and the change in host immune response after low-dose total-body irradiationin tumor-bearing rats." *Radiat Res.,* 151:717–724, 1999.

Hattersley, J.G. and Sprott, T.J. "Cause and prevention of cot death (SIDS)." *British Med Jour,* February 2003.

Hattori, S. "Using low-dose radiation for cancer suppression and vitalization." *21st Century Science & Technology,* 55, Summer 1997.

Haynes, R.M. "The distribution of domestic radon concentrations and lung cancer mortality in England and Wales." *Rad. Prot. Dosim.* 93 4, 1988.

Health Physics Society. *Radiation Risk in Perspective, Position Statement.* January 1996, and reaffirmed March 2001.

Henschler, D. "The origin of hormesis: historical background and driving forces." *Hum Exp Toxicol,* 25:347-351, 2006.

High Background Radiation Research Group. "Health survey in high background radiation areas in China." *Science.* 209:877–880, 1980.

Hileman, B. "Fluoridation of water." *Chemical & Engineering News,* 26-42, Aug 1, 1988.

Hiserodt, E. *Under-Exposed: What If Radiation is Actually Good for You?* Laissez Faire Books, 2005.

Hunter, D.J., Hankinson, S.E. et al. "Plasma organochlorine levels and the risk of breast cancer." *New Eng J Med,* 337; 18:1253-1258, 1997.

IAEA Digest Report. *The Chernobyl Forum, 2005.*

ICRP. *Recommendations of the international commission on radiological protection.* Publication No. 1, Pergamon press, London, 1959.

Ikushima, T., Aritomi, H., and Morisita, J. "Radioadaptive response: Efficient repair of radiation induced DNA damage in adapted cells." *Mutation research,* Vol. 358, 193-198, 1996.

Ina, Y. and Sakai, K. "Activation of immunological network by chronic low-dose rate irradiation in wild-type mouse strains: analysis of immune cell populations and surface molecules." *Int J Radiat Biol*, 81(10):72,9, Oct 2005.

Jaffe, S. "Foundations: Pauling, Meselson, and Socrates." *The Scientist* 17(20):11, 2003. (Ava Helen and Linus Pauling Papers at Oregon State University).

Jaworowski, Z. "Beneficial effects of radiation and regulatory policy." *Australian physical and engineering sciences in medicine,* Vol. 20, No.3, 1997.

——. "Radiation folly." *Environment & Health: Myths & Realities*. Okonski, K. and Morris, J., eds. Int. Policy Press, Chap.4:69-86, 2004.

Kathren, R.L. "Radiation protection." *Medical Physics Handbook* 16, 1985.

——. "Pathway to a paradigm: the linear nonthreshold dose response model in historical context." The American academy of health physics, 1995 radiology centennial Hartman Oraton; *Health Physics*, Vol. 70, No. 5, pp. 621-635, 1996.

Kato, F., Ootsuyama, A., and Norimura, T. "Dose rate effectiveness in radiation-induced teratogenesis in mice (2b-80)." Tenth International Congress of IRPA, Hiroshima, Japan, 2000.

Kelly, J.F. and Dowell, A. "Twelve-year review of x-ray therapy of gas gangrene." *Radiology*, 37, 421-39, 1941.

Kendall, G.M., Muirhead, C.R., MacGibbon, B.H., et al. "Mortality and occupational exposure to radiation: first analysis of the National Registry for Radiation Workers." *Brit Med J* ,304, 220, 1992.

Klein, D. "Policy speech of the Nuclear Regulatory Commission." June 27, 2007.

Kondo, S. "Health surveys of populations exposed to low level radiation." *Health Effects of Low-Level Radiation*, Kinki University Press, Osaka: Kinki University, 1993.

——. "Evidence that there are threshold effects in risk of radiation." *Journal of Nuclear Science and Technology*, Vol. 36, No. 1, 1-9, 1999.

——. "Apoptotic repair of genotoxic tissue damage and the role of P53 gene." *Mutation Research,* 402:311, 1998.

——. "Tissue repair error model for radiation carcinogenesis." *Proceedings of the 12th International Congress on Photobiology*, Milano, Italy, 1998.

Kronenfeld, J. and Wasner, C. "The use of unorthodox therapies and marginal practitioners." *Social Sciences and Medicine,* 16:1119, 1982.

Kumatori, T., Ishihara, T., Hirshima, K., Sugiyama, H., Ishii, S., and Miyoshi, K. "Follow up studies over a 25 year period on the Japanese fishermen exposed to radioactive fallout in 1954," pp. 35-54. Hubner, K.F. and Fry, A.A., eds., *The Medical Basis for Radiation Preparedness*, Elsevier, New York, 1980.

Lewis, W. *Arthritis and Radioactivity*. 4th Edition, revised by Patricia Lewis. [Originally published 1955]. Seattle: Peanut Butter Publishing, 1994.

Lipetz, P. Personal communication, January 2009.

Liu, S-Z. "Nonlinear dose-response relationship in the immune system following exposure to ionizing radiation: Mechanisms and Implications." *Nonlinearity in Biology, Toxicology and Medicine* 1(1):71-92, 2003.

Liu, S-Z., Liu, W.H., and Sun, J.B. "Radiation hormesis: its expression in the immune system." *Health Phys* 52(5):579, 1987.

Llope, W.J. "Radiation and radon from natural stone." *Consumer Reports*, May 7, 2008.

London Telegraph, March 8, 1998. Reported in Douglass WC, *Second Opinion*, Aug: 7, 1998.

Luckey, T.D. "Antibiotics in nutrition." H.S. Goldberg (ed.). *Antibiotics, Their Chemistry and Non-Medical Uses*. D. Van Nostrand Publisher, Princeton, 174-321, 1959.

——. "Physiological benefits from low levels of ionizing radiation." *Health Physics*, Vol. 43, pp. 771-789, 1982.

——. "Hormesis with ionizing radiation." CRC Press, Boca Raton, FL, 1980; *Radiation Hormesis*, 1991.

——. "Low dose radiation reduces cancer deaths." *Radiation Protection Management*, Vol. 11, No. 1, pp. 73-79, 1994.

——. "The evidence for radiation hormesis." *21st Century Science & Technology* 9(3):12, 1996.

——. "A Rosetta Stone for ionizing radiation." *Radiation Protection Management*, Vol. 14, No. 6, pp. 58-64, 1997.

Macklis, R.M. "The radiotoxicology of radithor, analysis of an early case of iatrogenic poisoning by a radioactive patent medicine." *JAMA*, Vol. 246, No. 5, 619-21, 1990.

——. "Radithor and the era of mild radium therapy." *JAMA*,Vol. 246, No. 5, 614-18, 1990.

Macklis, R.M. and Bresford, B. "Radiation hormesis." *J Nucl. Med.*,Vol. 32, 350-359, 1991.

Makinodan, T. and James, S.J. "T cell potentiation by low dose ionizing radiation: Possible Mechanisms." *Health Phys*, 59(1):29-34, 1990.

Matanoski, G.M., Abbey, H., Billings, C., et al. "Health effects of low-level radiation in shipyard workers." Final report. Report to the Department of Energy under contract DE-AC02–79 EV10095. Baltimore, MD: Department of Energy, 1991.

Mettler, F.A. Jr. and Upton, A.C. *Medical Effects of Ionizing Radiation*. 2nd ed. Philadelphia, PA: W.B. Saunders, 1995.

Mercola, J. Website: www.mercola.com.

Mifune, M., Sobue, T., Arimoto, H., Komoto, Y., Kondo, S., and Tanooka, H. "Cancer mortality survey in a spa region (Misasa, Japan) with a high radon background." *Japanese Journal of Cancer Research*, Vol. 83, No. 1, 1992.

Miller, C. "Radon and you: promoting public awareness of radon in Montana's air and ground water." Montana Bureau of Mines and Geology, 1998.

Mine, M., Okumura, Y., Ichimaru, M., Nakamura, T., and Kondo, S. "Apparently beneficial effect of low to intermediate doses of A-bomb radiation on human life span." *International Journal of Radiation Biology*, Vol. 58, 1035-1043, 1990.

Mitchel, R.E.J., Jackson, J.S., McCann, R.A., Boreham, D.R. "The adaptive response modifies latency for radiation-induced myeloid leukemia in CBA/H Mice." *Radiation Research*, 152, No.3, 273-279, 1999.

Moore, P.R., Evenson, A., Luckey, T.D., McCoy, E., Elvehjem, C.A., and Hart, E.B. "The use of sulfasuxadine, streptothrycin and streptomycin in nutritional studies with the chick." *J. Biol. Chem.*, 165, 437-441, 1946.

Muckerheide, J. "The health effects of low level radiation: science, data and corrective action." *Nuclear News* 38 (11):61, 1995.

——. "It's time to tell the truth about the health benefits of low-dose radiation." *21st Century Science & Technology*, 43-55, summer 2000.

Nair, K.M., et al. "Population study in the high natural background radiation area in Kerala, India." *Radiation Research*, 152, S145-S148, 1999.

Nambi, K.S. and Soman, S.D. "Environmental radiation and cancer in India." *Health Phys.*, 52:653–657, 1987.

Norimura, T., Nomoto, S., Katsuki, M., Gondo, Y., and Kondo, S. "P53-dependent apoptosis suppresses radiation-induced teratogenesis." *Nature Med.*, 2, 577-580, 1996.

Nuclear Regulatory Commission. "Medical use of byproduct materials." Title 10, Chapter 35, Section 35.69. Fed Reg. 67:20249–20397, 2002.

"Physiological Effects of X-Rays." *The Electrical Engineer*, Vol. XXII. No. 433, 183, August 19, 1896.

Pollycove, M. "The issue of the decade: hormesis." *Eur J Nucl Med* 22(5):399, 1995.

——. "Molecular biology, epidemiology and the demise of the linear no-threshold (LNT) hypothesis." *Proceedings of the International Symposium on Health Effects of Low Doses of Ionizing Radiation: Research into the New Millennium,* Ottawa: Canada, 1998.

——. "The rise and fall of the linear no-threshold (LNT) theory; theory of radiation carcinogenesis." *Annual Congress of the South African Radiation Protection Association*, Kruger National Park, South Africa, 1998.

——. "Radiobiological basis of low dose irradiation in prevention and therapy of cancer." *Proc 14th Pacific Basin Nucl Conf*, 647-653, Honolulu, HI, March 21-25, 2004.

Pollycove, M. and Feinendegen, L.E. "Radiation-induced versus endogenous DNA damage: possible effects of inducible protective responses in mitigating endogenous damage." *Human & Exp Tox,* 22:290, 2003.

Proceedings of 27th Annual Conference of the Canadian Nuclear Society, Toronto, June 11-14, 2006.

"Radiation Facts." From *Access to Energy*, PO Box 1250, Cave Junction, OR 97523, audio cassette.

Raloff, J. "Counterintuitive toxicity. Increasingly, scientists are finding that they can't predict a poison's low-dose effects." *Science News*, 171(3), Jan. 20, 2007.

Raman, E., Dulberg, C.S. and Spasoff, R.A. "Mortality among Canadian military personnel exposed to low-dose radiation." *Can. Med. Assoc. J.* 136, 1951-55, 1987.

Redpath, J.L. and Antonio, R.J. "Induction of an adaptive response against spontaneous neoplastic transformation in vitro by low dose gamma radiation." *Radiation Research*, 149, No.5, 517-520, 1998.

Richards, A. "The effect of x-rays on the action of certain enzymes." *Amer. Jour. Physiol.*, Vol. 35, 1914.

——. "The effect of x-rays on the rate of cell division in the early cleavage of planorbis." *Biol. Bull.*, Vol. 27, 1914.

——. "Recent studies on the biological effects of radioactivity." *Science,* Vol. XLII. No. 1079, 287-300, Sept 3, 1915.

——. "Note on the effect of radiation on fertilizin." *Biol. Bull.* V., 28, 1915.

Rigaud, O., Papadopoulo, O., and Moustacchi, E. "Decreased deletion mutation in radioadapled human lymphoblasts." *Radiat Res.* 133:94-101, 1993.

Robinette, C.D., Jablon, S., and Preston, T.L. "Studies of participants in nuclear tests." *National Research Council Final Report.* DOE/EVO1577, Washington, D.C., 1985.

Robinson, A.B. "Global Liars." *Access to Energy*. 4: 1-4, Dec; 25, 1997.

——. "Cancer postponement with radon." *Access to Energy,* 1997.

——. "Radiation Facts," from *Access to Energy*, audio cassette.

Rockwell, T. "What's wrong with being cautious?" *Nucl News*. 40(7):28, 1997.

——. *Creating the New World: Stories & Images from the Dawn of the Atomic Age,* 1st Books Library, Bloomington, Indiana, Fig 7.1, pp150, 2003.

——. Personal communication, Jan. 30, 2009.

Rodgers, B. "Cytogentic effects of exposure to Chernobyl radiation." Ph.D. dissertation, Texas Tech University, 1997, cited in *Avalanche-Journal*, Marlena Hartz. Thursday, October 16, 2008.

Russ, V. K. "Consensus of the effect of X-rays on bacteria." *Hygie*, Vol. 56, 341-344, 1909.

Sagan, L.A. "What is hormesis and why haven't we heard about it before?" *Health Phys.*, 52:521–525, 1987.

Sakai, K. "Biological responses to low dose radiation—hormesis and adaptive responses." *Yakugaku Zasshi*, 126(10):827-31, Oct 2006.

Sakamoto, K., Myogin, M., Hosoi, Y., et al. "Fundamental and clinical studies on cancer control with total and upper half body irradiation." *J Jpn Soc Ther Radiol Oncol,* 9:161-175, 1997.

Sato, F. "Experimental study on late somatic effects by continuous irradiation." *Proceedings of the Thirtieth NIRS Symposium on Radiation Effects, Supplement of Radiological Sciences*, Vol. 42, No. 6, 37-42, 1999.

Seabrook, Lochlainn. *Jesus and the Law of Attraction: The Bible-Based Guide to Creating Perfect Health, Wealth, and Happiness Following Christ's Simple Formula.* Franklin, TN: Sea Raven Press, 2013.

Shadley, J.D. and Wolff, S. "Very low doses of x-rays can cause human lymphocytes to become less susceptible to ionizing radiation." *Mutagenesis.* 2:95-96, 1987.

Shadley, J.D. and Dai, G.Q. "Cytogenic and survival adaptive responses in G-1 phase human lymphocytes." *Mutat Res*, 265:273-281, 1992.

Shimizu, Y., Kato, H., Schull, W.J., and Mabuchi, K. "Dose response analysis among atomic-bomb survivors exposed to low-level radiation." In Sugahara, T., Sagan, L., and Aoyama, T. (eds.), *Low Dose Irradiation and Biological Defense Mechanisms*, Exerpta Medical Publisher, Amsterdam, 71-74, 1992.

Simoncini, T. *Cancer is a Fungus,* Edizioni Lampis, 2005.

Smith, L.H. and Hattersley, J. *The Infant Survival Guide.* Petaluma, CA: Smart Publications, Chapter 9, 2000.

Smith, P.G. and Doll, R. "Mortality from all causes among British radiologists." *Br. J Radiol* 54:187-194, 1981.

Southam, C.M. and Ehrlich, J. "Effects of extract of western red cedar heartwood on certain wood decaying fungi in culture." *Phytopathol.* 33, 517-524, 1943.

"Sources and Effects of Ionizing Radiation: Adaptive Responses to Radiation in Cells and Organisms." UNSCEAR 1994 Report to the General Assembly with scientific annexes, Annex B.

Sponsler, R. and Cameron, J.R. "Nuclear shipyard worker study (1980–1988): a large cohort exposed to low-dose-rate gamma radiation." *Int. J. Low Radiation,* 1(4):463–478, 2005.

Stebbing, A. "Hormesis: the stimulation of growth by low levels of inhibitors." *The Science of the Total Environment,* 22:213, 1982.

Sugahara, T. "Epidemiological studies on low dose radiation exposure." *NSRA Primer No. 4*, 1998.

Sugahara, T., Sagan, L.A., and Aoyama, T. "Low dose irradiation and biological defense mechanisms." *Excerpta Medica* Publisher, Amsterdam, 1992.

Taleb, Nassim Nicholas. *Antifragile: Things That Gain from Disorder.* New York: Random

House, 2014.

Tamplin, A.R. and Gofman, J.W. *Population Control Through Nuclear Power.* Chicago: Nelson-Hall, 1970.

Tanooka, H., Yamada, T., et al. "Suppression of carcinogenic process by low dose rate irradiation." *Program and Abstracts of the Forty-third Annual Meeting of the Japan Radiation Research Society*, 3-C-13, Tokyo, Japan, August 30 – September 1, 2000.

Taylor, L.S. "The philosophy underlying radiation protection." *Am J. Roent.* 77, 914 (from address on 7 Nov. 1956), 1957.

——. "Radiation exposure and the use of radioisotopes." *Impact* 7, 210, 1957.

The Electrical Engineer. 1: "Experiments with x-rays upon germs." August 19, 1896.

"Of dirty bombs and the health" (*Townsend Letter*), in *Benefits of Low-Level Radiation and Toxins,* Joseph G. Hattersley.

The Wall Street Journal OnLine, February 24, 2007.

Thomas, T. and Goldsmith, R. "Department of energy radiation health studies: past, present, and future." *Radiation and Public Perception: Benefits and Risks,* American Chemical Society, Washington, D.C., 1995.

Travis, E.L. *Primer of Medical Radiobiology.* 2nd ed. Chicago: Year Book Medical Publishers; 1989:60.

Tschaeche, A.N. "There is no scientific basis for the linear no-threshold(LNT) hypothesis extension to low doses." *Presented at the Annual Congress of the South African Radiation Protection Association*, Kruger National Park, South Africa, 1998.

Tubiana, M. and Aurego, A. "Dose-effect relationship and estimation of the carcinogenic effects of low doses of radiation: the joint report of the Académie des Sciences (Paris) and of the Académie Nationale de Medicine." *Int J Low Rad,* 2(3/4):135-153, 2006.

United Nations Scientific Committee on the Effects of Atomic Radiation UNSCEAR; *Report to the General Assembly with Scientific Annexes, Sources and Effects of Ionizing Radiation,* 2000.

UNSCEAR. "Sources and effects of ionizing radiation." *United Nations Scientific Committee on the Effects of Atomic Radiation,* New York, 1994.

——. *Report of the United Nations Scientific Committee on the Effects of Atomic Radiation,* General assembly official records, Thirteenth session, Supplement No. 17, 1958.

U.S. Nuclear Regulatory Commission document NUREG-0713, Vol. 24, October 2003.

U.S. Dept. of Energy, Directive 5400.5. Published Feb. 8, 1990; revised Jan. 7, 1993.

Van Raamsdonk, J.M. and Hekimi, S. "Deletion of the mitochondrial superoxide dismutase sod-2 extends lifespan in caenorhabditis elegans." PLoS Genetics, 5 (2) 2009.

Voelz, G.L., Lawrence, J.N.P., and Johnson, E.R. "Fifty years of plutonium exposure to the Manhattan Project plutonium workers: an update." *Health Physics*, 73;4:611-618, 1997.

Wald, M.W. "Hanford exposure admitted." *Seattle Post-Intelligencer*, A1, A8. from *The New York Times*, Jan. 29, 2000.

Walker, D. *60 Minutes*, interview with Steve Kroft, July 8, 2007.

Wei, L. "Epidemiological investigation of radiological effects in high background radiation areas of Yangjiang China." *J. radiation research*, Vol.31, pp. 119-136, 1990.

Weinberg, A. M. Letter to editor, *Science* 174, 546, 1971.

Windham, C. "Study cites risks of full-body scans." *Wall Street Journal*, August 31, 2004.

Wolff, S. Failla Memorial Lecture. "Is radiation all bad? The search for adaptation." *Radiat Res.*, 131(2):117-23, 1992.

Wyngaarden, K.E. and Pauweles, E.K.J. "Hormesis; are low doses of ionizing radiation harmful or beneficial?" *European Journal of Nuclear Medicine*, Vol. 22, No. 5, 1995.

Yalow, R.S. "Concerns with low level ionizing radiation: Rational or phobic?" *J Nucl. Med.*, Vol. 31, 17A-18A, 1990.

Yamada, S., Nemoto, K., Ogawa, Y., Yakatou, Y., Hosi, A., and Sakamoto, K. "Anti-tumor effect of low dose total (or half) body irradiation and changes of the functional subset of peripheral blood lymphocytes in nonHodgkin's lymphoma patients after TBI." (HBI), 1992.

Yamamoto, O., Seyama, T., Ito, H., and Fujimoto, N. "Oral administration of tritiated water in mouse. III: Low dose-rate irradiation and threshold dose-rate for radiation risk." *Int. J. Radiat. Biol.*, 73, 535-541, 1998.

Yamaoka, K. "Increased SOD activities and decreased lipid peroxide in rat organs induced by low X-irradiation." *Free Radical Biol Med*, 11:3-7, 1991.

Yonezawa, M., et al. "Two types of X-ray-induced radio-resistance in mice: Presence of 4 dose ranges with distinct biological effects." *Mutat. Res.*, 358:237-243, 1996.

Young, R. Website: www.phmiracleliving.com

Zaichkina, S.I., et al. "Low doses of radiation decrease the level of spontaneous and gamma induced chromosomal mutagenesis in bone marrow cells of mice in vivo." *Rariats Biol Radioecol*, 43:153-155, 2003.

Zhang, H., Liu, B., Zhou, Q., et al. "Alleviation of pre-exposure of mouse brain with low-dose 12C6+ ion or 60Co gamma-ray on male reproductive endocrine damages induced by subsequent high-dose irradiation." *Int J Androl*, 29(6):592-6, Dec 2006.

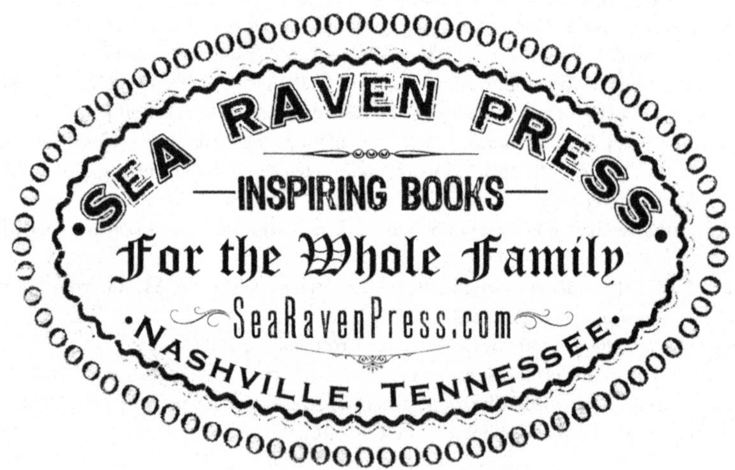

ANNOTATED BIBLIOGRAPHY

2000 to 2007

YEAR 2000

1. Liu SZ, Bai O, Chen D, Ye F. Genes and protein molecules involved in the cellular activation induced by low dose radiation. J Radiat Res Radiat Proc 2000, 18: 175-185. [Abstract] The effect of whole-body X-irradiation on the transcription and expression level of genes related to cell survival and cell cycle control, the transcription level of genes related to immune responses as well as the signal molecules of mouse thymocytes and / or splenocytes was reviewed. Opposite effects from low versus high doses of radiation were demonstrated in most of the parameters examined. The implications of these changes in connection with the cellular responses after different doses of ionizing radiation were analyzed.

2. Ju GZ, Fan C, Liu SZ. Metallothionein expression in mouse immune organs induced by radiation. J Radiat Res Radiat Proces. 2000, 18(4):308-311. [Abstract] To explore the effect of ionizing radiation on the expression of metallothionein (MT) in immune organs, the 109Cd-hamoglobulin affinity assay was employed to measure the content of MT in tissues. The dose effect relationship of the MT expression in mouse thymus and spleen was investigated 16 h after exposure to 0.5, 1, 2, 4 and 6 Gy whole body irradiation (WBI). And the time course changes in MT expression in mouse thymus and spleen were also determined at different time intervals after 4 Gy WBI. The results showed that the MT content in mouse thymus was significantly increased 16 h after 4 Gy and 6 Gy irradiation compared with that in sham-irradiated mice ($P<0.05$, respectively). And it was found that the MT content in mouse thymus was also increased significantly from 4 h to 48 h after 4 Gy irradiation compared with that in sham-irradiated mice ($P<0.05\sim P<0.001$). However there were no markedly changes for the MT expression in the mouse spleen after exposure to X-rays. These results mentioned above suggest that the MT expression in immune organs could be induced by X-rays which may be tissue-specific.

3. Wan H, Su X, Liu SZ Effect of low dose radiation on expression of Fos protein in mouse thymocytes. J Radiat Res Radiat Proc 2000 18 4 296-298 [Abstract] The purpose of the present study was to observe the changes of expression of Fos protein using immunohistochemistry and image analysis as well as flow cytometry. The results showed that the expression of Fos protein incresed rapidly in mouse thymocytes after whole body irradiation (WBI) with 75 mGy X rays. It reached the peak value at 24 h, and then gradually returned to the basic level. These findings were in accordance with our previous observation of the effect of low dose radiation on transcription level of c-fos mRNA in mouse thymocytes. The results indicate that low dose radiation could enhance the function of immune cells.

4. Ye F, Liu SZ. Effect of whole-body irradiation on cell cycle progression of thymocytes in mice. Radiat Protect 2000 20 189-192 [Abstract] The effects of whole-body X-irradiation (WBI) with various doses on cell cycle pogression of thymocytes in mice were investigated using flow cytometry. The results show that DNA synthesis was stimulated at 24~72 h after 75 mGy irradiation, reaching the level of sham-irradiated group on day 7. Meanwhile, after WBI with 2.0 Gy X-rays DNA synthesis was suppressed with significant G2 block beginning from 4 h and reaching its peak at 12 h, but the cell cycle progression was accelerated at 72 h and returned to the level of sham-irradiatied group on day 7. After WBI with 50 mGy X-rays, the progression of cell cycle of thymocytes from G0/G1 to S was promoted and DNA synthesis was enhanced. However, G1 block began to occur with 100 mGy. The number of S phase thymocytes decreased in a dose-dependent manner and the number of G0/G1 phase cells increased after WBI with 0.5 «4.0 Gy. In the same dose range, the number of G2/M phase cells increased in a dose-dependent manner. These data suggest that DNA synthesis is suppressed with occurrence of both G1 and G2 block. The study shows that the threshold dose for G1 block was 0.1 Gy in thymocytes after WBI and that for G2 block was 1 Gy.

5. Wu CM, Li XY, Liu SZ. Construction of pEgr.P-TNFá and its expression in NIH3T3 cells induced by ionizing irradiation. Chin J Radiol Med Radiol Prot 2001 21(5):332-334. [Abstract] Objective: To isolate and amplify Egr-1 promoter, construct pEgr.P-TNFá and study its response to different doses of ionizing radiation. Methods: Egr-1 promoter was isolated from genomic DNA by PCR to construct pEgr. P-TNFá expression plasmid. Plasmids were transfected into NIH3T3 cells with lipsome and the expression level of TNFá was detected by ELISA after irradiation with different doses of X-rays. Results: The sequence of Egr-1 promoter obtained was essentially the same as reported. Egr-1 promoter and TNFá cDNA was

inserted into expression vector correctly. Eight hours after irradiation with different doses (0.075~10 Gy) of X-rays, the expression level of TNFá was higher than that of non-irradiated group (P < 0.05 «0.001) . Conclusion: Egr-1 promoter can be activated by ionizing irradiation and regulate the expression of downstream gene. Low dose irradiation (0.075 Gy) is for the first time found to be able to induce gene expression downstream of Egr-1 promoter. The observation may be of potential significance in tumor therapy.

6. Fu HQ, Luo C, Fu SB and Ju GZ. Effect of ionizing radiation on the expression p53 and MDM2 in EL-4 cells. J Radiat Res Radiat Proces. 2000, 18(3):208-211. [Abstract] To explore the molecular mechanism of G1 arrest of EL-4 cells induced by whole body irradiation(WBI) flow cytometry (FCM) and Northern blot were used to analyze p53 MDM2 gene expressions of EL-4 cells after irradiation with X-rays. Results show that the p53 protein level of EI-4 cells increased from 2 to 24 h and the MDM2 protein level of EI-4 increased from 4 to24 h after 4 Gy irradiation with X-rays. Meanwhile, the MDM2 mRNA level was significantly increased 4 h after irradiation. Conclusion these results suggest that there was a feed back loop between p53 and MDM2 protein in EL-4 cells after irradiation with X-rays, which made G1 arrest cells reenter cell cycle.

7. Fu HQ, Ju GZ, Luo C, Fu SB. Effects of ionizing radiation on MDM2 mRNA and protein expressions of thymocytes and splenocytes in mice. J N Bethune Univ Med Sci. 2000, 26(3):226-228. [Abstract] Objective: To explore the molecular mechanism of G1 arrest of thymocytes and splenocytes in mice induced by whole body irradiation (WBI). Methods Flow cytometry (FCM) and dot blot were used to analyze MDM2 mRNA and protein expressions of thymocytes and splenocytes in Kunming mice after whole body irradiation (WBI) with x-rays. Results The expressions of MDM2 protein of thymocytes in mice increased from 4 h to 8 h after 2 Gy WBI. There were no significant changes of MDM2 mRNA level of thymocytes and splenocytes from 0 to 48 h after 75 mGy or 2 Gy WBI. No changes of MDM2 mRNA level were also found in thymocytes or splenocytes of mice 4 h after 0~6 Gy WBI. Conclusion These results suggest that ionizing radiation could induce MDM2 protein expression and make G1 arrest cells reenter cell cycle.

8. Sun YM, Liu SZ. Changes of IL-1b in mouse peritoneal macrophages after whole-body X-irradiation. Radiat Protec 2000 20 348-350 [Abstract] Bioassay was used to examine the activity of IL-2b in mouse peritoneal macrophages following whole-body irradiation (WBI) with 0.075 Gy and 2.0 Gy. The activity of IL-2b was increased to 1.72 fold of sham-irradiated control from 6 h to 24 h after WBI with 75 mGy and returned to the control level 7 days after irradiation. The biological activity of IL-2b reached its peak at 24 h after WBI with 2.0 Gy and it was significantly increased at 24 h after WBI with 0.075, 0.2, 0.5, 1.0, 2.0 and 4.0 Gy.

9. Sun YM, Liu SZ. Changes in tumor necrosis factor á (TNFá) expression in mouse peritoneal macrophages. J Radiat Res Radiat Proc 2000, 18: 236-239 [Abstract] The TNF-mediated L929 cell toxicity bioassay was used to examine the expression of TNFá in mouse peritoneal macrophages following whole-body irradiation (WBI). The expression of TNFá gradually increased after WBI with 0.075 Gy, reaching its peak at 12 h. The expression of TNFá gradually increased from 3 to 120 h after WBI with 2 Gy. The expression of TNFá was significantly increased at 24 h after WBI with 0.05, 0.075, 0.1, 0.2, 0.5, 1.0 and 2.0 Gy. The expression of TNFá increased most markedly in the group irradiated with 0.5 Gy. WBI with 4.0 and 6.0 Gy caused significant suppression of TNFá by the peritoneal macrophages.

10. Sun YM Liu SZ. Effect of whole body X-irradiation on production of nitric oxide in peritoneal macrophages of mice. Chin J Radiol Med Radiol Protec 2000, 20: 232-234 [Abstract] Objective: To disclose the changes of nitric oxide (NO) in murine peritoneal macrophages at different time intervals after whole body irradiation (WBI) with 75 mGy and 2.0 Gy X-rays and the changes of NO and inducible nitric oxide synthase (iNOS) 24 hours after WBI with 0.05-6.0 Gy X-rays. Methods Immunohistochemistry and spectophotometry were used. Results: The expression of iNOS and the production of NO increased in a dose-dependent manner after irradiation. The production of NO increased from 6 h to 48 h and reached its peak at 48 h which was 3.8-fold of sham-irradiated control. Conclusion Ionizing radiation stimulates expression of iNOS and production of NO in peritoneal macrophages of mice.

11. Liu SZ, Xie F. Adenylate cyclase signaling in the activation of thymocytes in response to whole-body irradiation with low dose X-rays. Chin Med Sci J, 2000, 15: 1-7 [Abstract] Objective: To study the molecular mechanism of the stimulatory effect of low dose radiation (LDR) on T cell activation. Methods. Thymocytes from Kunming mice exposed to whole-body irradiation (WBI) with different doses of X-rays were analyzed for the changes in signal molecules of the phospholipase C-phosphatidylinositol biphosphate (PLC-IP2) and G protein-adenylate cyclase (AC) pathways. Results: It was found that [Ca2+]i

increased in response to doses within 0.2 Gy which was most marked after 0.075 Gy and the increase was accentuated in the presence of Con A. The changes in CD3 and calcineurin (CN) expression of the thymocytes followed the same pattern as the alterations in [Ca2+]i after I.DR. The expression of á, â1 and â2 isoforms of protein kinase C (PKC) was all up-regulated after 0.075 Gy with the increase in PKC-â1 expression being most marked. The eAMP/cGMP ratio and PKA activity of the thymocytes was lowered after low dose radiation and increased after doses above 0.5 Gy in a dose-dependent manner, thus giving rise to J-shaped dose-response curves. The Ca antagonist TMB-8 and cAMP stimulant cholera toxin suppressed the augmented thymocyte proliferation induced by LDR. Conclusion. Data presented in the present paper suggest that activation of the PLC/PIP2 signal pathway and suppression of the AC-cAMP signal pathway are involved in the stimulation of the thymocytes following WB1 with low dose X rays.

12. Liu SZ, Bai O. On mechanistic studies of immune responses following low-dose ionizing radiation. Biological Effects of Low Dose Radiation (Eds. Yamada T, Mothersill C, Michael BD and Potten CS), Amsterdam: Elsevier, 2000, 129-135. (Excerpta Medica International Series 1211) [Abstract] The present paper reviews the low-dose radiation (LDR)-induced intercellular reactions in the immune organs and their molecular basis. There exist delicate interactions between the lymphocytes and the accessory cells by direct contact via surface molecules as well as by paracrine and autocrine action via secretion of cytokines and growth factors. These events were found to be activated after LDR. The multiple signal transduction pathways activated in the immune cells led to positive and negative regulation of cellular processes forming a complex signal transduction network. Whole-body irradiation (WBI) with low-dose X-rays caused facilitation of these pathways with enhanced expression or increased activity of some important signal molecules and suppression of others leading to induction of genes related to lymphocyte survival and proliferation. The present state of knowledge indicates that more work has to be done on the effect of different doses of ionizing radiation on these regulatory mechanisms within the immune system. It is emphasized that in a complex organism there exist defense and adaptive mechanisms at the molecular and cellular (as well as systemic) levels which produce a response to ionizing radiation, and these have to be considered as a whole in mechanistic studies of the biological effects of low level exposures.

13. Chen SL, Cai L, Meng QY, Su X, Wan H, Liu SZ. Low-dose whole-body irradiation (LD-WBI) changes protein expression of mouse thymocytes: Effect of a LD-WBI-enhanced protein RIP10 on cell proliferation and spontaneous or radiation-induced thymocyte apoptosis. Toxicol Sci 2000 55, 97-106. [Abstract] Low-dose radiation (LDR) can potentiate cellular metabolic activities or immune functions in vivo (hormesis), and can render cells resistant to DNA or chromosome damage caused by subsequent high-dose radiation (adaptive response). Protein synthesis was required for these cellular responses to LDR. In the present study, the early expression of proteins by thymocytes in response to low-dose whole-body irradiation (LD-WBI) was investigated. The expression of novel and previously existing proteins was found in the nucleus, cytoplasm, and extracellular fluid of thymocytes at 4 hours after WBI with 75-mGy X-rays. A 10 kD protein (RIP10) was seen in the cytoplasm of thymocytes after LD-WBI was further investigated. The fraction containing RIP10 separated by Sephadex G 100 gel filtration potentiated spontaneous thymocyte, and mitogen-induced splenocyte, proliferation. Western blotting demonstrated that an anti-RIP10 antibody could react with a 10-kD cytoplasm protein and also with a 13-kD nuclear protein in thymocytes at 4 h after LD-WBI. Immunocytochemical staining showed the existence of RIP10 in several immune tissues including thymus, spleen, and lymph node. RIP10 expression, as determined by immunocytochemical staining and flow cytometry, was enhanced at 4-8 h after LD-WBI. Cell-cycle arrest (G0/G1 block with decreased percentage of S-phase cells), and increased levels of spontaneous or radiation-induced apoptosis were observed in thymocytes incubated with RIP10 antibody in vitro for 4 h or 24 h. These results directly demonstrated the role of RIP10 in modulating cell proliferation and apoptosis. This finding is important to understand the mechanisms underlying LDR-induced hormesis and adaptive response.

14. Chen SL, Meng QY, Liu SZ. Effect of ionizing radiation on protein expression in murine thymocytes. J NBUMS 2000 26 1 4-6 [Abstract] Objective: Alterations of protein expression in cytosol and extracellular fluid and exchanges between intracellular and extracellular proteins of thymocytes in mice 4 hours after whole-body irradiation with 75 mGy X-rays were investigated. Methods: Two dimensional electrophoresis was used. Results: It was found that alterations of 12 proteins ranging in size from 10 to 53 kD with their pI distribution from 5.0 to 8.2 were displayed in the cytoplasmic fraction of thymocytes in irradiated mice, of which there were 5 novel proteins, 4 up-regulated proteins and 3 down-regulated proteins, and 5 proteins ranging in size from 32 to 67 kD with their pI distribution from 5.8 to 7.7 disappeared after irradiation. Alterations of 3 proteins ranging in size from 15 to 67 kD with their pI distribution from 5.1 to 8.2 were displayed in the extracellular fluid of thymocytes in irradiated mice, of

which there were one novel protein, one up-regulated protein and one down-regulated protein, and 3 proteins ranging in size from 13 to 69 kD with their pI distribution from 5.0 to 8.0 disappeared after irradiation. It was shown that a protein molecule in the sham-rradiated cytosol of thymocytes appeared in the extracellular fluid after irradiation and a protein molecule in the sham-irradiated cytosol was decreased after irradiation and increased in the extracellular fluid. Two proteins in sham-irradiated extracellular fluid appeared in the thymocyte cytosol after irradiation. Conclusion. The results suggest that alterations of protein expression and exchanges of protein molecules occurred between intracellular and extracellular compartments after irradiation. These findings may have implications in the mechanism of immunoenhancement and adaptive response induced by low dose radiation. The elucidation of the nature and mode of action of these protein molecules remains to be clarified in future studies.

15. Gong SL, Liu SC, Liu JX, Zhang YC, Liu SZ. Dose-effect of adaptive response in apoptosis and cell cycle progression of thymocytes induced by low dose X-irradiation in mice. Radiat Protect, 2000, 20 (5): 294-298. [Abstract] In the present study, male Kunming mice irradiated by whole-body with X-rays were used to observe the dose-effect of adaptive response in apoptosis and cell cycle progression of thymocytes induced by low dose radiation. The mice were irradiated with inductive doses (D1) of 25, 50, 75, 100 or 200 mGy and challenge dose (D2) of 1.0, 1.5 or 2.0 Gy, and divided randomly into 3 groups, namely, sham-irradiation, D2 and D1 + D2 groups. The results showed that for D1 + D2 group, the percentages of apoptotic bodies in thymocytes reduced in varying degrees. The G1 arrest and G2 arrest diminished and the number of cells with DNA synthesis of S phase increased, as compared with D2 group. When D1 reached 200 mGy, the adaptive response in apoptosis and cell cycle progression of thymocytes were no longer induced by low dose radiation. The results mentioned above indicate that when the mice were irradiated with 25~100 mGy (D1, 12.5 mGy/min) at 6 h before 1.0~2.0 Gy (D2, 0.287 Gy/min) exposure, the adaptive response in apoptosis and cell cycle progression of thymocytes may be induced under the condition of whole-body irradiation.

16. Meng QY, Chen SL, Liu SZ. Expression of proteins in mouse splenic cells after low dose radiation and their biological activity. Chin J Radiol Med Radiol Protec 2000, 20 228-231 [Abstract] Objective: In order to investigate the mechanisms of the hormetic effect of low dose ionizing radiation, the induction of protein expression in mouse splenic cells after whole-body irradiation was studied. Methods Expression of proteins and their biological activity was detected using gel filtration and high performance liquid chromatography (HPLC) as well as mouse splenic lymphocyte proliferation with 3H-TdR incorporation and chromosome aberrations of human lymphocytes were observed. Results: The changes in expression of three polypeptides with MW 18.5 kD, 17 kD and 50 kD were respectively detected in the crude extracts of the whole cell, cytoplasm and nucleus using HPLC. The 17 kD and 18.5 kD molecules were down-regulated, while the 50 kD molecule was up-regulated by low dose X-irradiation. The proliferative response of splenic lymphocytes from normal mice to Con A was significantly enhanced after the addition of protein fractions containing the reduced amount of 17 kD and 18.5 kD molecules, but not after the addition of the fraction containing increased amount of 50 kD molecules. The fractions with down-regulated expression of 18.5 kD protein and with up-regulated expression of 50 kD protein showed a protective effect on the chromosome damage caused by radiation. Conclusion. The changes in expression of protein molecules might play an important role in the mechanism of radiation hormesis.

YEAR 2001

17. Ju GZ, Fu HQ, Fu SB, Liu JX, Liu SZ. G1 arrest and relative protein expressions in mouse thymocytes induced by whole body X-ray irradiation. Biomed Environ Sci. 2001, 14(4):278-282. [Abstract] Objective: To investigate the molecular regulation of G1 arrest of mouse thymocytes induced by ionizing radiation. Methods Cell cycle was analyzed by flow cytometry (FCM) following staining of cells with propidium iodide. Fluorescent staining and flow cytometry analysis were employed for measurement of protein expression. Results It was demonstrated that G1 phase of mouse thymocytes increased significantly at 12 h after whole body irradiation (WBI) with the doses of 0.5, 1.0 and 2.0 Gy, and at 24 h following 2.0 Gy exposure, measured by FCM. In the time course experiment, it was found that G1 phase of thymocytes increased significantly at 4 h, reached a peak level at 24 h and came down toward 48 h after WBI with 2.0 Gy X-rays. The results also showed that after 2.0 Gy exposure, the expression of proteins in mouse thymocytes increased significantly from 1 h to 8 h for p53, for p21 from 4 h to 48 h, and for MDM2 at 4 h and 8 h, as measured by FCM. But no change was found for GADD45 protein expression. Conclusion These results suggest that G1 arrest could be induced by a single dose of 0.5 Gy, 1.0 Gy or 2.0 Gy, and its

molecular control might be established through the p53-p21 pathway.

18. Ju GZ, Fu HQ, Luo C, Fu SB. G1 arrest and the expressions of relative proteins in EL-4 cells induced by ionizing radiation. J Radiat Res Radiat Proces. 2001, 19(1):67-70. [Abstract] To investigate G1 arrest and the expressions of relative proteins in EL-4 cells induced by ionizing radiation, flow cytometry (FCM) was used to analyze cell cycle through staining cells with propidium iodide (PI) . And FCM was also employed to analyze protein expression of EL-4 cells stained with monoclonal and polyclonal antibodies for their immunofluorescence. It was found that the number of EL-4 cells in G1 phase increased significantly 12-72 h after X-irradiation with doses of 2.0Gy and 4.0Gy. The results also showed significant increases of p53 protein expression at 2 h to 24 h ($P<0{\cdot}05$-$P<0{\cdot}001$), p21 protein expression at 2 h to 48 h ($P<0{\cdot}05$-$P<0{\cdot}001$), GADD45 protein expression at 2 h to 48 h ($P<0{\cdot}05$- $P<0{\cdot}001$), and MDM2 protein expression at 4 h to 24 h ($P<0{\cdot}05$-$P<0{\cdot}001$) after 4.0Gy X-irradiation. These results suggest that G1 arrest of EL-4 cells could be induced by ionizing radiation and the expression of p53, p21 and GADD45 proteins may play an important role in the mechanism.

19. Wu CM, Li XY, Liu SZ. Study on cloning of the Egr-1 promoter and its radiation-inducible property. J N. Bethune Univ Med Sci. 2001 27(1):6-8. [Abstract] Objective: Egr-1 promoter was amplified and Egr-PGL plasmid was constructed to study the expression of luciferase in transfected NIH3T3 cells after different doses of X-ray irradiation. Methods: Egr-1p was amplified by PCR and inserted into PGL 3-E vector. The expression of luciferase induced by X-rays was studied by measuring the light of luciferase and substrate. Results: Egr-1 cDNA was obtained by PCR and was sequenced. The results indicated that the sequence was the same as reported in literature except G®C at 393 bp. The Egr-1p was connected with PGL 3 vector and was detected by electrophoresis. The constructs were used to transfect mouse NIH3T3 cells to characterize the regulatory function of Egr-1p after exposure to X-irradiation. The results indicate that the expression of luciferase of all groups irradiated (0.075 to 10 Gy) is highter than that of 0 Gy group. The expression in irradiated groups is 5-7.5 times greater than that of 0 Gy group. Conclusion: Egr-1p obtained can induce the expression of its downstream gene after different doses of X-ray irradiation. The effect of low dose irradiation on Egr-1 induction may be important in tumor gene therapy.

20. Wu CM, Li XY, Liu SZ. Experimental study on anti-tumor effect of pcEgr-IFNã gene-radiotherapy. Chin J Radiol Med radiol Prot 2001 21(4):236-238. [Abstract] Objective: To study the anti-tumor effect of IFNã gene-radiotherapy on murine melanoma and its immunologic mechanism. Methods: pcEgr-IFNã plasmids were injected locally into tumor and 36 hours later the tumors were given 20 Gy X-ray irradiation. Tumor growth at different times, IFNã expression on day 3 and immunologic indexes on day 15 were detected. Results: The tumor growth rate 3 - 15 days after pcEgr-IFNã gene-radiotherapy was significantly slower than that of the group with irradiation alone and the group with gene therapy alone. Tumor IFNã expression was higher than that of plasmid treatment alone group on day 3. NK activity as well as IL-2 and IFNã secretion were significantly higher than those in the groups with genetherapy alone and with irradiation alone. Conclusion. The anti-tumor effect of IFNã gene-radiotherapy is better than that of either of them applied solely. Its mechanism might be related with the activation of anti-tumor immunologic functions, especially with higher expression of IFNã induced by irradiation in the tumors.

21. Lv Z, Liu SC, Sun ZY, Fu SB, Gong SL. Time-effect of adaptive response of thymocyte apoptosis and cell cycle progression induced by low dose ionizing radiation in mice. Chin J Radiol Med Protect, 2001, 21 (4): 276-278. [Abstract] Objective: In the present study we observed the general pattern of the adaptive response of thymocyte apoptosis and cell cycle progression induced by low dose radiation. Methods Kunming male mice were irradiated with the inductive dose (D1, 75 mGy) and the challenging dose (D2, 1.5 Gy). The intervals between D1 and D2 were 3, 6, 12, 24 and 60 hours separately. The changes of thymocyte apoptosis and cell cycle progression were measured with flow cytometry. Results: When the intervals between D1 and D2 were 3, 6 and 12 hours, the percentages of apoptotic cells in D1 + D2 groups were significantly lower than those in D2 groups ($P < 0.05$), and the percentages of G0/G1 and G2 + M phase cells decreased in varying degrees, while the percentages of S phase cells increased significantly ($P < 0.05$ or $P < 0.01$). Conclusion. The results mentioned above indicate that when the mice were irradiated with 75 mGy (D1, 12.5 mGy/min) 3 – 12 hours before 1.5 Gy (D2, 0.287 Gy/min) exposure, the adaptive response of thymocyte apoptosis and cell cycle progression could be induced under the condition of whole-body irradiation.

22. Fu HQ, Ju GZ, Su X, Fu SB. Effect of ionizing radiation on p53 gene. Radiation Protection. 2001, 21(2):89-92. [Abstract] To elucidate the molecular mechanism of G1 arrest induced by ionizing radiation, flow cytometry (FCM) and Northern blot were used to analyze p53 gene mRNA and protein

expressions of thymocytes and splenocytes in Kunming mice after whole body irradiation (WBI) with x-rays. The results indicated that the percentages of p53+ cells of thymocytes in mice increased at 1 h to 8 h after 2.0 Gy WBI. There were not significant changes of p53 mRNA level of thymocytes and splenocytes from 1 h to 48 h after 75 mGy or 2.0 Gy WBI. No dose-dependent effect was found of p53 mRNA level of thymocytes or splenocytes in mice 4 h after from 0.5 to 6. 0 Gy WBI. These results suggested that ionizing radiation could induce p53 protein expression via post-transcriptional mechanism.

23. Fu HQ, and Ju GZ. The role of [Ca2+]i mobilization of splenocytes in immune adaptive response induced by low dose radiation. Radiat Protec. 2001, 21(2):115-118. [Abstract] To elucidate the role of [Ca2+]i mobilization of splenocytes in immune adaptive response induced by low dose radiation , dose effects and adaptive response of intracellular [Ca2+]i of splenocytes in Kunming mice following whole body irradiation (WBI) with X-rays were studied by using fura-2 as a fluorescent indicator. Results indicated that WBI with 1.0~6.0 Gy X-rays could decrease the [Ca2+]i of splenocytes in a dose-dependen manner 24 h after irradiation in mice. However, [Ca2+]i of splenocytes in mice irradiated with 0.075~0.2 Gy X-ray WBI was significantly higher than that irradiated with 0 Gy. Pre-irradiation with 0.075 Gy WBI could markedly reduce the inhibition of [Ca2+]i in splenocyte by 2.0 Gy WBI. In conclusion, [Ca2+]i mobilization in T lymphocyte might play an important role in immune adaptive response induced by low dose radiation.

24. Ye F, Liu SZ. Effect of whole-body irradiation with X-rays on cyclin B1 and cdc2 transcription level of splenocytes in mice. J Radiat Res Radiat Proc 2001 19 181-185 [Abstract] The changes in cyclin B1 and cdc2 transcription level of splenocytes in mice were observed after WBI with low and high doses of X-rays. The results showed that cyclin B1 mRNA expression slightly increased at 2 h and 12 - 24h after 75 mGy X rays, being 1.25, 1.27 and 1.22 times of sham-irradiated group, returning to sham - irradiated level at 48 h. However, cyclin B1 mRNA began to decrease at 4 h after irradiation with 2.0 Gy X rays, reaching its lowest level at 12 h, with a decrease of 39%, and gradually returning to the level of sham-irradiated control. In addition, we observed the time course of cdc2 mRNA expression. The results showed that there were no changes in cdc2 mRNA expression at 2 ~48 h after 75 mGy WBI, but the time course of cdc2 mRNA expression with 2.0 Gy WBI was the same as cyclin B1 after the same dose. The results indicated that low dose irradiation could induce an increase in cyclin B1 transcription level, accelerating the progression of cell cycle, but did not affect the expression of cdc2 gene. In contrast, high dose irradiation could induce the decrease in expression of the above two factors, with marked G2 arrest.

25. Ye F, Liu SZ. Effect of whole-body irradiation with X-rays on cyclin B1 and p34cdc2 protein expression in mouse thymocytes. Radiat Protect 2001 21 365-368 [Abstract] The effects of whole-body X-irradiation (WBI) with low and high doses on Cyclin B1 and p34cdc2 protein expression in the thymocytes of mice were studied using immunohistochemistry. The results showed that in comparison with the control group cyclin B1 protein expression increased at 8 h after WBI with 75 mGy, reaching its peak at 12 h followed by its return to normal level at 48 h. Cyclin B1 protein expression decreased at 4 h after WBI with 2 Gy, reaching its lowest level at 12 h, followed by a return to the control level at 48 h. At the same time, the changes of p34cdc2 protein expression were observed. In comparison with the control group, there were no changes in p34cdc2 protein expression after WBI with 75 mGy, the time course of p34cdc2 protein expression after WBI with 2 Gy was the same as cyclin B1 after the same dose. The results indicated that low dose radiation could induce the increase of cyclin B1 protein expression accompanied with acceleration of cell cycle progression. In contrast, high dose irradiation could induce a decrease of expression of both proteins finally resulting in G2 arrest.

26. Liu SZ, Jin SZ, Liu XD, Sun YM. Role of CD28/B7 costimulation and IL-12/IL-10 interaction in the radiation-induced immune changes. BMC Immunology. 2001, 2: 8 (http://www.biomedcentral.com/1471-2172/2/8) [Abstract] Background: The present paper aims at studying the role of B7/CD28 interaction and related cytokine production in the immunological changes after exposure to different doses of ionizing radiation. Results: The stimulatory effect of low dose radiation (LDR) on the proliferative response of lymphocytes to Con A was found to require the presence of APCs. The addition of APCs obtained from both low- and high-dose-irradiated mice to splenic lymphocytes separated from low-dose-irradiated mice caused stimulation of lymphocyte proliferation. B7.1/2 expression on APCs was up-regulated after both low and high doses of radiation. There was up-regulation of CD28 expression on splenic and thymic lymphocytes after LDR and its suppression after high dose radiation (HDR), and cytotoxic T lymphocyte-associated antigen 4 (CTLA-4) expression showed changes in the opposite direction. IL-12 secretion by macrophages was stimulated after both low and high doses of radiation, but IL-10 synthesis by splenocytes was suppressed by low dose radiation and up-regulated by high dose radiation. Conclusion: The status of CD28/CTLA-4 expression on T lymphocytes in the presence of up-regulated B7 expression

on APCs determined the outcome of the immune changes in response to radiation, i.e., up-regulation of CD28 after LDR resulted in immunoenhancement, and up-regulation of CTLA-4 associated with down-regulation of CD28 after HDR led to immunosuppression. Both low and high doses of radiation up-regulated B7.1/2 expression on APCs. After LDR, the stimulated proliferative effect of increased IL-12 secretion by APCs, reinforced by the suppressed secretion of IL-10, further strengthened the intracellular signaling induced by B7-CD28 interaction.

27. Jin SZ, He SJ, Liu SZ. Effect of different doses of X-rays on the expression of CD80 and CD86 on mouse macrophages. J Radiat Res Radiat Proc 2001, 19:153-157 [Abstract] The effect of X-irradiation on CD80 and CD86 expression on peritoneal macrophages of mice after whole-body irradiation (WBI) and in J774A.1 mouse macrophage cells line irradiated in vitro was studied with immunohistochemistry (ABC method). Results showed that the up-regulation of CD80 expression induced by WBI and in vitro irradiation with 2 Gy X-rays appeared earlier than that with 0.075 Gy X-rays, but no significant difference was found in the response of CD86 to these doses. The study on the dose-effect relationship showed that the expression of both CD80 and CD86 reached its peak at 0.075 Gy after WBI as well as in vitro irradiation with X-rays. The doses inducing the second peak of CD80 and CD86 upregulation were higher in the case of WBI in comparison with the in vitro irradiation. The results suggested that the up-regulation of expression of B7 molecules after irradiation may be an important factor involved in the enhancing effect of low dose radiation on immunity.

28. He SJ, Liu SZ. The relation between activation of different dimers of NF-kB and radiation-induced apoptosis. Foreign Med: Radiat Med & Nucl Med 2001£¬25: 74-77 [Abstract] NF-kB used to be considered as a surviving factor, conferring vigorous resistance to cells against radiation-induced apoptosis. However, recent research gradually disclosed that combination of different subunits of NF-kB may have different, even opposite, effects. Further investigation in more depth would undoubtedly provide theoretical basis for the understanding of the mechanism of the depressive effect of medium to high doses of radiation on immunity and valuable new information for clinical radiotherapy of tumors.

29. He SJ, Xie F, Liu SZ. Activation of CREB induced by X-rays and its relation with cAMP signal pathway. J Radiat Res Radiat Proc 2001, 19: 138-140 [Abstract] To measure the changes in DNA binding activity of CREB and the ratio of cAMP/cGMP in thymocytes after whole body irradiation (WBI) with X rays, as well as to discuss the relationship of the activation of CREB with cAMP signal pathway. Changes in DNA binding activity of CREB and the concentration of cAMP and cGMP in mouse thymocytes were respectively assayed by electrophoresis mobility shift assay (EMSA) and competitive protein binding assay. The activity of CREB DNA-binding was upregulated after irradiation with larger doses of X rays (0.5~6.0 Gy), with the upregulation being most significant after irradiation with 2.0 Gy X rays. Following WBI with 0.075Gy, there was only a brief decrease followed by slight increase in the DNA binding activity of CREB, while the decrease in cAMP/cGMP ratio reached the lowest value at 24h. These results suggested that the slight increase in the DNA binding activity of CREB observed after irradiation with 0.075 Gy may not involve the cAMP signal pathway, while the latter was probably involved in the marked increase in the DNA binding activity of CREB induced by WBI with higher doses of X rays.

30. Liu XD , Liu SZ , Ma SM , Liu Y. Changes in opposite directions for the expression of IL-10 and IL-12 after low dose irradiation. J Radiat Res Radiat Proc 2001, 19: 283-288 [Abstract] To observe the effects of LDR on the synthesis of IL-10 in splenocytes and the secretion of IL-12 by peritoneal macrophages. Northern blot and flow cytometry were adopted to detect the changes of IL-10 at mRNA and protein level, respectively. Northern blot and ELISA were used respectively to examine the changes of IL-12p35/p40 mRNA and IL-12p70 protein levels. In splenocytes IL-10 mRNA decreased significantly, while both IL-12 p35 and p40 subunits in macrophages increased after WBI with 75 mGy X rays. Meanwhile, IL-10 synthesis in splenocytes decreased beginning from 4 h after exposure and remaining at low level up to 48 h, and IL-12 secretion by macrophages was found to take an opposite direction. WBI with 75 mGy X rays may suppress IL-10 both at the mRNA level and protein level and stimulate IL-12 expression simultaneously, and this would lead to a shift of the immune response in favour of TH1 differentiation.

YEAR 2002

31. Ju GZ, Ma SM, Fu SB and Liu SZ. Effect of X-irradiation on bone marrow cell cycle. Chin J Prev Med. 2002, 3(2):87-88. [Abstract] Objective: To investigate the effect of whole body X-irradiation with different doses on bone marrow cell cycle. Methods Cell cycle was analyzed by flow cytometry (FCM) following staining of cells with propidium iodide (PI). Results It was found that G1 and G2 phases of bone

marrow cells increased significantly at 12 h after whole body irradiation (WBI) with the doses of 1.0 , 2.0, 4.0 and 6.0 Gy, whereas S phase cells decreased at the same time. However, S phase was increased significantly at 72 h following 0.05, 0.075, 0.1 and 0.2 Gy low dose X-irradiation. Conclusion These results suggest that G1 and G2 arrest could be induced by X-irradiation with the doses above 0.5 Gy. S phase was found to be stimulated by low dose X-rays below 0.2 Gy.

32. Ju GZ, Ma SM, Fu SB and Liu SZ., Effect of ionizing radiation on bone marrow cell cycle and Its molecular regulation. Chin J Radiol Med Prot. 2002, 22(5):342-343. [Abstract] Objective: To investigate the effect of ionizing radiation on bone marrow cell cycle and its molecular regulation. Methods Cell cycle was analyzed by flow cytometry (FCM) following staining of cells with propidium iodide (PI). Fluorescent staining and flow cytometry analysis were employed for measurement of protein expression. Results It was found that G1 and G2 phase cells of bone marrow cells increased significantly at 12 h after whole body irradiation (WBI) with the doses of 1.0 , 2.0, 4.0 and 6.0 Gy. It was also shown that with the increase of G1 phase cells the protein expressions of p53 and p21 also increased significantly following 2.0 Gy WBI X-irradiation, whereas the protein expressions of cyclin D1 and CDK4 decreased significantly. Conclusion These results suggest that G1 arrest could be induced by X-rays and its molecular control might be established through the p53-p21 pathway.

33. Jin SZ, Liu SZ. Effect of whole-body X-irradiation on the expression of costimulatory molecules on immune cells Chin J Radiol Med Protect 2002 22 256-259 [Abstract] Objective: To study the effect of ionizing radiation on costimulatory molecules on immune cells. Methods Flow cytometry (FCM) was used to detect the changes in the expression of CD28/CTLA-4 of thymocytes and splenocytes after whole-body irradiation (WBI) with different doses of X-rays. Immunohistochemistry (IHC, ABC method) was used to detect the changes in the expression of B7.1 and B7.2 on peritoneal macrophages after WBI with different doses of X-rays. Results: The results showed that 0.075 Gy X-rays caused significant up-regulation of CD28 on both thymocytes and splenocytes and down-regulation of CTLA-4 expression, which was more significant on the splenocytes. After 2 Gy irradiation the expression of CTLA-4 on both thymocytes and splenocytes was significantly up-regulated with down-regulation of CD28 expression, which was more significant on the splenocytes. The dose-effect studies showed that there was no change in the expression of CTLA-4 on the thymocytes 72 h after LDR, while 2 and 4 Gy caused apparent increase in the expression of CTLA-4 ($P<0.05$, $P< 0.01$). For splenocytes, LDR caused no changes in the expression of CTLA-4 4 h after irradiation, while higher doses could increase the expression of CTLA-4 significantly ($P<0.05$, $P<0.01$). The expression of B7.1 and B7.2 on peritoneal macrophages increased after both 0.075 Gy and 2 Gy X-rays. The increase in B7.2 expression preceded that of B7.1 expression after 0.075 Gy and lasted longer than that after 2 Gy irradiation. Conclusion Up-regulation of expression of costimulatory molecules CD28 and B7 after whole-body X-irradiation may be an important factor involved in the enhancing effect of low dose radiation on immunity.

34. Liu XD ,Ma SM ,Liu SZ. Effects of ionizing radiation on IL-12 and NF-êB activities in peritoneal macrophages of mice. Chin J radiat Med Radiat Protec 2002 22 1 7-10 [Abstract] Objective: To observe the changes of IL-12 and NF-êB in murine peritoneal macrophages after whole-body irradiation (WBI) with different doses of X-rays. Methods Enzyme-linked immunosorbent assay (ELISA) and electrophoresis mobility shift assay(EMSA) were used to detect the secretion of IL-12 and the DNA-binding activity of NF-êB, respectively. Results: ELISA data indicated both 0.075 Gy and 2 Gy increased the secretion of IL-12 and the latter seemed to increase IL-12 more than the former. EMSA showed two bands representing p65/p50 and p50/p50 respectively. 0.075 Gy increased the p65/p50 activity and showed little effect on p50/p50 while 2 Gy increased both the two dimers. Conclusion: The results suggested that NF-êB activation might be involved in the radiation-induced changes of IL-12.

35. He SJ, Jin SZ, Liu SZ Effect of X-irradiation on DNA binding activity of NF-YMBOL 107 \f "Symbol" \s 12B in EL-4 cells. Radiat Protec 2002, 22: 20-25 [Abstract] Changes in time course of the DNA-binding activity of NF-kB as well as the subcellular localization of p65 subunit and expression of IkBá in EL-4 cells after irradiation with 2 Gy and 0.075 Gy X-rays were examined using electrophoresis mobility shift assay (EMSA) and immunohistochemistry (IHC), respectively. Results showed that the increases in DNA-binding activity of NF-kB p50/p50 and p50/p65 were induced by both 0.075 Gy and 2 Gy X-rays. However, the amplitude of the increase in activity of the two dimers was different after irradiation with the two doses of X-rays. After irradiation with 0.075 Gy, the increase in p50/p65 activity was higher than that of p50/p50 activity. After irradiation with 2 Gy, the situation was reversed. Irradiation with both 2 Gy and 0.075 Gy induced an increase in the rate of p65 nuclear translocation and the degradation of IkBá before the increase of its expression, but the degree of these changes after different doses of irradiation was different.

These results suggest that the transcriptional regulation of NF-kB changes with irradiation dose and results in the difference in responses of the cells.

36. Liu GW, Li PW, Liu SC, Gong SL. Adaptive response of spermatogenic cell apoptosis induced by low dose X-ray irradiation in mice. Chin J Radiol Med Protect, 2002, 22 (5): 322-325. [Abstract] Objective: To study the adaptive response of spermatogenic cell apoptosis induced by whole-body X-ray irradiation with low doses in male Kunming mice. Methods: The spermatogenic cell apotosis induced by 75 mGy X-ray irradiation during spermatogenic cell cycle was measured by using the methods of terminal deoxyribonucleotide transferase-mediated dUTP-bictin nick end labeling (TUNEL) and HE staining. Results: When an inductive dose (D1) of 75 mGy was given or not at 6 h before the challenging dose (D2) of 1.0, 2.0 or 3.0 Gy, the apoptotic percentages of the spermatogonia and spermatocytes in the D1 + D2 groups were declined rapidly as compared with those in the D2 alone groups, and the apoptotic percentages of spermatids showed no significant changes. When the inductive dose (D1) 75 mGy was given at 3, 6, 12 and 24 h before the challenging doses (D2) of 1.0, 1.5, 2.0, 2.5 and 3.0 Gy, the apoptotic percentages in spermatogonia and spermatocytes reduced early and significantly and continued for a longer duration under smaller D2 doses (1.0, 1.5 and 2.0 Gy). However, the apoptotic percentages reduced only at 6 h after whole-body irradiation under larger D2 doses (2.5 and 3.0 Gy), and were not significant. Conclusions: The adaptive response of apoptosis in spermatogonia and spermatocytes could be induced by low dose X-ray irradiation. The effect could closely relate to D2 doses and the interval time between D1 and D2.

37. Jin SZ , Liu XD, Liu SZ. Effects of Different Doses of X-Irradiation on NF-êB Expression in Peritoneal Macrophages of Mice. J Jilin Univ (Med Ed), 2002, 28(4): 335-337. [Abstract] Objective: To study the effect of different doses of X-irradiation on NF-êB activation in peritoneal macrophages of mice. Methods Electrophoresis mobility shift assay (EMSA) was used to separate the bands of NF-êB protein combined with isotope-labeled DNA probe, the results were analysized by PhosphorImager scaning system. Results: The binding activities of NF-êB protein to DNA began to increase 4 h after whole-body irradiation (WBI) with 0.075 Gy X-rays, followed by gradual return to the sham-irradiation level at 48 h while after the treatment of 2 Gy X-rays, the binding activities of NF-êB protein to DNA began to increase at 8 h, sustaining at higher level up to 48 h. Conclusion: Both low dose and high dose irradiation could induce the NF-êB activation in peritoneal macrophages of mice.

38. He SJ, Ye F, Liu SZ. Relationship between X-ray-induced activation of transcription factors and apoptosis. Chin J Radiol Med Radiol Protec 2002 22 4-6 [Abstract] Objective: To investigate the role of activation of transcription factors in the induction of apoptosis of immune cells after whole-body irradiation (WBI) with X-rays by comparing the time course of the changes of DNA-binding activity of several transcription factors and that of apoptosis in mouse thymocyte after 2 Gy X-rays. Methods The dynamic changes of the activity of transcription factors NF-êB, CREB and OCT-1, as well as thymocyte apoptosis after whole body irradiation with 2 Gy X-rays were respectively examined with electrophoresis mobility shift assay (EMSA) and flow cytomentry (FCM) . Results: There was a significant distinction between the changes of DNA-binding activity of the two dimers of NF-êB (p50/p50 and p50/p65) in thymocytes after WBI with 2 Gy X-rays, with significant increase in the binding activity of NF-êB homodimer p50/p50. In addition, the activity of CREB and OCT-1 also increased significantly. Their activity peaks at 4-12 h after WBI coincided well with the peaking time of thymocyte apoptosis. Conclusions: WBI with 2 Gy X-rays mainly induces the activation of NF-êB homodimer p50/p50. The results suggest that the three transcription factors including NF-êB p50/p50, CREB and OCT-1 might act synergistically in the induction of apoptosis in thymocytes after WBI with 2 Gy X-rays.

YEAR 2003

39. Jin GH, Tian M, Jin SZ, Liu SZ. Cloning and Sequencing of Mouse IL-18 and Construction of Recombinant Plasmid pIRES- IL-18-B7.1. J Jilin Univ (Med Ed) 2003 29 125-127 [Abstract] Objective: To clone the sequence of the cDNA of mouse IL-18 coding area and construct its expression vector. Methods: Using mouse splenocyte mRNA as template to obtain full length mIL-18 with the technique of RT-PCR followed by automatic sequencing of pMD18T-mIL-18 and to construct a recombinant plasmid containing mIL-18 and B7.1 genes with recombinant DNA technique. Results: Sequencing proved the cloned mIL-18 cDNA to be completely identical with that reported in the literature and the recombinant plasmid containing mIL-18 and B7.1 was constructed successfully. Conclusion: mIL-18 cDNA was successfully cloned and an expression vector pIRES-IL-182B7.1 was constructed.

40. Liu SZ. Nonlinear Dose-Response Relationship in the Immune System Following Exposure

to Ionizing Radiation: Mechanisms and Implications Nonlinearity in Biol Toxicol Med, 2003, 1: 71-92. [Abstract] The health effects of low-dose radiation (LDR) have been the concern of the academic spheres, regulatory bodies, governments, and the public. Among these effects, the most important is carcinogenesis. In view of the importance of immune surveillance in cancer control, the dose-response relationship of the changes in different cell types of the immune system after whole-body irradiation is analyzed on the basis of systemic data from the author's laboratory in combination with recent reports in the literature. For T lymphocytes J- or inverted J-shaped curves are usually demonstrated after irradiation, while for macrophages dose-response curves of chiefly stimulation with irregular patterns are often observed. The intercellular reactions between the antigen presenting cell (APC) and T lymphocyte (TLC) in the immunologic synapse via expression of surface molecules and secretion of cytokines by the two cell types after different doses of radiation are illustrated. The different pathways of signal transduction thus facilitated in the T lymphocyte by different doses of radiation are analyzed to explain the mechanism of the phenomenon of low-dose stimulation and high-dose suppression of immunity. Experimental and clinical data are cited to show that LDR retards tumor growth, reduces metastasis, increases the efficacy of conventional radiotherapy and chemotherapy as well as alleviates the suppression of immunity due to tumor burden. The incidence of thymic lymphoma after high-dose radiation is lowered by pre-exposure to low-dose radiation, and its mechanism is supposed to be related to the stimulation of anticancer immunity induced by low-dose radiation. Recent reports on lowering of standardized cancer mortality rate and all cause death rate of cohorts occupationally exposed to low-dose radiation from the US, UK, and Canada are cited.

41. Liu SZ. On radiation hormesis expressed in the immune system. Crit Rev Toxicol. 2003;33:431-441 [Abstract] Radiation hormesis is reviewed with emphasis on its expression in the immune system. The shape of the dose-response relationship of the immune functions depends on a number of factors, chiefly the target cell under study, experimental design with emphasis on the dose range, dose spacing, dose rate and temporal changes, as well as the animal strain. For mouse and human T lymphocyte functions in the dose range of 0.01 to 10 Gy a J or inverted J-shaped curve is usually observed. For the more radioresistant macrophages, stimulation of many of their functions is often observed in the dose range up to a few grays. The cellular and molecular mechanisms of the enhancement of immunity induced by low-dose radiation were analyzed on the basis of literature published in the last decade of the past century. Intercellular reactions among the APCs and lymphocytes via distinct changes in expression of relevant surface molecules and secretion of regulatory cytokines in response to different doses of radiation were described. The major signal transduction pathways activated in response to these intercellular reactions were illustrated. The suppressive effect of low-dose radiation on cancer induction, growth, and metastasis and its immunologic mechanisms were analyzed. The present status of research in this field gives strong support to radiation hormesis in immunity with low-dose radiation as one of the mechanisms of cancer surveillance. Further research with new techniques using microarray with biochips to fully elucidate the molecular mechanisms is suggested.

42. Jin SZ, He SJ, Liu SZ. Experimental studies on the activation of NF-êB and its signal pathway induced by low dose radiation. Chin J Radiol Med Radiol Protec 2003, 23: 408-410 [Abstract] Objective: To observe the effect of low dose radiation (LDR) on the activation of NF-êB and the possible mechanism of its signal transduction. Methods: Electrophoretic mobility shift assay (EMSA) and immunohistochemistry were used to detect the changes of DNA-binding activity of NF-êB and the nuclear translocation of p65 in EL-4 cells, respectively. LipofectAMINE-mediated transient transfection was used to carry vacant plasmid and NF-êB-luciferase-containing plasmid into NIH3T3 cells, with and without the addition of PKC-specific blocking agent Calphostin C, to detect the expression of luciferase after irradiation. Results: X-irradiation with 0.075 Gy increased the activities of p50/p65 and p50/p50 dimers, especially the former. The translocation of p65 into nuclei increased and IêBá exhibited the opposite changes. Calphostin C reversed the effect of 0.075 Gy radiation on the activity of NF-êB. Conclusion The activation of NF-êB induced by LDR might be effected via the PKC pathway resulting in the facilitation of the expression of cytokines and up-regulation of immune functions, which might be involved in the mechanisms of the hormetic effects of LDR.

43. Liu XD, Ma SM, Liu SZ Changes of CD2 and CD48 expression in EL-4 and J774A.1 cell lines after different doses of X-irradiation. Chin J Radiol Med Radiol Protec 2003, 23 241-243 [Abstract] Objective: To observe the changes in the expression of CD2 on EL-4 and CD48 on J774A.1 cells after different doses of X-irradiation with time-course and dose-effect studies. Methods: Flow cytometry (FCM) was adopted to detect the changes of CD2 and CD8 expressions. Results: FCM data showed increased CD2 expression on EL-4 cells beginning from 4 h reaching its peak at 8-16 h after 0.075 Gy irradiation, while 2

Gy suppressed its expression from 4 h reaching its minimum at 8 h. Dose-effect results of CD2 expression revealed that 0.050 Gy and 0.075 Gy up-regulated its expression while 1~6 Gy induced reverse changes 8 h after exposure. Simultaneously, CD48 expression on J774A. 1 cells showed an earlier increase (4 h) and a later decrease (16~48 h) after 0.075 Gy irradiation, whereas 2 Gy irradiation led to a sustained decrease up to 48 h. Dose-effect studies of CD48 expression showed that 0.05-0.10 Gy up-regulated the expression of CD48 while 1~6 Gy down-regulated its expression significantly. Conclusion The different changes of CD2 expression on EL-4 cells and CD48 expression on J774A.1 cells after different doses of X-irradiation indicate that LDR exhibits an opposite effect to that of HDR.

44. Ju GZ, Wang XM, Fu SB and Liu SZ. Effect of ionizing radiation on p16 gene transcription and protein expression. Chin J Radiol Med Prot. 2003, 23(1): 4-6. [Abstract] Objective: To investigate the effect of ionizing radiation on p16 gene transcription and protein expression. Methods Northern blot was employed to determine p16 mRNA level. Flow cytometry was used to measure p16 protein expression. Results It was demonstrated that p16 mRNA level was markedly increased at 2-24 h in thymocytes and at 2-8 h in splenocytes, and p16 protein expression increased significantly at 8-48 h for thymocytes ($P<0{\cdot}05$ to $P<0{\cdot}01$) and at 24 h for splenocytes ($P<0{\cdot}05$) after whole body X-irradiation with 2·0 Gy in mice. In the dose-effect experiments, it was found that p16 mRNA level increased with the increase of doses in thymocytes and splenocytes and the p16 protein expression was also increased significantly with the doses from 1.0 to 4.0 Gy for both thymocytes and splenocytes ($P<0.05$ to $P<0.01$). Conclusion p16 gene transcription and protein expression could be up-regulated by X-rays and the tendency of increase varied with the radiation dose and cell type.

45. Ju GZ, Ma SM, Ye F, Fu SB and Liu SZ. Effect of different dose x-rays on cell cycle. Chin J Radiol Med Prot. 2003, 23(6):415-417. [Abstract] Objective: To investigate the effect of different dose x-rays on cell cycle. Methods Cell cycle was analyzed by flow cytometry (FCM) following staining of cells with propidium iodide (PI). Results It was found that the number in G1 and G2 phase cells of thymocytes, splenocytes and bone marrow cells increased significantly at 12-24 h after whole body irradiation (WBI) with the doses of 0.05-6.0Gy ($P<0.05$- $P<0.001$), whereas the number in S phase cells was decreased significantly at the same times ($P<0.05$- $P<0.001$). However, the number in S phase cells of thymocytes, splenocytes and bone marrow cells were increased significantly at 24-72 h following 0.05 and 0.075Gy low dose X-irradiation ($P<0.05$- $P<0.01$). Conclusion These results suggest that G1 and G2 arrest of thymocytes, splenocytes and bone marrow cells could be induced by X-rays with the doses above 0.5Gy. And the proliferation of thymocytes, splenocytes and bone marrow cells could be stimulated by low dose X-rays with the doses of 0.05Gy and 0.075Gy.

46. Ju GZ, Wang XM, Fu SB and Liu SZ. Effect of ionizing radiation on the protein expressions of p16, CyclinD1 and CDK4 of thymocytes and splenocytes in mice. Chin J Radiol Med Prot. 2003, 23(6):399-401. [Abstract] Objective: To investigate the effect of ionizing radiation on the expressions of p16, CyclinD1 and CDK4 in thymocytes and splenocytes in mice. Methods Fluorescent staining and flow cytometry analysis were employed for measurement of protein expressions. Results It was found in time course experiments that the expression of p16 protein increased significantly at 8, 24 and 48 h in thymocytes ($P<0.05$, $P<0.01$ and $P<0.05$, respectively) and at 24 h in splenocytes ($P<0.05$) after whole body irradiation (WBI) with 2.0 Gy X-rays. However, the expression of CDK4 protein decreased significantly from 8 to 24 h in thymocytes ($P<0.05$~ $P<0.01$) and from 8 to 72 h in splenocytes ($P<0.05$~$P<0.01$). In dose effect experiments, it was found that the expression of p16 protein in thymocytes and splenocytes increased significantly at 24 h after WBI with the doses of 1.0, 2.0 and 4.0Gy ($P<0.05$~$P<0.01$), whereas the expression of CDK4 protein decreased significantly with the dose of 2.0Gy for thymocytes ($P<0.05$) and with the doses from 0.5~6.0Gy in splenocytes ($P<0.05$~$P<0.01$). The expression of CyclinD1 protein decreased markedly in both thymocytes and splenocytes after exposure. Conclusion The results indicated that the expression of p16 protein in thymocytes and splenocytes could be induced by ionizing radiation. And the p16-CyclinD1/CDK4 pathway may play an important role for G1 arrest of thymocytes induced by X-rays.

47. Zhang X, Gong SL, Zhang M, Liu SZ Protective effect of melatonin against damage of immune functions in C57BL/6J mice irradiated with ionizing raidaiton. J Radiat Res Radiat Proc 2003, 21: 202-205 [Abstract] The aim of the present work is to explore the effects and the mechanism of melatonin (MLT) on the damage of immune functions in mice induced by ionizing radiation. MLT was given to C57BL/6J mice through intraperitoneal injection 1 h before whole-body irradiation with 2 Gy X-rays. Twenty four hours after irradiation, the number of thymocytes and splenocytes, 3H-TdR incorporative rate (HTIR) of thymocytes and T and B lymphocyte transforming rates (TLTR and BLTR) induced by Con A and LPS were observed. The number of thymocytes and splenocytes, HTIR, TLTR and BLTR of the irradiated

mice were significantly lower than those of the sham-irradiation group (P<0.001). For all groups injected with 0.5~10 mg·kg-1 of MLT, the number of thymocytes and splenocytes were significantly higher than that in 0 mg group (simple irradiation), with the 0.5 mg•kg-1 MLT group being the highest. HTIR of thymocytes also increased significantly (P<0.01 or P<0.001), with the 0.5 mg•kg-1 MLT group being the highest. TLTR induced by Con A in the 0.5 mg•kg-1 MLT group increased most significantly, while BLTR in 10 mg•kg-1 MLT group increased most significantly. In addition, 2.5 mg•kg-1 of MLT enhanced splenocyte LTR without the stimulation of the mitogens. It is concluded that MLT can reduce the damage to lymphocytes of the irradiated mice and has a protective effect on immune functions.

48. Ju GZ, Shen B, Sun SL, Yan FQ and Fu SB. Effect of X-rays on the expression of caspase-3, p53 in EL-4 Cells and its biological implications. Biomed and Environ Sci. 2003, 16(1):47-52. [Abstract] Objective: To investigate the effect of X-rays on the expression of caspase-3, p53 protein in EL-4 cells and its implications in the induction of apoptosis and polyploidy cells. Methods Mouse lymphoma cell line, EL-4 cells, was used. Fluorescent staining and flow cytometry analysis were employed for measurement of protein expression, apoptosis, cell cycle and polyploid cells. Results It was found that the expression of caspase-3 protein increased significantly at 8 h and 12 h compared with sham-irradiated control (P<0.05, respectively) and the expression of p53 protein increased significantly at 2 4 8 12 and 24 h compared with sham-irradiated control (P<0.05~P<0.01) in EL-4 cells after 4.0 Gy X-irradiation. The results showed that apoptosis of EL-4 cells was increased significantly at 2 4 8 12 24 48 and 72 h after 4.0Gy exposure compared with sham-irradiated control (P<0.05~P<0.001). The results also showed that G2 phase cells were increased significantly at 4 8 12 24 48 and 72 h (P<0.05~ P<0.001), however, no marked change in the number of 8 C polyploidy cells was found from 2~48 h after 4.0Gy exposure. Conclusion Our results indicated that the expressions of caspase-3 and p53 protein in EL-4 cells could be induced by X-rays, which might play an important role for the induction of apoptosis, and the molecular pathway for polyploid formation might be p53-independent.

49. Meng QY, Chen SL, Liu SZ. Effect of low dose radiation on thymocyte cytosol and nuclear protein synthesis in mice. Chin J Radiol Med Radiol Protec 2003 23 14-16 [Abstract] Objective: To observe the effect of low dose radiation on thymocyte cytosol and nuclear protein synthesis in mice. Methods: The expression of proteins was analyzed by gel filtration with Sephadex G-100 and HPLC separation of proteins on thymocyte cytosol and nuclei after whole-body irradiation with 75 mGy X-rays and sham-irradiation, and their biological activity was examined by mouse splenocyte proliferation and chromosome aberration of human peripheral blood lymphocytes. Results: HPLC analysis showed that there was a marked increase in expression of 61.4 kD protein in the extract of thymocyte cytosol and 30.4 kD protein in the extract of thymocyte nuclei in comparison with the corresponding fractions from the sham-irradiated control mice. These protein fractions from the thymocyte cytosol and nuclei of the irradiated mice showed both stimulating effect on normal T cell proliferation and protective effect on chromosome damage induced by high dose radiation. Conclusion: These findings might have implications in the exploration of the mechanism of immunoenhancement and cytogenetic adaptive response induced by low dose radiation.

50. Li XJ, Song XF, Yang W, Tian M, Yang X, Liu LL, Li XY. Expression Property and Antitumor Effect of pEgr-angiostatin Induced by Ionizing Radiation. J Jilin Univ (M ed Ed) 2003 29(5):543-546. [Abstract] Objective: To study the exp ression and antitumor effect of pEgr-angiostatin induced by ionizing radiation. Methods: Mouse angiostatin cDNA was amplified with RT-PCR. The pEgr-angiostatin recombinant plasmid was constructed and was then transfected into B16 cells with liposome. The cells were irradiated and the exp ression of angiostatin mRNA in B16 cells was detected. Finally, the antitumor effect of pEgr-angiostatin was studied in a mouse model. Results: The sequence of mouse angiostatin cDNA was identical to that as previously reported. Egr-1 promoter and angiostatin cDNA was inserted correctly into expression vector. The expression property of pEgr-angiostatin was examined by ionizing radiation. The gene-therapy with pEgr-angiostatin showed remarkable antitumor effect. Conclusion: Mouse angiostatin cDNA was successfuly cloned in the study. The expression property and the antitumor effect of pEgr-angiostatin induced by ionizing radiation were observed. The present study provides the basis for multi-gene-radiotherapy of tumor.

51. Li XJ, Li XY, Tian M, Yang W. Expression of pEgr-ssEndostatin in tumor induced by radiation and its anti-tumor effect. Chin J Radiol Med Prot 2003 23(3):148-150. [Abstract] Objective: To observe the antitumor effect of pEgr-ssEndostatin gene-radiotherapy in murine melanoma and the expression of Endostatin gene in tumor induced by radiation. Methods: pEgr-ssEndostatin plasmids were injected locally into the B16 tumor in mice, and 42 h later the tumors of half of the mice were given 20 Gy X-irradiation. The tumor growth at different times and Endostatin expression 2 days after irradiation were detected.

Results: Endostatin gene-radiotherapy could enhance the curative effect of radiotherapy. Both pEgr-ssEndostatin group and pEgr-ssEndostatin + 20 Gy group showed Endostatin mRNA expression, but the mRNA level of pEgr-ssEndostatin + 20 Gy group was higher than that of pEgr-ssEndostatin group. Conclusion: The antitumor effect of pEgr-ssEndostatin gene-radiotherapy is better than that of radiotherapy alone and gene therapy alone.and Endostatin expression in tumor is enhanced after irradiation.

52. Tian M, Liu LL, Li XY.Cloning and Sequencing of the Human Tumor Suppressor Gene PTEN/MMAC1 by RT-nested PCR and Construction of its Expression Vector. J Jilin Univ (Med Ed) 2003 29(1):9-12. [Abstract]: Objective: To clone the cDNA of the human tumor suppressor gene-PTENöMMAC1 and construct its expression vector. Methods: About 1 200 bp DNA fragment was amplified from human placenta tissue by using RT-nested PCR and was cloned into pUCm-T vector after automatic sequencing, and the fragment was linked with expression vector pcDNA 3. 1. Results: The PTENöMMAC1 cDNA was cloned correctly and it s expression vector pcDNA-w P was constructed. Conclusion: Human tumor suppressor gene-PTENöMMAC1 cDNA was cloned by RT -nested PCR and its expression vector was constructed successfully. The result lays the foundation for further study on the tumor suppression function of PTENöMMAC1.

53. Liu GW, Wang CY, Lv Z, Liu SC, Gong SL. Effect of Bcl-2/Bax gene expression on apoptosis of apermatogenic cells of mouse testes induced by low dose radiation. Radiat Protect, 2003, 23 (6): 244-248, 354. [Abstract] The different kinds of spermatogenic cells were separated using density gradient centrifugation and their apoptosis and Bcl-2 and Bax protein expression were measured with flow cytometry and immunohistochemical method, respectively. The results showed the apoptosis in all kinds of spermatogenic cells induced by low dose radiation (LDR) had an obvious regularity. When the doses were 0.025 and 0.05 Gy, spermatogone apoptosis was dominant. With the increase of irradiation dose (0.075 – 0.2 Gy), spermatocytes also showed an apoptotic change, but the apoptotic percentage of spermatogonia was significantly higher than that of spermatocytes. Moreover, the apoptosis of spermatids and spermatozoa scarcely occurred after LDR. Bax protein was primarily expressed in spermatogonia and spermatocytes, and the former was siginificantly higher than that of the latter after LDR. With the increase of irradiation doses, Bax protein expression showed a upgrading tendency, but that of spermatids and spermatozoa scarcely occurred. Bcl-2 protein was primarily expressed in spermatids and spermatozoa, but the Bcl-2 protein expressions of spernatogonia and spermatocytes scarcely occurred after LDR. These results imply that the interacting regulation of Bcl-2 and Bax gene expression might be involved in selective apoptosis of spermatogenic cells induced by LDR, which provided an experimental evidence for further exploring the apoptotic mechanism of adaptive response of spermatogenic cells by LDR.

54. Liu GW, Lu WT, Wang ZQ, Lv Z, Liu SC, Gong SL. Apoptosis and expression of p53 mRNA and protein in mouse spermatogenic cells induced by low dose ionizing radiation. Chin J Pathophysiol, 2003, 19 (12): 1618-1622. [Abstract] Aim: The effect of low dose radiation (LDR) with different doses of X-rays on apoptosis and its related gene p53 expression were studied in spenmatogenic cells of male Kunming mouse testis. Methods: The different kinds of spenmatogenic cells were separated using density gradient centrifugation and their apoptosis was measured by flow cytometry. At meantime, p53 mRNA and protein were measured with immunohistochemical SABC and in situ hybridization, respectively. Results: The apoptosis in all kinds of spenmatogenic cells induced by LDR had a remarkable regularity. When the doses were 0.025 and 0.05 Gy, spermatogone apoptosis was dominant. With the increase in irradiation dose (0.075 – 0.2 Gy), spermatocytes also showed an apoptotic change, but the apoptotic percentage of spermatogonia was significantly higher than that of spermatocytes. Moreover, the apoptosis of spermatids and spermatozoa scarely occurred after LDR. p53 protein expression in spematogonia and spermatocytes in varying degrees, and the former was significantly higher than that of the latter after LDR. With the increase in irradiation doses, p53 protein expression showed a upregulated tendency, but that of spermatids and spermatozoa scarcely occurred. p53 mRNA primarily expressed in spermatids and spermatocytes when the dose was 0.025 Gy. With the increase in irradiation doses (0.05 – 0.2 Gy), that of spermatogonia also showed an enhancement. p53 mRNA expression in spermatogonia and spermatocytes showed a remarkable dose-effect relationship. Conclusion: The apoptosis of spermatogenic cells was selectively induced by LDR of X-rays, which had remarkable dose- and time-effect relationships. The mechanism of the selective apoptosis in spermatogenic cells by LDR is closely related to the upregulation of p53.

55. Liu GW, Dong LH, Liu Y, Lv Z, Liu SC, Gong SL. Adaptive response of spermatogenic cell apoptosis selectively induced by low dose X-ray irradiation in mice. Chin J Radiol Med Protect, 2003, 23 (6): 405-408. [Abstract] Objective: The adaptive response of spermatogenic cell apoptosis induced by whole-body X-ray irradiation at low doses was studied in mice. Methods: Kunming male mice were

irradiated with an inducitive dose (D1: 75 mGy) and/or a challengine dose (D2: 1.0, 2.0 or 3.0 Gy). Different kinds of spermatogenic cells were separated using density gradient centrifugation and their apoptotic percentages were analysed using flow cytometry (FCM). Results: When the mice were irradiated with D1 6 h before irraditation with D2, the apoptotic percentages of the spermatogonia and spermatocytes declined rapidly as compared with those in the groups irradiated with D2 only, and those of spermatids and spermatozoa showed no significant changes. When the interval times between D1 and D2 was 3, 6, 12 or 24 h, the apoptotic percentages in spermatogonia and spermatocytes reduced early, significantly and continued for a longer duration after smaller D2 (1.0 and 2.0 Gy) irradiation, while the apoptotic percentages did not change after larger D2 (3.0 Gy) irradiation. Conclusion: The adaptive response of apoptosis in spermatogonia and spermatocytes could be selectively induced by low dose X-ray irradiation. The adaptive response could be closely related to the D2 dose and interval time between D1 and D2.

56. Liu GW, Liu SC, Lv Z, Gong SL. Effect of low dose X-ray irradiation on apoptosis in spermatogenic cells of mouse testes. J Radiat Res Radiat Process, 2003, 21 (2): 148-153. [Abstract] To study the effects of low dose radiation (LDR) with different doses of X-rays on the apoptosis in spermatogenic cells of male Kunming mouse testes. The time- and dose-effects of apoptosis in the different stages of spermatogenic cell cycles of mouse testis after LDR with different doses of X-rays were studied with light microscope using the methods of TdT-mediated dUTP nick end labeling (TUNEL) and HE staining. The apoptosis of spermatogenic cells induced LDR had a remarkable regularity in cell types. When the dose was 0.025 Gy, spermatogonium apoptosis was taken as main. With the dose increase of irradiation (0.025 - 0.2 Gy), spermatocytes also showed an apoptotic change, but the apoptotic rate of spermatogonia was significantly higher than that of spermatocytes. Moreover, the apoptosis of spermatids and spermatozoa scarcely occurred after irradiation with low dose. The apoptosis of spermatogenic cells induced by LDR has a regular change, which provides a further experimental evidence for the mechanism study of hormesis by LDR.

57. Gong SL, Lv Z, Liu SC, Liu Y, Wang ZQ, Liu GW, Liu SZ. Adaptive response of thymocyte cycle progression induced by low dose ionizing radiation in mice. Chin J Radiol Med Protect, 2003, 23 (6): 413-415. [Abstract] Objective: The dose-, dose rate- and time-effect of adaptive response of thymocyte cycle progression induced by low dose radiation were observed. Methods: Kunming mice were irradiated with inductive doses (doses of D1 were 25, 50, 100 and 200 mGy, dose rate was 12.5 mGy/min; dose of D1 was 75 mGy, dose rates were 6.25, 12.5, 25, 50, 100 and 200 mGy/min) and challenging doses (doses of D2 were 1.0, 1.5 and 2.0 Gy, dose rate was 287 mGy/min), the intervals between D1 and D2 were 3, 6, 12, 24 and 60 h. The thymocyte apoptosis was measured with flow cytometry and the DNA fragmentation was measured fluorospectrophotometry. Results: When the doses of D1 were 25, 50 and 100 mGy and the dose rate was 12.5 mGy/min (the interval between D1 and D2 was 6 h) , or the dose of D1 was 75 mGy and the dose rates were 6.25, 12.5 and 25 mGy/min (the intervals between D1 and D2 were 3, 6 and 12 h), and the doses of D2 were 1.0, 1.5 and 2.0 Gy, the D2/sham-irradiation ratio of G0/G1 and G2 + M phase thymocytes increased significantly ($P < 0.05$ or $P < 0.01$), while that of S phase thymocytes decreased significantly ($P < 0.05$ or $P < 0.01$) however the (D1 + D2)/D2 ratio in G0/G1 and G2 + M phase thymocytes decreased in varying degrees while that in S phase thymocytes increased significantly ($P < 0.05$ or $P < 0.01$). Conclusion : The results suggest that when the mice were irradiated with 25~100 mGy (dose rates: 6.25~25 mGy/min) 3 ~12 h before 1.0~2.0 Gy (dose rate: 287 mGy/min) exposure, the adaptive response of thymocyte cycle progression could be induced under the condition of whole-body irradiation.

58. Tian M, Jin GH, Piao CJ, Liu LL Li XY. Study on construction of pEgr-hPTEN expression vector and its anti-tumor effect induced by irradiation in vitro. Chin J Radiol Med Prot 2003 23 6 423-426. [Abstract] Objective: To clone the cDNA of human tumor suppressor gene PTEN and construct pEgr-hPTEN expression vector as well as study its inhibitory effect on proliferation of malignant glioma cell line SHG44 with stable transfection of pEgr-hPTEN after different doses of X-ray irradiation. Methods: A DNA fragment about 1 200 bp, PTEN was amplified from human placenta tissue by using RT-nested PCR and was cloned into pUCm-T vector after automatic sequencing, then the fragment was inserted into a vector pcDNA3.1-Egr to construct an expression vector pEgr-hPTEN. pEgr-hPTEN was transfected into SHG44 cells in vitro. Stably transfected cell line SHG44-sPTEN was selected through G418. The inhibitory effect on SHG44-sPTEN was observed after different doses of X-ray irradiation in vitro. Results: The PTEN cDNA was cloned correctly and its expression vector pEgr-hPTEN was constructed. Growth of SHG44 cells was inhibited significantly by stable pEgr-hPTEN transfection combined with X-ray irradiation. With the increase of dose, the inhibitory effect was enhanced within 5 Gy. Conclusion: Human tumor suppressor gene-PTEN cDNA was cloned and its expression vector was constructed. Tumor growth was inhibited significantly by

gene-radio-therapy in vitro. The result provides theoretical and experimental basis for improvement of clinical radiotherapeutic effect on tumors.

YEAR 2004

59. Liu SZ. Radiation-induced changes in lymphocyte proliferation and its neuroendocrine regulation; dose-response relationship and pathophysiological implications. Nonlinearity Biol Toxicol Med 2004, 2: 133-243 [Abstract] Cellular activities are regulated by intracellular signals initiated by stimulation from the external and internal environments. Different signal pathways are involved in the initiation of different eellular functions. In connection with cell proliferation in response to mitogenic stimulation, the dose-effect relationship of the magnitude of 3H-TdR incorporation into lymphocytes after exposure to different concentrations of concanavalin A (Con A) showed an inverted U-shaped curve in the concentration range 2-30 ìg/ml. In previous studies it has been observed that the stimulatory effect of Con A (5 ìg/ml) on lymphocyte proliferation was potentiated by whole-body irradiation (WBI) with low dose (0.075 Gy) and suppressed by WBI with high dose (2 Gy). When different concentrations of corticosterone, ranging from I0-12 to 10-7 M, were added to the Con A-stimulated lymphocytes, low-concentration stimulation and high-concentration suppression of lymphocyte proliferation were demonstrated. In the presence of 5×10-12 M (subphysiological concentration) of corticosterone the proliferation of thymocytes and splenic T cells in response to Con A was further up-regulated after low-dose radiation. Low-dose radiation (0.075 Gy) caused lowering of serum ACTH and corticosterone concentration as well as down-regulated transcription of the hypothalamic proopiomelanocortin gene. The present paper intends to show that multiple neurohormonal factors, including the pineal gland and neurotrausmitters, in addition to the hypothalamic-pituitary-adrenocortical axis, are involved in the stimulation of immune responses indueed by low-dose ionizing radiation. The complex nature of the interrelationship between the intracellular signaling of lymphocytes and the neuroendocrine regulation after WBI is discussed.

60. Liu SZ, Jin SZ, Liu XD. Radiation-induced Bystander Effect in Immune Response. Biol Environ Sci 2004 17: 40-46 [Abstract] Objective: Since most reports on bystander effect have been only concerned with radiation-induced damage, the present paper aimed at disclosing whether low dose radiation could induce a stimulatory or beneficial bystander effect. Methods A co-culture system containing irradiated antigen presenting cells (J774A.1) and non-irradiated T lymphocytes (EL-4) was established to observe the effect of J774A.1 cells exposed to both low and high doses of X-rays on the unirradiated EL-4 cells. Incorporation of 3H-TdR was used to assess the proliferation of the EL-4 cells. Expression of CD80/86 and CD48 on J774A.1 cells was measured with immunohistochemistry and flow cytometry, respectively. No release from J774A.1 ceils was estimated with nitrate reduction method. Results Low dose-irradiated J774A.1 cells could stimulate the proliferation of the unirradiated EL-4 cells while the high dose-irradiated J774A.1 cells exerted an inhibitory effect on the proliferation of the non-irradiated EL-4 ceils. Preliminary mechanistic studies illustrated that the differential changes in CD48 expression and NO production by the irradiated J774A.1 cells after high and low dose radiation might be important factors underlying the differential bystander effect elicited by different doses of radiation. Conclusion Stimulatory bystander effect can be induced in immune cells by low dose radiation.

61. Wang XM, Ju GZ, Mei SJ, Fu SB and Liu SZ. Changes in expressions of p16, Cyclin D, CDK4 in splenocytes after 2Gy X-irradiation in mice. Chin J Radiol Health. 2004, 13(1):10-12. [Abstract] Objective: To study the effect of ionizing radiation on gene transcription and protein expression of p16, Cyclin D and CDK4 in splenocytes in mice. Methods Northern blot was employed to determine p16 and CDK4 mRNA level. RT-PCR method was employed to check Cyclin D mRNA level. Flow cytometry was used to measure their protein expression. Results p16 mRNA level in splenocytes was markedly increased at 2~8 h, and p16 protein expression was significantly elevated at 24 h ($P<0.05$). Cyclin D mRNA level and protein expression showed little reduction after irradiation. CDK4 mRNA level began to decrease from 2 h and was reduced to 55.9% of normal level at 72 h. CDK4 protein level was also dramatically reduced at 8~72 h ($P<0.05$~$P<0.01$). Conclusion Ionizing radiation induces increase of p16 and reduction of CDK4 gene transcription and protein expression in splenocytes in mice.

62. Wang XM, Ju GZ, Mei SJ, Fu SB and Liu SZ. p16 gene transcription and protein expression in EL-4 cells irradiated with X-rays in vitro. J Radiat Res Radiat Proc. 2004, 22(2):123-125. [Abstract] To investigate the effect of ionizing radiation on p16 gene transcription and protein expression in EL-4 cells in vitro, RT-PCR semi-quantitative method was used to determine the p16 mRNA level and immunocytochemistry (ICC) was employed to measure the p16 protein expression. The time-course

experiments showed that the p16 mRNA level increased at 2-48 h and the p16 protein expression increased significantly at 12 h (P<0.01) in EL-4 cells after 2.0 Gy X-irradiation. The dose-effect experiments showed that the p16 mRNA level increased with the increase of dose, and the p16 protein expression increased significantly (P<0.01) with doses of 2.0-6.0 Gy. The results suggested that the increase of p16 gene transcription and protein expression in EL-4 cells might play a role in G1 arrest induced by ionizing radiation in vitro.

63. Yang Y, Liu SZ, Fu SB. Anti-tumor Effects of pNEgr-mIL-12 Recombinant Plasmid Induced by X-irradiation and Its Mechanisms. Biomed Environ Sci 2004 17(2): 135-143 [Abstract] The present paper aims at the effect of gene radiotherapy applying intratumor injection of recombinant plasmid pNEgr-mIL-12 followed by local X-irradiation on cancer growth and the elucidation of the mechanisms of tumor inhibition. Alkaline lysis was used to extract the plasmid and polyethylene glycol 8000 (PEG 8000) was used to further purify the plasmid. Enzyme-linked immunoadsorbent assay (ELISA) was used to detect the expression of IL-12 protein. C57BL/6J mice were subcutaneously inoculated with B16 melanoma cells and the plasmid was injected directly into the tumor. Changes in immunologic parameters of tumor-bearing mice were detected with relevant immunologic assays. Gene-radiotherapy with pNEgr-mIL-12 recombinant plasmid and X-irradiation was given three times to C57BL/6J mice bearing B16 melanoma and the results showed significant decrease in tumor growth rate (P<0.05-0.001). Immunologic studies showed significant increase in CTL and NK cytolytic activity (P<0.05-0.001) and up-regulated secretion of IFN-g and TNF-a (P<0.01-0.001). Moreover, the expression of mIL-12 in B16 melanoma cells of the treated tumor-bearing mice was found to be higher than that of control. The results demonstrated that pNEgr-mIL-12 combined with X-irradiation could increase tumor control and the mechanism of increased tumor inhibition was related to the enhancement of anticancer immunity in tumor-bearing mice.

64. Wang XM, Ju GZ, Fu HQ, Mei SJ and Liu SZ. Changes in mRNA levels of cyclin B1 and cdc2 of EL-4 cells after 4Gy X-ray irradiation. J Radiat Res Radiat Proc. 2004, 22(1):43-46. [Abstract] To explore the molecular mechanism of G2 arrest in EL-4 cells induced by X-irradiation, flow cytometry (FCM) and semi-quantitative RT-PCR methods were used to observe the time-course changes in cell cycle and the mRNA levels of cyclin B1 and cdc2 of EL-4 cells after 4Gy X-rays irradiation. Results showed that the cells in G2/M phase increased at 2 h and reached the maximum at 4-8 h after irradiation (P<0.001). The cyclin B1 mRNA level of El-4 cells began to decrease at 1 h, reaching the minimum at 24 h after irradiation. Meanwhile, the cdc2 mRNA level also declined at 12 h to 48 h, reducing to 59.2% and 58.9%, respectively, as compared with that of the control group, and recovered at 72 h after irradiation. The results suggest that reduction of MPF (M phase promoting factor) activity resulting from inhibition of cdc2 and cyclin B plays a critical role in G2 arrest induced by X-ray irradiation in EL-4 cells.

65. Tian M, Piao CJ, Li XY. Effect of stable transfectopn of pEgr-hPTEN on the cell cycle progression and proliferation of SHG44 human glioma cells. Chin J Lab Diagn, 2004, 8(1):1~3. [Abstract] Objective: To investigate the effect of exogenous wild type PTEN gene transfer on the cell cycle progression and proliferation of SHG44 human glioma cells and explore the mechanism of the inhibitory effect of PTEN gene on the proliferation of tumor cells. Methods: pEgr-hPTEN recombinant plasmids were packed with liposome to transfect glioma cell line SHG44 which contains the endogenous mutant PTEN gene. The cells with stable expression of pEgr-hPTEN were selected with G418. The proliferation of tumor cells were examined by cell counting and the changes of cell cycle progression were observed by flow cytometry with FACscan. Results: After selection with G418 for 10 to 20 days, stably expressing cells were obtained. Growth of SHG44 was inhibited significantly by stable transfection with pEgr-hPTEN in vitro. The progression of cell cycle was found to be arrested from G1 to S phase. Conclusion: The cell cycle of SHG44 glioma cells is arrested at G1 phase by exogenous PTEN gene transfer to inhibit their proliferation.

66. Li XJ, Li ZG, Tian M, Yang W, Liu LL, Li XY. Construction of pEgr-ssEndostatin and in vitro expression of mouse endostatin induced by ionizing radiation. J Radiat Res Radiat Proc, 2004, 22(1):35-38. [ABSTRACT] Objective: To study the regularity of mouse endostatin expression in B16 cells transfected by pEgr−ssEndostatin after different doses of X-ray irradiation and different time after the irradiation. Methods: Mouse endostatin cDNA was amplified by RT−PCR and signal peptide was ligated to it. The pEgr−ssEndostatin recombinant plasmid was constructed and transfected into B16 cells with liposome and cells were irradiated. The expression of endostatin in the supernatant medium of B16 cells was detected by ELISA. Results: The results showed that the cDNA sequence of mouse secretable endostatin is identical with that reported in literature. Egr−1 promoter and secretable endostatin cDNA were inserted into expression vectors correctly. pEgr−ssEndostatin had the expression property induced by radiation. Conclusion: It suggests that the Egr−1 promoter can be activated by ionizing irradiation and expression of

downstream gene can be regulated.

67. Wu CM, Li XY. Construction of pEgr-TNF plasmid and experimental study on the effect of gene-radiotherapy on mouse melanoma Chin J Oncol , 2004,26(3):143~145. [Abstract] Objective: The pEgr-TNFá plasmid was constructed to investigate the effect of gene-radiotherapy on melanoma and host immune system. Methods: pEgr-TNFá plasmids was constructed and injected into tumor tissue, 36 hours later, the tumors were given 20 Gy X-ray irradiation. Tumor growth at different time points was recorded and immunologic parameters were detected 15 days later. Results: From 3 to 15 d after pEgr-TNFá gene-radiotherapy the tumor growth was significantly slower than irradiation or genetherapy alone. NK activity, IL-2, TNFá and IL-1â secretion activities of pEgr-TNFá gene-radiotherapy group and pEgr-TNFá gene group were significantly higher than those of irradiation alone group. Conclusion: The anti-tumor effect of pEgr-TNFá gene-radiotherapy is better than that of either one applied solely, and it can alleviate the lesion caused by radiation therapy.

68. Liu LL, Yang W, Wu CM, Tian M, Piao CJ, Li XY. Cloning and sequencing of mouse IFNã and construction of radiation- inducible expression plasmid pIRESEgr-IFNã J Jilin Univ (Medicine Edition) 2004,30(2):166-68. [Abstract] Objective: To clone the sequence of the cDNA of mouse interferon-gamma coding area and construct radiation-inducible expression plasmid pIRESEgr-IFN Ccontaining Egr-1 p romoter. Methods: With the technique of RT-PCR, mouse splenocyte mRNA was used as template to obtain full length mouse IFNC. The pGEMT-IFNC was sequenced automatically and radiation-inducible expression plasmid pIRESEgr-IFN C containing Egr-1 promoter was constructed with gene recombinant technique. Results: The sequencing p roved the cloned mouse IFNCcDNA to be completely identical with that reported in the literature and the radiation-inducible exp ression plasmid pIRESEgr-IFNC containing Egr-1 p romoter was constructed successfully. Conclusion: Mouse IFNC cDNA was cloned and the radiation-inducible expression plasmid pIRESEgr-IFNC containing Egr-1 promoter was constructed successfully.

69. Wu CM Li XY Huang TH. Anti-tumor effect of pEgr-IFNã gene-radiotherapy in B16 melanoma-bearing mice. World J Gastroenterol, 2004,10(20):3011-3015. [Abstract] AIM: To construct a pEgr-IFNã ?plasmid and to investigate its expression properties of interferon-ã (INF-ã) induced by irradiation and the effect of gene-radiotherapy on the growth of melanoma. Methods: A recombined plasmid, pEgr-IFNã, was constructed and transfected into B16 cell line with lipofectamine. The expression properties of pEgr-IFNã ?were investigated by ELISA. Then, a B16 melanoma-bearing model was established in mice, and the plasmid was injected into the tumor tissue. The tumor received 20 GyX-ray irradiation 36 h after injection, and IFN-ã ?expression was detected from the tumor tissue. A tumor growth curve at different time points was determined. Results: The eukaryotic expression vector, pEgr-IFNã was successfully constructed and transfected into B16 cells. IFN-ã expression was significantly increased in transfected cells after X-ray irradiation in comparison with 0 Gy group (77.73-94.60 pg/mL, P<0.05-0.001), and was significantly higher at 4 h and 6 h than that of control group after 2 Gy X-ray irradiation (78.90-90.00 pg/mL, P<0.01-0.001). When the transfected cells were given 2 Gy irradiation 5 times at an interval of 24 h, IFN-ã ?expression decreased in a time-dependent manner. From d 3 to d 15 after IFNã ?gener-adiotherapy, the tumor growth was significantly slower than that after irradiation or gene therapy alone. Conclusion: The anti-tumor effect of pEgr-IFNã ?gene-radiotherapyis was better than that of genetherapy or radiotherapy alone for melanoma. These results may establish an important experimental basis for gene-radiotherapy of cancer.

70. Yang W, Liu LL, Sun T, Li XJ, Tian M, Piao CJ, Pan Y, Li XY. Cloning and sequencing of mouse endostatin and construction of recombinant plasmid pEgr- IFNã-mEndostatin. J Jilin Univ (M edicine Edit ion) 2004, 30(1):17-19. [Abstract] Objective: To clone the sequence of the cDNA of mouse endostatin (mEndostatin) coding area and construct an expression vector containing Egr-1 promoter, IFNã and endostatin genes. Methods: Full length mEndostatin was obtained with the technique of RT -PCR and using mouse hepatocyte mRNA as template, pMD18T-mEndostatin was sequenced automatically and an expression vector containing Egr-1 promoter, IFNã, and endostatin genes was cons ructed with gene recombinant technique. Results: It was proved that the cloned mEndostatin cDNA to be completely identical with that reported in the literature and the recombinant plasmid containing Egr-1 promoter, IFNã, and endostatin genes was constructed successfully. Conclusion: mEndostatin cDNA was cloned and the expression vector pEgr-IFNã-mEndostatin was constructed successfully.

71. Zhang X, Gong SL, Wang ZQ, Lu Z, Liu Y, Zhang M, Liu SZ. Effect of melatonin on apoptosis of lymphocytes in mice induced by ionizing radiation. Chin J Pathophysiol 2004, 20: 1702-1705 [Abstract] AIM: To explore the effect of melatonin (MLT) on the apoptosis of thymocytes and splenocytes in mice induced by ionizing radiation and its mechanism. Methods: The percentages of apoptotic bodies and the DNA fragmentation rates of thymocytes and splenocytes in mice in vitro and in vivo were detected with

flow cytometry and fluorospectrophotometry, respectively. Results: The apoptosis of mouse thymocytes and splenocytes in vitro increased dose-dependently after 0.5~6.0 Gy X-irradiation. When MLT of 2 mmol·L-1 was added to thymocytes or splenocytes in vitro before irradiation with 0.5~6.0 Gy X-rays, the percentages of apoptotic bodies and the DNA fragmentation rates all decreased significantly as compared with those in the group with irradiation only. The percentages of apoptotic bodies in these two kinds of cells were 86.25% and 89.22% of those in the irradiation group, respectively, and the DNA l fragmentation rates were 87.23% and 89.16%, respectively. When MLT was injected into intraperitonium in mice 60 min before whole-body irradiation with 2 Gy X-rays, the percentages of apoptotic bodies and the DNA fragmentation rates were significantly lower than those in the group with irradiation only, and near to or lower than those in the sham-irradiation group. MLT of 0.1~2.5 mg/kg decreased the lymphocyte apoptosis, but without significant dose-dependence. Conclusion: The protective effects of MLT on mouse lymphoctes damaged by irradiation in vivo are more obvious than those in vitro.

72. Yang JZ, Jin GH, Tian M, Pan XN, Jin SZ, Liu SZ Cloning and sequencing of mouse B7.2 gene and construction of its recombinant plasmids. J Jilin Univ (Med Ed) 2004, 30(3): 333-335 [Abstract] Objective: To clone the sequence of the cDNA of mouse B7.2 gene and construct its expression vectors. Methods: Using mouse splenocyte mRNA as template to obtain full length B7.2 with the technique of RT-PCR followed by automatic sequencing of pMD18T2B7.2 and to construct recombinant plasmids containing CMV, Egr-1 and B7.2 genes with recombinant DNA technique. Results: Sequencing proved the cloned B7.2 cDNA to be essentially identical with that reported in the literature and the recombinant plasmids containing CMV, Egr-1 and B7.2 genes were constructed successfully. Conclusion: B7.2 cDNA was successfully cloned and two expression vectors pcDNA3.-CMV-B7.2 and pcDNA3.1-Egr-B7.2 were constructed.

73. Ju GZ, Fu SB , Yan FQ. Experimental study on cell cycle uncoupling induced by ionizing radiation.Chin J Radiol Med Radiol Prot. 2004, 24: 295-296. [Abstract] Objective: To investigate whether or not cell cycle uncoupling could be induced by ionizing radiation. Methods Cell cycle was analyzed by flow cytometry (FCM) following staining of cells with propidium iodide (PI) and polyploid cells were analyzed. Results It was found that 24 h after exposure with X-rays to SKOV-3 cells with the doses of 1.0, 2.0, 4.0 or 6.0 Gy, the 2N cells were decreased significantly ($P<0.01$), whereas 4N cells were increased significantly ($P<0.01$) and 8N cells were also increased significantly ($P<0.01$). Conclusion The results suggest that cell cycle uncoupling could be induced by ionizing radiation.

74. Fan C, Zhang JJ, Li XL, Xu L, Chen WH, Ju GZ. Effect of ionizing radiation on MT-1 mRNA expression of mouse tissues. Chin J Radiol Med Prot. 2004, 24(6):525-526 [Abstract] Objective: To investigate the effect of whole body X-irradiation (WBI) on metallothionein-(MT-1) gene transcription level in mouse tissues and its dose-effect relationship. Methods MT-1 mRNA level in mouse liver, brain, thymus and spleen were measured using Northern blot assay. Results Time-course experiment showed that MT-1 mRNA levels in mouse liver and thymus gradually increased and reached its peak at 4 h after WBI, then recovered to normal level at 24 h. MT-1 mRNA levels in mouse liver and thymus increased with the increase of irradiation dose at 4 h after 0·5~6 Gy X-rays WBI. But there was no obvious change of MT-1 mRNA levels in mouse brain and spleen. Conclusion MT-1 mRNA levels in mouse liver and thymus significantly increased after WBI and showed a dose-dependent trend. But there was no obvious change in MT-1 mRNA levels in mouse brain and spleen. These results indicate that the increase of MT-1 mRNA in mouse tissue after WBI is tissue-specific, and MT protein synthesis is regulated through MT-1 gene transcriptional elevation.

75. Lv Z, Liu Y, Wang ZQ, Ma SM, Liu GW, Sun YH, Gong SL. p53, Bcl-2 and Bax protein expression of apoptosis-associated gene in adaptive response of thymocyte apoptosis in mice induced by low dose radiation. J Jilin Univ (Med Ed), 2004, 30 (6): 850-852. [Abstract] Objective: To explore the regulative mechanism of apoptosis-associated gene proteins on the adaptive response of thymocyte apoptosis in mice induced by low dose radiation. Methods: Kunming male mice were irradiated with the inductive doses (D1: 25, 50, 75, 100 and 200 mGy; dose rate: 12.5 mGy · min–1) and the challenging dose (D2: 1.5 Gy; dose rate: 287 mGy · min–1). The time interval between D1 and D2 was 6 h. The expressive levels of thymocyte apoptosis-associated gene proteins were measured with flow cytometry. Results: As compared with the sham-irradiation, the positive percentage of thymocyte Bcl-2 protein expression decreased significantly in D2 group ($P < 0.05$), Bax increased significantly ($P < 0.05$), and Bcl-2/Bax decreased significantly ($P < 0.001$); p53 increased significantly ($P < 0.001$). As compared with D2 group, the positive percentage of thymocyte Bcl-2 protein expression increased in varying degree in D1 + D2 group of 25 – 75 mGy D1, Bax decreased in varying degree, and Bcl-2/Bax increased significantly ($P < 0.01$); p53 decreased significantly ($P < 0.001$).

Conclusion: The apoptotic thymocytes in the adaptive response of thymocyte apoptosis in mice induced by irradiation with 25 – 75 mGy decrease significantly due to the increase of apoptosis-associated gene Bcl-2 protein expression and Bcl-2/Bax, the decrease of Bax and p53 protein expressions.

76. Gong SL, Lv Zhe, Liu SC, Wang ZQ, Liu Y, Liu GW, Liu SL Adaptive response of thymocyte cycle progression induced by low dose ionizing radiation in mice. J Radiat Res Radiat Process, 2004, 22 (3): 176-180. [Abstract] Objective: The dose-, dose rate- and time-effect of adaptive response of thymocyte cycle progression induced by low dose radiation were observed. Methods: Kunming mice were irradiated with inductive doses (doses of D1 were 25, 50, 100 and 200 mGy, dose rate was 12.5 mGy/min; dose of D1 was 75 mGy, dose rates were 6.25, 12.5, 25, 50, 100 and 200 mGy/min) and challenging doses (doses of D2 were 1.0, 1.5 and 2.0 Gy, dose rate was 287 mGy/min), the intervals between D1 and D2 were 3, 6, 12, 24 and 60 h. The tymocyte apoptosis was measured with flow cytometer and the DNA fragmentation was measured fluorospectrophotometry. Results: When the doses of D1 were 25, 50 and 100 mGy and the dose rate was 12.5 mGy/min (the interval between D1 and D2 was 6 h) , or the dose of D1 was 75 mGy and the dose rates were 6.25, 12.5 and 25 mGy/min (the intervals between D1 and D2 were 3, 6 and 12 h), and the doses of D2 were 1.0, 1.5 and 2.0 Gy, the D2/sham-irradiation ratio in G0/G1 and G2 + M phase thymocytes increased significantly ($P<0.05$ or $P<0.01$), while that in S phase thymocytes decreased significantly ($P < 0.05$ or $P < 0.01$) however the D1 + D2/D2 ratio in G0/G1 and G2 + M phase thymocytes decreased in varying degrees while that in S phase thymocytes increased significantly ($P < 0.05$ or $P < 0.01$). Conclusion: The results suggest that the mice were irradiated with 25 – 100 mGy (dose rates: 6.25 – 25 mGy/min) 3 – 12 h before 1.0 – 2.0 Gy (dose rate: 287 mGy/min) exposure, the adaptive response of thymocyte cycle progression could be induced under the condition of whole-body irradiation.

77. Liu GW, Dong LH, Wang ZQ, Piao CN, Zhao HG, Zhou LF, Gong SL Effect of low dose radiation on p53 and Bcl-2 protein expression in spermatogenic cells of mouse testis. J Jilin Univ (Med Ed), 2004, 30 (1): 85-88. [Abstract] Objective: To investigate the effect of low dose radiation (LDR) with different doses of X-rays on p53 and Bcl-2 protein expression in spermatogenic cells of male Kunming mouse testis. Methods: The relationships between time- and dose-effects of p53 and Bcl-2 protein expression positive rates in spermatogenic cells of mouse testis after LDR with different doses of X-rays were studied with immunohistochemical technique (SABC). Results: p53 and Bcl-2 proteins expressed in spermatogonia and spermatocytes in varying degrees, the positive rate of spermatogonia was obviously superior to that of spermatocytes. With the increase of irradiation dose, the expression of p53 protein showed a increasing tendency, however, the p53 protein expression of spermatozoa scarcely occurred after LDR. Bcl-2 protein was primarily expressed in spermatozoa. With the increase of irradiation doses, the positive rate of Bcl-2 protein expression showed a downregulated tendency. However, the Bcl-2 protein expression of spermatogonia and spermatocytes scarely occurred after LDR. Conclusion : The expressions of p53 and Bcl-2 may have regular changes in mouse testis induced by LDR, which may provide a experimental evidence for the mechansis study of spermatogonic cell apoptosis induced selectively by ionizing radiation.

78. Dong LH, Liu GW, Piao CN, Lv WT, Zhao HG, Jia XJ, Zhao Y, Zhao SL Effect of signal factors on lymphocyte apoptosis in mouse thymus induced by ionizing radiation in vitro. Chin J Radiol Med Protect, 2004, 24 (5): 399-402. [Abstract] Objective: To observe the effects of corticosterone (CS), cAMP, cGMP, Ca2+ and protein kinas C (PKC) signal factors on lymphocyte apoptosis in mouse thymus induced by ionizing radiation with X-rays of 4 Gy in vitro. Method: The DNA lytic rate of lymphocytes in thymus was measured with fluorospectrophotometry. Results: The DNA lytic rates of lymphocytes in thymus 4 – 8 h after irradiation with 2 – 8 Gy were significantly higher than that in the control. As compared with the control, the DNA lytic rates of lymphocytes in 0.01 mol/L CS ($P < 0.01$), 50 ng/ml cAMP ($P < 0.01$), 0.05 – 0.4 g/ml ionomycin (Iono, $P < 0.05$ or $P < 0.01$) and 0.05 – 0.4 ng/ml phorbol myristate acetate (PMA, $P < 0.05$ or $P < 0.01$) groups, respectively, all increased significantly, while the rate in 50 ng/ml cGMP did not significantly. The DNA lytic rates of lymphocytes in 0.01 mol/L CS ($P < 0.01$), 50 ng/ml cAMP ($P < 0.01$), 0.2 and 0.4 ìg/ml Iono ($P < 0.05$) and 0.2 and 0.4 ng/ml PMA ($P < 0.05$) plus 4 Gy-irradiation groups, respectively, were significantly higher than that in simple 4 Gy-irradiation group, while that in 50 ng/ml cGMP plus 4 Gy-irradiation group was not. As both Iono and PMA were combined to act to the lymphocytes, the DNA lytic rate of only in 0.4 ìg/ml Iono and 0.4 ng/ml PMA group was significantly higher than that in the control $P < 0.01$ the rate in 0.4 ìg/ml Iono and 0.4 ng/ml PMA plus 4 Gy-irradiation group was significantly higher than that in the simple 4 Gy-irradiation group ($P < 0.05$), but was not significantly than that in the 0.4 ìg/ml Iono plus 4 Gy-irradiation group or 0.4 ng/ml PMA plus 4 Gy-irradiation group. Conclusion: There are the promoting effect of CS, cAMP, Ca2+ and PKC signal factors in some dose ranges on lymphocyte apoptosis in mouse thymus induced by ionizing radiation with larger dose X-rays.

YEAR 2005

79. Liu SZ. Research in Radiation Immunology: Present Status and Prospects. Chin J Radiol Med Radiol Protec 2005, 25: 193=200 [Abstract] In this paper the following topics are reviewed: 1. Response of innate and adaptive immunity to radiation; 2. Reaction of thymocytes to radiation; 3. Reaction of splenocytes to radiation; 4. Radiation effect of expression of surface molecules on immune cells and its influence on intercellular reactions; 5. Studies of molecular mechanisms of immunologic effects induced by radiation; 6. The dose-effect relationship of the reaction of immune cells to radiation; 7. The neuroendocrine regulation of radiation immune effects. 8. A final section on future studies in the field of radiation immunology was briefly outlined.

80. Zhang X, Gong SL, Zhang M, Liu SZ Protective effect of melatonin damage of splenocytes in mice. Radiat Protec 2005, 25: 31-35. [Abstract] The aim of the present paper is to explore the effect of melatonin (MLT) on the damage of mouse splenocytes induced by whole-body irradiation (WBI) and its mechanism. MLT was administered to Kunming mice by peritoneal injection 60 min before WBI with 1.0~4.0 Gy X-rays. For consecutive administration of MLT, changes in splenocyte number were observed 24 h after WBI; for single administration of MLT, apoptotic body percentage (ABP) and cell percentages of cell cycle phases in splenocytes were determined with flow cytometry, and DNA fragmentation rate (DFR) was assayed by fluorescence spectrophotometry. The number of splenocytes increased significantly after consecutive daily administration of MLT for 1 week, in 0.1 mg•kg-1 (BW) group (P<0.01). The number of splenocytes 24 h after irradiation with 1~4 Gy decreased in a dose-dependent manner (P<0.01). The number of splenocytes increased significantly with daily consecutive administration of MLT (0.1 mg•kg-1 •d-1) for 1 week before WBI (P<0.05). ABP and DFR of splenocytes increased significantly 12 h after WBI with 2 Gy (P<0.01), and the percentages of G0/G1 and G2+M phase splenocytes increased significantly (P<0.05), indicating G1 and G2 arrests. When MLT was administered once before irradiation, ABP and DFR of splenocytes decreased significantly (P<0.05 or P<0.01), G1 arrest was attenuated while G2 arrest became more serious. The administration of MLT to mice before WBI has protective effect on immunity as evidenced by decreased damage of splenocytes after WBI.

81. Jin GH£¬Jin SZ£¬Liu Y£¬Xu RM£¬Yang JZ£¬Pan XN£¬Liu SZ Therapeutic effect of gene therapy in combination with local X-irradiation in a mouse malignant melanoma model. Biochem Biophys Res Commun 2005, 330: 975-981 [Abstract] Plasmid containing mIL-18 and B7.1 genes downstream of Egr-1 promoter was constructed and used in gene radiotherapy on malignant melanoma in C57BL/6J mice implanted with B16 cells followed by exploration of the immunologic mechanism of the therapeutic effect. The treatment with plasmid pEgr-IL-18-B7.1 plus local X-irradiation showed more effective suppression of tumor growth than the treatment with radiation alone, pEgr-IL-18-B7.1 alone, or single gene pEgr-IL-18 (or pEgr-B7.1) combined with local X-irradiation. Anticancer immunity was found to be significantly upregulated in tumor-bearing mice treated with pEgr-IL-18-B7.1 plus local X-irradiation. IL-18 showed no direct killing effect on malignant melanoma cells in vitro and the mechanism of the combined therapy with pEgr-IL-18-B7.1 and local X-irradiation was apparently related with the stimulation of host anticancer immunity by increased secretion of IL-18 and upregulated immunogenecity of the tumor cells by increased expression of B7.1 on their surface in addition to the direct effect of local X-irradiation on the tumor cells.

82. Liu SZ. Nonlinear dose-effect relationship of different parameters in cancer cell lines. Critical Reviews in Toxicology, 35:595–597, 2005 [Abstract] The dose-effect curves of most parameters in cancer cell lines in response to x-irradiation or toxic agents are usually nonlinear. Such a nature is demonstrated in this article with cell lines of the immune system. However, the shape of the nonlinear dose-effect curves was found to be different for lymphocytes (EL-4) and macrophages (J774A.1). The mechanisms and implications are briefly discussed.

83. Yang W, Li XY. Anti-tumor effect of pEgr-IFNã-Endstatin gene-radiotherapy in mice bearing Lewis lung carcinoma and its mechanism. Chin Med J, 2005, (4):296-301. [Abstract] AIM Gene-radiotherapy, the combination of gene therapy and radiation therapy, is a new paradigm for cancer treatment. To enhance anti-tumor effect of gene-radiotherapy, in this study we construct a radiation-inducible dual-gene co-expression vector pEgr-interferon (IFN)-gamma-endostatin and studied the anti-tumor effect of pEgr-IFN-gamma-endostatin gene-radiotherapy in mice bearing Lewis lung carcinoma and its mechanism. Methods: Gene recombinant technique was used to construct dual-gene co-expression plasmid pEgr-IFN-gamma-endostatin, and single-gene expression plasmid pEgr-IFN-gamma and pEgr-endostatin. The plasmids packed by liposome were injected locally into the tumors of the mice, and the tumors were irradiated with 5 Gy X-ray 36 hours later. The tumor growth rate at different time and

mean survival period of the mice were observed. Cytotoxic activity of splenic cytotoxic T-lymphocyte (CTL), natural killer (NK) cell and tumor necrosis factor (TNF)-alpha secretion activity of peritoneal macrophages of the mice in various groups were evaluated 15 days after irradiation. The intratumor micro-vessel density was evaluated by immunohistochemical staining 10 days after irradiation. Results: The tumor growth rate of the mice in dual-gene-radiotherapy group was significantly lower than those in control group, 5 Gy group and single-gene-radiotherapy group at different time after gene-radiotherapy, and the mean survival period of which was longer. Cytotoxic activity of splenic CTL, NK and TNF-alpha secretion activity of peritoneal macrophages of the mice in dual-gene-radiotherapy group were significantly higher than those in control group, 5 Gy X-ray irradiation group and pEgr-endostatin gene-radiotherapy group 15 days after irradiation. The intratumor micro-vessel density of the mice in dual-gene-radiotherapy group was significantly lower than those in control group, 5 Gy X-ray irradiation group and pEgr-IFN-gammagene-radiotherapy group. Conclusion: The anti-tumor effect of dual-gene-radiotherapy was significantly better than that of single-gene-radiotherapy by combining the enhancement of anti-tumor immunologic function induced by IFN-gamma with the anti-angiogenesis function of endostatin.

84. Tian M, Piao CJ, Li XY, Yang W. Study on enhancement of anti-tumor effect of pEgr-hPTEN expression induced by ionizing radiation in vitro. J Jilin Univ (Medicine Edition) 2005 31 3 330-333. [Abstract] Objective: To investigate the effect of pEgr-hPTEN stable transfer combined with irradiation on the proliferation and apoptosis of SHG44 human glioma cells in vitro. Methods: pEgr-hPTEN vector containing the exogenous wild type PTEN gene was transfected into SHG44 cells under mediation of lipofectamine in vitro, positive cell clones were selected and amplified. Western blotting was used to detect the properties of PTEN expression induced by X-ray irradiation. Flow cytometry and cell growth curve were adopted to measure the effects of PTEN gene transfer combined with different doses of X-ray irradiation on cell proliferation and apoptosis of the transfected SHG44 cells. Results: Expression of PTEN protein could be enhanced by X-ray irradiation in SHG44-hPTEN stable transfer cells. Expression of PTEN protein relative level was increased in a dose-dependent manner after irradiation within 5 Gy. pEgr-hPTEN stable transfer combined with X-ray irradiation could significantly inhibit the proliferation and induce apoptosis of SHG44 cells. On the 8th day after irradiation with different doses of X-rays, the numbers of SHG44-hPTEN stable transfer cells were only 30.0% - 50.0% of that of SHG44-hPTEN /0 Gy group and 7.7% - 13.0% of SHG44/0 Gy group. The percentage of early apoptotic cells of SHG44-hPTEN group after irradiation with X- rays were 1.5-2.3 times as much as that of SHG44-hPTEN/ö0 Gy group, 1.9- 4.4 times as much as that of SHG44 irradiated group and 3.4- 5.1 times as much as that of SHG44/0 Gy group. Conclusion: The apoptosis of tumor cells could be significantly enhanced and its growth could be significantly inhibited by gene-radiotherapy with pEgr-hPTEN in vitro.

85. Piao CJ, Tian M, Liu LL, Yang W, Li XY. Construction of pEgr-hTRAIL expression vector induced by irradiation and apoptosis in tumor cells in vitro. J of Jilin Univ (Medicine Edition) 2005,31(2):169-172. [Abstract] Objective: To construct the radiation-inducible expression vector pEgr-hTRAIL containing human TNF related apoptosis inducing ligand (hTRAIL) gene and study its expression and function of inducing apoptosis in A549 human lung adenocarcinoma cells. Methods: Expression vector pEgr-hTRAIL was constructed with DNA recombinant technique. pEgr-hTRAIL plasmids were packaged with lipofectamine to transfect A549 cells in vitro. Stably transfected cell line A 549-shTRAIL was selected through G418. The expression of hTRAIL gene was detected by RT-PCR. The early stage apoptosis of A 549 cells was detected by Annexin-V-FITC apoptosis detecting kit. Results: Expression vector pEgr-hTRAIL was constructed correctly by identification with restriction enzyme digestion. The expression of hTRAIL mRNA in stably transfected cell line A 549-shTRAIL was increased significantly. The percentage of apoptotic A549-shTRAIL cells was increased significantly; being 1.8 times as much as A549 cells (P < 0105). Conclusion: Expression vector pEgr-hTRAIL was constructed successfully, which can increase the apoptosis of the stably transfected cell line A5492shTRAIL significantly.

86. Yang W, Piao CJ, Liu LL, Tian M Pan Y, Li XY. Expression of a recombinant dual-gene co-expressing plasmid pEgr-IFNã-endostatin in Lewis lung cancer cells induced by radiation Chin J Radiol Med Radiool Prot 2005, 25(3):210-212. [Abstract] Objective: To construct a recombinant dual-gene co-expressing plasmid pEgr-IFNã-endostatin and detect its radiation-induced expression in Lewis lung cancer cells. Methods: The recombinant plasmid pEgr-IFNã-endostation containing Egr-1 promoter, IFNã and endostatin genes was constructed with gene recombination technique. The plasmid was transferred into Lewis lung cancer cells by liposome in vitro. The correlation of dose and effects and the time-course patterns of the expressions of IFNã and endostatin genes induced by different doses of X- rays were detected by ELISA. Results: Identification with enzymes proved that Egr-1 promoter , IFNã and endostatin genes were

inserted into the dual-gene co-expressing vector pIRESlneo correctly. After different doses of X-irradiation, the expressions of IFNã and endostatin the supernatant of cultured Lewis lung cancer cells transfected by pEgr- IFNã-endostatin were significantly higher than those in 0 Gy group. After 5 Gy X-irradiation, the expressions of IFNã and endostatin were the highest, being 4.14 and 2.92 times as much as those in 0 Gy group, respectively. The concentrations of IFNã and endostatin in the supernatant increased after 2 Gy X-irradiation, being 3.75 and 3.02 times as much as those in 0 Gy group, respectively, 36 h after irradiation ($P < 0.001$). Conclusion: The dual-gene co-expressing plasmid pEgr-IFNã-endostatin has been constructed successfully, and it has the property of enhancing the co-expression of IFNã and endostatin genes induced by irradiation.

87. Wu CM, Li XY and Tian.M. Effect of pEgr-TNFá gene radiotherapy on mice melanoma. Melanoma Res, 2005, 15:185 – 90. [Abstract] AIM: In the present study, we constructed a pEgr-tumour necrosis factor-alpha (TNFalpha) plasmid and investigated its expression properties in B16 cells on exposure to ionizing irradiation and, furthermore, the effect of gene radiotherapy on a melanoma model. Methods: Firstly, the recombinant pEgr-TNFalpha plasmid was constructed and transfected into B16 cells with liposomes to investigate its expression properties on exposure to X-irradiation. The melanoma-bearing model was then established and the tumour tissue was injected locally with the pEgr-TNFalpha plasmid and exposed to 20 Gy of X-irradiation. The tumour growth curve at different time points was described. At day 3, TNFalpha transcription in the tumour tissue was detected by reverse transcriptase-polymerase chain reaction (RT-PCR). Results: The results showed that: (1) the eukaryotic expression vector pEgr-TNFalpha was successfully constructed and transfected into B16 cells; (2) TNFalpha expression was significantly increased in the transfected cells after X-irradiation, in contrast with that of the pCMV-TNFalpha group or the pEgr-TNFalpha group that received 0 Gy of irradiation; (3) after pEgr-TNFalpha gene radiotherapy, tumour growth was significantly slower than in those groups receiving irradiation or gene transfer alone. The TNFalpha concentration in the peripheral blood of tumour-bearing mice that received an injection of pEgr-TNFalpha and 20 Gy of irradiation was higher than that of the control group. Only in pEgr-TNFalpha and pEgr-TNFalpha + 20 Gy groups was TNFalpha messenger RNA (mRNA) detected in the tumour tissue. Conclusion: We conclude that pEgr-TNFalpha gene radiotherapy may significantly inhibit tumour growth, and that the anti-melanoma effect is superior to that of either gene therapy or radiotherapy alone. Our work provides the theoretical basis for further study on the gene radiotherapy of this tumour.

88. Yang W, Piao CJ, Liu LL, Tian M Lu Z Li XY. Anti-tumor effect of IFNã endostatin gene-radiotherapy in vivo and its mechanism Chin J Radiol Med Prot 2005, 25(4):325-8. [Abstract] Objective: To study the anti-tumor effect of pEgr-IFNã-endostatin gene-radiotherapy in mice bearing Lewis lung carcinoma and its mechanism. Methods: The plasmids packed by liposome were injected locally into the tumors of the mice, and the tumors were irradiated with 5 Gy X-rays 36 hours later. The tumor growth rate at different times and the mean survival period of the mice were observed. Cytotoxic activity of splenic CTL, NK and TNFá secretion activity of peritoneal macrophages of the mice in various groups were evaluated 15 days after irradiation. The intratumor microvessel density was evaluated by immunohistochemical staining 10 days after irradiation. Results: The tumor growth rate of the mice in double-gene-radiotherapy group was significantly lower than that of the control group, 5 Gy X-irradiation alone group and single-gene-radiotherapy group 6-18 days after gene-radiotherapy, and the mean survival period of which was longer. The tumor growth rate in mice treated with pEgr-IFNã-endostatin and 2.5 Gy X-ray irradiation for four times was lower significantly than that in mice treated with pEgr-IFNã-endostatin and 10 Gy X-irradiation for once only 12-18 days after therapy, and the mean survival time of mice was longer. Cytotoxic activity of splenic CTL , NK and TNFá secretion activity of peritoneal macrophages of the mice in the double-gene-radiotherapy group were significantly higher than those in the control group, 5 Gy X-irradiation alone group and pEgr-endostatin gene-radiotherapy group 15 days after irradiation. The intratumor microvessel density of the mice in double-gene-radiotherapy group was significantly lower than that in the control group, 5 Gy X-irradiation alone group and pEgr-IFNã gene-radiotherapy group. Conclusions: The anti-tumor effect of double-gene-radiotherapy is significantly better than that of single-gene-radiotherapy. Its mechanism is perhaps associated with the expressions of IFNã and endostatin induced by X-ray irradiation, which enhance anti-tumor immunologic function and anti-angiogenesis function. The anti-tumor effect of repeated lower dose double-gene-radiotherapy is better than that of higher dose double-gene-radiotherapy for once only.

89. Yan FQ, Wang JQ, Fu SB and Ju GZ. Effects of ionizing radiation on the expression of P21 protein in EL-4 mouse lymphoma cells. Chin J Radiol Med Prot. 2005, 25(6):514-516. [Abstract] Objective: To explore the effects of ionizing radiation on the expression of P21 protein. Methods

Immunocytochemistry and flow cytometry were used to measure the changes in the expression of P21 protein in EL-4 cells along with the increment of time and radiation doses. Results After 4·0 Gy X-rays irradiation, marked elevation of P21 protein level was found to increase in EL-4 cells at 2-72 h with immunocytochemical method and at 8-72 h with flow cytometry (P<0·01 or P<0·001, respectively). On the other hand, it was observed that the level of P21 protein increased evidently after exposure to 0·5-6·0 Gy X-rays by using immunocytochemical method and after exposure to 1·0-4·0 Gy X-rays by using flow cytometry in EL-4 cells at 24 h after irradiation. Conclusion The P21 protein expression could be increased by X-irradiation in time-and dose-dependent manners.

90. Sun ZY, Fu JY, Liu SC, Lv Z, Sun LG, Li XY, Zhao Y, Gong SL Influences of low dose radiation on inhibitory effects of tumor-associated antigen peptide extract of H-22 hepatocarcinoma in mice. J Jilin Univ (Med Ed), 2005, 31 (4): 539-542. [Abstract] Objective: To investigate the influences of low dose radiation (LDR) on the inhibitory effects of tumor-associated antigen peptide (TAP) extract of H-22 hepatocarcinoma in mice. Methods: Mild acid elution method was applied to prepare TAP extract (MW £ 3 000) from tumor cell membrane. The mice were given by whole-body irradiation (WBI) with 75 mGy X-rays 12 h before immunization with TAP extract. After immunization, the cell cycle progression of the thymocytes was detected with flow cytometry, the response of splenocytes to Con A and the percentage of T cell subsets in splenocytes were analyzed. Meantime, the tumor-inhibited effect was observed in vivo. Results: The present experiment showed that the TAP extract reduced the incidence of the transplanted tumor, delayed the average development time and decreased the growth speed of the tumor. The response of the splenocytes to Con A increased significantly as compared with that in the control group after mice were immunized with TAP extract, but there were no changes in the cell cycle progression of thymocytes. WBI with 75 mGy X-rays given to the mice 12 h before immunization can enhance the inhibitory effects of TAP extract, the percentage of S phase increased significantly as compared with that in the TAP extract group, and the percentage of the CD8+ splenocytes increased. Conclusion: The results suggest that LDR can efficiently activate the function of immune system, and enhance the inhibitory effects of the TAP extract.

91. Ju GZ, Yan FQ, Fu SB, Li PW. P21 protein expression induced by ionizing radiation and its effect in cell cycle uncoupling. J Radiat Res Radiat Proces. 2005, 23(4):251-253. [Abstract] To investigate whether P21 protein expression could be induced by ionizing radiation and the effect on cell cycle uncoupling. Immunocytochemistry assay was used to measure P21 protein expression. Polyploid was analyzed by FCM following staining of cells with propidium iodide (PI). The results showed that P21 protein expression of EL-4 cells was increased significantly 2-72h following 4.0Gy X-irradiation (P<0.05-P<0.001). In dose-effect experiments it was found that P21 protein expression also increased significantly 24h after exposure to 0.5-6.0Gy X-rays of EL-4 cells (P<0.01-P<0.001). However, 8N cells were not changed in EL-4 cells irradiated with doses of 1.0-6.0Gy X-rays compared with sham-irradiated control (P>0.05). These results demonstrated that P21 protein expression. But not cell cycle uncoupling, of EL-4 cells could be induced by ionizing radiation. It suggested that P21 might not play an important role in cell cycle uncoupling.

YEAR 2006

92. Shen B, Ju GZ, Liu Y. Survivin and chromosome instability induced by X-irradiation. Chin J Radiol Med Prot. 2006, 26(2):129-132. [Abstract] Objective: To explore the biological effect of survivin on chromosome instability induced by X-rays. Methods Immunocytochemistry was used to detect the expression of survivin in HeLa cells. Carrier pSUPER-SVV was transfected into HeLa cells to interfere the expression of survivin. Flow cytometry assay was applied to detect the occurrence of polyploid at 0 h, 4 h, 12 h, and 48 h after the HeLa cells transfected with pSUPER-SVV and irradiated with 4 Gy X-rays, and compared with the group irradiated with 4 Gy X-rays but no transfection. Results: The expression of survivin was down-regulated by transfecting with small hairpin RNA, and its depression rate was estimated to be about 32·16% at 48 h after transfection. The occurrence of polyploid gaint cells was higher in the 4 Gy X-ray irradiated group at 48 h after the irradiation than that in control group (P<0·001). With expression of survivin interfered, the occurrence of polyploid gaint cells at 12 h or 48 h after irradiation, however, was about two times higher than that in the control group. Conclusion X-ray irradiation can induce chromosome instability in HeLa cells and the effect could be enhanced by interfering the expression of survivin. It was suggested that survivin plays an important role in maintaining the stability of chromosome.

93. Ju GZ, Sun SL, Fu SB, Yan FQ, Liu Y, Li PW. Effect of ionizing radiation on caspase-3 protein expression in EL-4 cells in mice. Journal of Jilin University Medicine Edition. 2006, 32(2):179-181.

[Abstract] Objective: To investigate the effect of ionizing radiation on caspase-3 protein expression of EL-4 cells Methods Mouse lymphoma EL-4 cell line was used. Flow cytometry (FCM) was used to examine caspase-3 protein expression and apoptosis. For dose-effect experiment, caspase-3 protein expression and apoptosis were measured 24 h after X-irradiation with doses of 0·5, 1·0, 2·0, 4·0 and 6·0 Gy. For time course experiment, caspase-3 protein expression was measured at 2, 4, 8, 12, 24 and 72 h after 4.0 Gy X-irradiation. Results In dose-effect experiment, it was demonstrated that the caspase-3 protein expression of EL-4 cells was increased significantly 24 h after X-irradiation with the doses of 0·5, 2·0, 4·0 and 6·0 Gy compared with sham-irrad (P<0·05 or P<0·01). It was also shown that apoptosis of EL-4 cells was induced significantly 24 h after X-irradiation with the doses 0·5, 1·0 and 4·0 Gy compared with sham-irrad (P<0·05 or P<0·01). In time course experiment, the results showed that the caspase-3 protein expression of EL-4 cells was increased significantly 8, 12 and 24 h after 4·0 G X-irradiation compared with sham-irrad (P<0.01 or P<0.001). Conclusion: Caspase-3 protein expression and apoptosis in EL-4 cells could be induced by X-rays.

94. Tian M, Piao CJ, Zhao BF, Li XY, Su X. Construction of human soluble TRAIL expression vector and its effect on apoptosis of tumor cells. Chin J Gerontol, 2006 11 1495-1497 [Abstract] Objective: To construct soluble TNF related apoptosis inducing ligand (TRAIL) expression vector and investigate the apoptotic effect of TRAIL transient transfer on EJ human bladder cancer cells. Methods: Human soluble TRAIL containing TNF-á signal was cloned by gene splicing by overlap extension (SOE) method and then was linked with T-vector1 After sequenced, the expression vector pcD-NA3.1-sTRAIL was constructed and was transfected into EJ cells under mediation of GeneCompanionTM in vitro. The expression of TRAIL was detected by RT-PCR and Western blot. The early and late apoptosis of transfected cells was detected by flow cytometry. The cell survival level was determined by colony formation assay. Results: The expression vector pcDNA3.1-sTRAIL was successfully constructed.The percentage of apoptotic cells in pcDNA3.1-sTRAIL transfected cells was significantly increased compared with that of non-transfected cells and pcDNA3.1 cells. The rate of clone formation of pcDNA3.1-sTRAIL transfected cells (51.34%) was significantly lower than that of non-transfected cells and pcDNA3.1 transfected cells. Conclusions: Expression vector pcDNA3.1-sTRAIL transiently transfected can induce apoptosis and obviously inhibit cell survival.

95. Tian M, Piao CJ, Liu LL, Yang W, Li XY. Apoptosis and down-regulated expression of Bcl-2 in SHG44 glioma cells induced by pEgr-hPTEN stable transfection in combination with X-ray irradiation. Chin J Radiol Med Radiol Prot 2006 26(2):106-109. [Abstract] Objective: To investigate the apoptotic effect and the changes of Bcl-2 protein expression of pEgr-hPTEN stable transfection in SHG44 human glioma cells in combination with irradiation. Methods: pEgr-hPTEN vector containing the exogenous wild type PTEN gene was transfected into SHG44 cells under mediation of lipofectamine in vitro; the positive cell clones called SHG44-hPTEN were selected and amplified by using G418. Transmission electron microscope was used to detect the cell ultrastructural changes and flow cytometry to measure the apoptotic effect and Bcl-2 expression of SHG44- hPTEN cells after X-ray irradiation at different doses. Results: Many degenerative changes and early apoptotic changes including chromosome condensation around the nuclear envelope were observed in SHG44- hPTEN cells. pEgr-hPTEN stable transfection in combination with X-ray irradiation can significantly induce apoptosis of SHG44 cells. The percentage of early apoptosis of SHG44-hPTEN cells irradiated with X-rays at different doses was 1.5-2.3 times as much as that of SHG44-hPTEN/0 Gy group, 1.9-4.4 times as much as that of SHG44 irradiated group , and 3.4-5.1 times as much as that of SHG44/0 Gy group. The expression of Bcl-2 proteins decreased in a dose-dependent manner. Conclusion: PTEN stable transfection in combination with irradiation can significantly induce apoptosis of tumor cells and significantly down-regulate the expression of Bcl-2 protein.

96. Wang ZC, Zhao HG, Piao CN, Liu GW, Liu SC, Lv Z, Gong SL. Effect of low dose radiation on cytochrome c and caspase-3 protein expressions in spermatogenic cells of mouse testis. Chin J Radiol Med Protect, 2006, 26 (2): 151-154. [Abstract] Objective: To investigate the effect of low dose radiation on the expressions of cytochrome c (Cyt c) and caspase-3 proteins in spermatogenic cells of mouse testis. Methods: The relationships of dose- and time-effect of Cyt c and caspase-3 protein expressions after low dose radiation with different dose X-irradiation were observed in the spermatogenic cells of mouse testis with immunohistochemical technique (SABC). Results: After irradiation with 0, 0.025, 0.05, 0.075, 0.1 and 0.2 Gy, Cyt c and caspase-3 proteins expressed in all kinds of spermatogenic cells in different degrees, and principally in spermatogonia and spermatocytes, but less in spermatids and spermazoa. And the expressions increased with the increasing of irradiation doses. The expressions of Cyt c and caspase-3 proteins after irradiation with 0.075 Gy increased with time prolongation and reached to the peak at 12 h late, then descreased. Conclusion: The expressions of Cyt c and caspase-3 proteins in spermatogenic cells of mouse

testis induced by low dose radition have dose- and time-effect regularity.

97. Wu N Liu YZ Xu RM Liu Y Jin SZ. Effects of whole-body irradiation with X-rays on apoptosis in mouse splenocytes and peritoneal macrophages J Jilin Univ (Med Ed) 2006, 32(6): 950-952. [Abstract] Objective: To study the effects of whole-body irradiation WBI with different doses of X-rays on apoptosis in mouse splenocytes and peritoneal macrophages. Methods: The apoptosis percentages of mouse splenocytes and peritoneal macrophages were detected with flow cytometry FCM at different times after the whole-body X-irradiation using the staining of Annexin-V and PI. Results: As compared with the control the percentage of apoptosis in mouse splenocytes began to increase gradually 24 h after WBI with 2 Gy X-rays < 0.05 and the increase of the percentage of apoptosis in mouse peritoneal macrophages arose 4 h after 2 Gy irradiation sustaining at higher level up to 48 h < 0.05 < 0.01 < 0.001 . After WBI with 0.075 Gy X-rays the percentage of apoptosis in mouse splenocytes reduced at 24 h < 0.05 and the percentage of apoptosis of peritoneal macrophages significantly reduced from 2 h to 16 h < 0.05 as compared with the control. Conclusion High dose irradiation induces apoptosis in mouse splenocytes and peritoneal macrophages while low dose irradiation causes an opposite effect suppressing immunocyte apoptosis.

98. Yang W, Sun T, Liu SC, Piao CJ, Lian GS, Li XY, Gong SL. Anti-tumor effect of repeated low dose of pEgr-IFNã-Endostatin gene-radiotherapy on mice bearing Lewis lung carcinoma. J Jilin Univ (Medicine Edition) 2006 32 4 547-549. [Abstract] Objective: To study the anti-tumor effect of repeated low dose pEgr-IFNã-Endostatin gene-radiotherapy on mice bearing Lewis lung carcinoma. Methods: Mice bearing Lewis lung carcinoma were divided randomly into control , 10 Gy, 4 ×2.5 Gy, 4 ×P, P + 10 Gy and 4 × (P + 2.5 Gy) groups. The pEgr-IFNã-Endostatin plasmid packaged with liposome was injected into tumors which were irradiated by X-ray 36 h later. Tumor growth rates at different times were observed after gene-radiotherapy. Number of lung metastatic nodes and tumor weight of the mice were detected 18 d after gene-radiotherapy. Results: Tumor growth rate of the mice in gene-radiotherapy for four-times group was significantly lower than that for only once group 12-18 d after gene-radiotherapy. Number of lung metastatic nodes and tumor weight of the mice in gene-radiotherapy for four-times group were significantly lower than those for only once group 18 d after gene-radiotherapy. Conclusion: Anti-tumor effect of repeated low dose pEgr-IFNã-Endostatin gene-radiotherapy is better than that of high dose for only once.

YEAR 2007

99. Liu SZ. Cancer control related to stimulation of immunity by low dose radiation. Dose-Response, 2007, 5: 39-47 [Abstract] Previous studies showed that low dose radiation (LDR) could stimulate the immune system in both animal and human populations. This paper reviews the present status of relevant research as support to the use of LDR in clinical practice for cancer prevention and treatment. It has been demonstrated that radiation-induced changes in immune activity follows an inverse J-shaped curve, i.e., low dose stimulation and high dose suppression. The stimulation of immunity by LDR concerns most anticancer parameters, including antibody formation, natural killer activity, secretion of interferon and other cytokines as well as other cellular changes. Animal studies have revealed that LDR retards tumor growth, decreases cancer metastasis, and inhibits carcinogenesis induced by high dose radiation. These effects of LDR on cancer control were found to be related to its stimulation on immunity. The experimental data may well explain the efficacy of the clinical trial of LDR in the treatment of cancer.

100. Jin S.Z., Pan X.N., Wu N., Jin G.H., Liu S.Z. Whole-body low dose irradiation promotes the efficacy of conventional radiotherapy for cancer and possible mechanisms. Dose response 2007, 5: 349-358. [Abstract] The purpose of the present study was to explore the possibility of establishing cancer radiotherapy protocols that could promote treatment efficacy at a reduced radiation dose. Mouse models of melanoma (B16) and Lewis lung carcinoma (LLC) were used in the experiments. Conventional local radiotherapy was combined with low dose whole-body irradiation (LDWBI) in the presence or absence of gene therapy by intratumor injection of a recombinant plasmid Egr-mIL-18-B7.1 (E18B). After a number of trials with different combinations it was found that a protocol of 2-week treatment with 2 x (E18B + 2 Gy + 0.075 Gy x 2) was found to be able to promote treatment efficacy at a reduced radiation dose. In this protocol local irradiation with 2Gy was administered 24h after intratumor injection of 10 ìg of the plasmid E18B followed by LDWBI with 0.075 Gy every other day for 2 sessions in 1 week, and the procedure was repeated for another week. When this combined treatment was compared with conventional radiotherapy, i.e., 2Gy every other day 3 times in one week repeated for 2 weeks, the treatment efficacy was improved, as judged by increased average survival rate, reduced mean tumor weight, reduced pulmonary metastasis and

suppressed intratumor capillary growth with a 2/3 reduction of radiation dose. Immunologic studies showed stimulated natural killer (NK) and cytotoxic T lymphocyte (CTL) activity as well as increased interferon-ã (IFN- ã) secretion in this combined treatment group as compared with the group receiving local treatment alone. It is suggested that up-regulation of host anticancer immunity by LDWBI and the initiation of expression of immune genes by both the local large dose and LDWBI are important factors in the realization of improved cancer control.

101. Xu RM, Wu N, Liu Y, Jin SZ. Effect of whole-body X-irradiation on the expression of protein kinase C è in immune cells. Chin J Radiol Med Prot. 2007, 27(1): 60-62. [Abstract] Objective: To study the effect of ionizing radiation on protein kinase Cè (PKCè) expression in immune cells from thymus and spleen. Methods: Immunohistochemistry (IHC, ABC method) was used to detect the cytoplasmic expression and membrane translocation of PKCè in the splenocytes and thymocytes at 24 h after whole body irradiation (WBI) with different doses of X-rays. Results: The results show that both LDR and HDR caused significant up-regulation of PKCè in the cytoplasm and on the membrane of splenocytes and thymocytes, being more significant and, more in a dose-dependent manner for the thymocytes. The cytoplasmic expression of PKCè in the thymocytes peaks with 2Gy irradiation and that in the splenocytes has not attained to the significant peak in the whole course, but with higher expression in both organs than control. The ratio of PKCè membrane-positive cells in the thymus begins to rise dose-dependently from 0.1Gy, peaks at 2Gy and then declines dose-dependently until 10Gy; with the effect in the spleen being much more marked than that in the thymus in the range of 0.075Gy 0.5Gy, but much lower in the range of 0.5Gy 10Gy. Conclusion: Under the effect of ionizing radiation the expression of PKCè in the cytoplasm and on the plasma membrane is up-regulated significantly.

102. Wu N Liu YZ Jin SZ The effect of low dose whole-body X-irradiation on the efficacy of pEgr-IL18-B7.1 gene-radiotherapy. Chin J Radiol Med Protec, 2007,27(3): 223-225. [Abstract] Objective: To observe the therapeutic effect of whole-body irradiation with low dose X-rays in mice bearing Lewis lung carcinoma under recombinant plasmid pEgr-IL18-B7.1 gene-radiotherapy. Methods: The pEgr-IL18-B7.1 recombinant plasmids mediated by polyethylenimine were injected locally into tumors of the mice with gene-radiotherapy and then the tumors received different therapeutic regimens including local X-irradiation with 2 Gy and whole-body X-irradiation with 0.075 Gy, respectively. The anti-tumor effects of low dose X-rays in optimizing the protocol of E18B gene-radiotherapy on the tumor-bearing mice were observed. Results: As compared with repeated high dose local X-irradiation alone single time high dose local X-irradiation in combination with repeated low dose whole-body X-irradiation showed more significant inhibition of tumor growth under pEgr-IL18-B7.1 gene-radiotherapy. Conclusion: Low dose whole-body X-irradiation superimposed upon a local high dose could significantly enhance the anti-tumor effect in the protocol of pEgr-IL18-B7.1 gene-radiotherapy.

103. Tian M, Wu CM, Liu LL, Piao CJ, Li XY. Effects of PTEN transfer on cell cycle progression and expression of P27kip1 following X-ray irradiation. J Jilin Univ (Med Ed) 2007 33 2 195-199 [Abstract] Objective: To investigate the effect s of p Egr-hPTEN stable transfer combined with irradiation on the cell cycle progression and the expression of cell cycle kinase inhibitor P27kip1 protein of SHG44 human glioma cells. Methods: pEgr-hPTEN vector containing the exogenous wild type PTEN gene was transfected into SHG44 cells under mediation of lipofectamine in vitro, the positive cell clones were selected and amplified by using G418. Western blotting was used to measure the expression of PTEN protein. Transmission electron microscopy was adopted to detect the cell ultrastructural changes and flow cytometry was adopted to analyze the changes of cell cycle progression and the expression of P27kip1 in SHG44-sPTEN cells followed by different doses of X-ray irradiation. Results: Egr-1 promoter could be induced and activated by irradiation enhancing the expression of downstream PTEN gene within 5Gy. The ultrastructure of SHG44-sPTEN cells had many degenerative changes and many early apoptotic changes including chromosome condensation around the nuclear envelope. pEgr-hPTEN stable transfer combined with X-ray irradiation could significantly induce G1 arrest. The expression of P27kip1 proteins increased in SHG44-sPTEN stable transfected cells. Conclusion: PTEN stable transfer combined with irradiation can significantly induce G1 arrest . The molecular basis may be correlated with the enhanced expression of PTEN induced by irradiation and increased expression of cell cycle kinase inhibitor P27kip1.

104. Yang JZ Jin GH, Liu XD, Liu SZ. Therapeutic effect of pEgr-IL18-B7.2 gene radiotherapy in B16 melanoma-bearing mice. Human Gene Therapy 2007, 18 (4): 323-332. [Abstract] To evaluate the antitumor role of genes B7.2 and IL18, the radiation-inducible dual-gene coexpression plasmid pEgr-IL18-B7.2 was constructed and its effects on tumor were detected both in vitro and in vivo. After the introduction of pEgr-IL18-B7.2 into B16 melanoma cells, followed by X-ray irradiation, higher expression

levels of B7.2 and IL18 compared with control were found both by flow cytometry and enzyme-linked immunosorbent assay. It was shown that even low-dose irradiation was able to induce their expression, which could be tightly regulated either by giving cells different doses of radiation or the same dose at different time points. pEgr-IL18-B7.2 was then packaged with liposome and injected into melanoma tumor-bearing mice. The tumors received 5 Gy of local X-ray irradiation every other day for a total of five treatments. B16 tumor growth slowed significantly when treated with pEgr-IL18-B7.2 plus X-radiation versus either treatment separately. Both 1 and 3 days after the last irradiation the group of mice with combined gene and radiation therapy showed significantly higher tumor necrosis factor (TNF)-alpha secretion in peritoneal macrophages, upregulated splenic cytotoxic T lymphocytes (CTLs) and natural killer (NK) cells, and higher interferon (IFN)-alpha secretion than those in either individual treatment group or the control group. The stimulation of host anticancer immunity by increased secretion of IL-18 and upregulated immunogenicity of the tumor cells by increased expression of B7.2 on their surface, in addition to the direct effect of local X-irradiation on the tumor cells, may contribute to the novel effect of the combined therapy.

105. Shan YX, Jin SZ, Liu XD, Liu Y, Liu SZ. Ionizing radiation stimulates secretion of pro-infammatory cytokines. Radiat Environ Biophys 2007, 46:21–29. [Abstract] In previous studies we showed a marked increase in secretion of infammatory cytokines TNFa and interleukin (IL)-1b by mouse macrophages in response to different doses of ionizing radiation (IR). Here we show the stimulation of IL-12 and IL-18 secretion by mouse peritoneal macrophages after whole-body irradiation with exploration of the possible mechanisms and implications in cancer radiotherapy. Both low (0.075 Gy) and high (2 Gy) doses of IR were found to cause sustained stimulation of IL-12 and IL-18 secretion by mouse macrophages; this paralleled the activation of NF-kB as well as up-regulated expression of CD14 and TLR4–MD2 on the macrophage surface and MyD88 in the cytoplasm. The expression of CD14, TLR4–MD2 and MyD88 increased in a dose-dependent manner from radiation doses between 0.05 and 2 Gy. The secretion of IL-12 and IL-18 showed a dose-dependent increase from doses between 0.05 and 4 Gy. It is concluded that IR can stimulate the secretion of IL-12 and IL-18 presumably via activation of the Toll signaling pathway in macrophages. The potential harmful effect of repeated doses of radiation used in radiotherapy for certain cancers is discussed.

106. Jin GH, Liu Y, Jin SZ, Liu XD, Liu SZ. UVB induced oxidative stress in human keratinocytes and protective effect of antioxidant agents. Radiat Environ Biophys (2007) 46:61–68. [Abstract] This study aims at exploring the oxidative stress in keratinocytes induced by UVB irradiation and the protective effect of nutritional antioxidants. Cultured Colo-16 cells were exposed to UVB in vitro followed by measurement of reactive oxygen species (ROS), endogenous antioxidant enzyme activity, as well as cell death in the presence or absence of supplementation with vitamin C, vitamin E, or Ginsenoside Panoxatriol. Intracellular ROS content was found significantly reduced 1 h after exposure, but increased at later time points. After exposure to 150–600 J m-2 UVB, reduction of ROS content was accompanied by increased activity of catalase and CuZn-superoxide dismutase at early time points. Vitamins C and E, and Ginsenoside Panoxatriol counteracted the increase of ROS in the Colo-16 cells induced by acute UVB irradiation. At the same time, Ginsenoside Panoxatriol protected the activity of CuZn-superoxide dismutase, while vitamin E showed only a moderate protective role. Vitamins C and E, and Ginsenoside Panoxatriol in combination protected the Colo-16 cells from UVB-induced apoptosis, but not necrosis. These findings suggest that vitamins C and E as well as Ginsenoside Panoxatriol are promising protective agents against UVB-induced damage in skin cells.

107. Ju GZ, Shen B, Sun SL, Yan FQ and Fu SB. Effect of X-rays on the expression of caspase-3, p53 in EL-4 cells and its biological implications. Biomed and Environ Sci. 2007, 20: 456-459. [Abstract] Objective: To investigate the effect of X-rays on the expression of caspase-3, p53 protein in EL-4 cells and its implications in the induction of apoptosis and polyploidy cells. Methods Mouse lymphoma cell line, EL-4 cells, was used. Fluorescent staining and flow cytometry analysis were employed for the measurement of protein expression, apoptosis, cell cycle and polyploidy cells. Results It was found that the expression of caspase-3 protein increased significantly at 8 h and 12 h compared with sham-irradiated control ($P<0.05$, respectively) and the expression of p53 protein increased significantly at 2, 4, 8, 12 and 24 h compared with sham-irradiated control ($P<0.05 \sim P<0.01$) in EL-4 cells after 4.0 Gy X-irradiation. The results showed that apoptosis of EL-4 cells was increased significantly at 2 4 8 12 24 48 and 72 h after 4.0Gy exposure compared with sham-irradiated control ($P<0.05 \sim P<0.001$). The results also showed that G2 phase cells were increased significantly at 4, 8, 12, 24, 48 and 72 h ($P<0.05 \sim P<0.001$), however, no marked change in the number of 8 C polyploidy cells was found from 2~48 h after 4.0Gy exposure. Conclusion Our results indicated that the expressions of caspase-3 and p53 protein in EL-4 cells could be induced by X-rays, which

might play an important role for the induction of apoptosis and the molecular pathway for polyploid formation might be p53-independent.

108. Cheng GH, Zhao HG, Li YB, Guo W, Gong SL Change of p53 protein in adaptive respone of EL-4 cells induced by low dose ionizing radiation. Tumor, 2007, 27 (4): 269-271. [Abstract] Objective: To investigate the expression of p53 protein in the adaptable reaction of EL-4 cells induced by low dose radiation (LDR), which may provide the experimental clues for studying the repair mechanism of DNA damage in the adaptable reaction of EL-4 cells induced by LDR. Methods: EL-4 cells were divided into control, irradiation (the irradiation doses were 1, 2 and 3 Gy) and adaptable radiation groups (75 mGy + 1 Gy, 75 mGy + 2 Gy and 75 mGy + 3 Gy). The p53 mRNA and protein expressions in EL-4 cells were measured by flow cytometry and RT-PCR methods, respectively. Results: The expression levels of p53 protein in the three adaptive radiation groups were significantly higher than that in the normal control group ($P < 0.01$). 75 mGy induced the adaptive reaction of EL-4 cells and decreased the expression level of p53 protein as compared with that in the control group ($P < 0.01$). The expression level of p53 mRNA showed the same change as its protein level in EL-4 cells. Conclusion: The expression level of p53 protein decreased in the adaptive radiation group, which suggests that p53 might play an important role in the adaptive response of EL-4 cells induced by LDR.

109. Du X, Zhao HG, Wang W, Guo W, Gong SL Effects of 3-AB on PARP expression, apoptosis and cell cycle progression of Hela cells after X-ray irradiation. J Jilin Univ (Med Ed), 2007, 33 (3): 418-421. [Abstract] Objective: To study the changes of apoptosis and cell cycle progression of Hela cells after the poly (ADP-ribose) polymerase (PARP) inhibited by its inhibitor 3-aminobenzamid (3-AB) and the effect mechanisms of PARP on Hela cells damaged by irradiation. Methods: Flow cytometry (FCM) was used to examine the PARP expression, the percentage of apoptotic cells and cell cycle progression. Results: The percentage of Hela cells with positive expression of PARP protein 2, 4, 8 and 12 h after administration with 3-AB was significantly lower than that in the control ($P < 0.01$). The percentage of apoptotic cells in the 3-AB plus irradiation group 2, 8, 12 and 24 h after 2 Gy irradiation was higher than that in the irradiation group ($P < 0.01$ or $P < 0.05$), and the percentage of G2 cells decreased significantly ($P < 0.01$ or $P < 0.05$). Conclusion: 3-AB could rapidly inhibit the PARP expression of Hela cells, enhance the apoptosis, and block G2 arrest induced by irradiation.

110. Du X, Wang ZC, Wang H, Li YB, Gong SL. Radiosensitization effect of PARP inhibitor 3-AB and its mechanism. Chin J Radiol Med Protect, 2007, 27 (4): 409-410. [Abstract] Objective: To investigate the radiosensitization effect of the 3-aminobenzamid (3-AB) which is the inhibitor of poly (ADP-ribose) polymerase (PARP) and explore its mechanisms. Methods Hela cells were damaged with 0 – 4 Gy irradiation after administrated with 5 mmol/L 3-AB and investigated the survival fraction with MTT. The change of the Hela cells damaged 0 – 12 h after irradiation with X-rays was investigated with single cell gel electrophoresis (SCGE). Results: the survival fraction in the 3-AB group decreased significantly. The damage Hela cells at different times after irradiation of different doses after administrated with 5 mmol/L 3-AB were higher than those in the radiation groups. Conclusion 3-AB as a PARP inhibitor can aggravate the irradiation-induced damage. And this may be one of the mechanisms that 3-AB could enhance the cell radiosensitivity.

111. Wang ZC, Li YB, Guo W, Zhao HG, Jiang XY, Lu WT, Gong SL. Effects of low dose radiation on activity of reactive oxygen species and mitochondrion membrane potential in spermatogenic cells of mouse testes. J Jilin Univ (Med Ed), 2007, 33 (5): 786-789. [Abstract] Objective: To investigate the effects of low dose X-ray radiation on the activity of the reactive oxygen species (ROS) and mitochondrion membrane potential (Δm) in spermatogenic cells of mouse testes. Methods: The ROS activity and Δm in the cells were measured indirectly by flow cytometry with 2',7'-dichlorofluorescin diacetate (DCFH-DA) and Rhodamine 123 probes. Results: The ROS activity increased with the increase of irradiation doses 12 h after irradiation as compared with that in the 0 Gy group ($P < 0.05$); but the Δm decreased with the increase of irradiation ($P < 0.05$). After irradiation with 0.075 Gy X-ray, the ROS activity increased with time prolongation as compared with that in the 0 h group ($P < 0.05$), reached the peak at 12 h later, and kept the higher level; but Δm decreased with the time prolongation ($P < 0.05$), and reached the lowest level at 12 h later, then recovered graduatlly to the normal level. Conclusion: Low dose radiation can induce the increase of ROS and the decrease of Δm in spermatogenic cells of mouse testes in the pattern of dose- and time-effect.

112. Xu RM Wu N, Liu YZ Jin SZ. Change in expression of LAMP-1 on the splenocytes after WBI of mice with X-rays. Chin J Radiol Med Prot. 2007, 27(2): 121-124. [Abstract] Objective: To study the effect of mice WBI with X-rays on the expression of LAMP-1 on the splenocytes. Methods: The LAMP-1 positive cells from mouse splenocytes were detected by flow cytometry (FCM) with immunofluorescence

at different times (0, 2, 4, 8, 16, 24 and 48 h) after whole body irradiation (WBI) with X-rays of 0.075 Gy and 2.0 Gy. Results LAMP-1 expression on the splenocytes was significantly inhibited 8, 16, 24 h after WBI by 2. 0 Gy X-rays while the LAMP-1 expression was markedly enhanced 2 h and suppressed 48 h after WBI with 0.075 Gy X-rays. Conclusion: LAMP-1 which plays an important role in immune activity is differentially affected by low versus high dose of radiation. High dose radiation inhibits the LAMP-1 expression and the low dose radiation possibly causes the opposite biological effect in the early phase after WBI.

113. Yang W, Sun T, Gong PS, Li XY, Gong SL. Construction of recombinant plasmid pIRESEgr-IFNã and its expression in Lewis lung carcinoma induced by irradiation. J Jilin Univ (Med Ed) 2007 33 5 790-793 [Abstract] Objective: To construct the recombinant plasmid pIRESEgr-IFNã and detect its expression in Lewis lung carcinoma induced by irradiation in vitro. Methods: The recombinant plasmid pIRESEgr-IFNã containing Egr-1 promoter and IFNã gene was constructed with gene recombinant technique. The plasmid was transferred into Lewis lung carcinoma by liposome in vitro. The correlations of dose- and time- effects in the expression of IFNã gene induced by X-ray were detected by ELISA. Results: The identification with enzymes proved that Egr-1 promoter and IFNã gene were inserted into vector pIRES1neo correctly. After X-ray irradiation with different doses, the expression of IFNã in the supernatant of Lewis lung carcinoma transfected by pIRESEgr-IFNã was significantly higher than that in 0 Gy group ($P < 0.001$). After 5 Gy X-ray irradiation, the expression of IFNã was the highest , being 4.39 times as much as that in 0 Gy group. The expression of IFNã in the supernatant increased 36 h after irradiation after 5 Gy X-ray irradiation , being 6.27 times as much as that in 0 h group. Conclusion: The recombinant plasmid pIRESEgr-IFNã is constructed successfully, and it has the property of enhancing the expression of IFNã gene induced by irradiation.

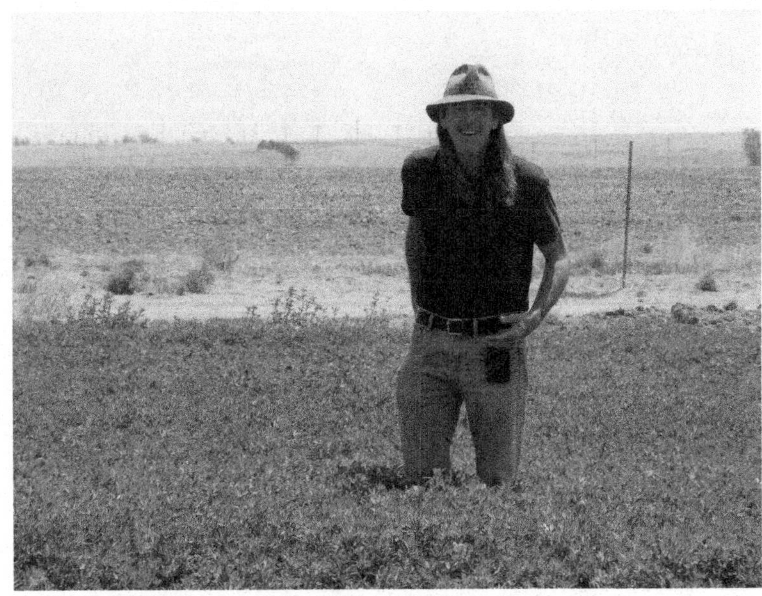

Jay Gutierrez, Medicine Man and radiation hormesis expert.

INDEX

A-bomb, 59-62, 120
Abelson, Philip, 71
abnormal cells, 155, 187
absorption of nutrients, 142, 160
abstinence, 153
acid, 4, 162-164, 173, 179, 279
acid condition, 163, 164
acid foods, 163
acid/alkaline balance, 163, 164
acid/alkaline ratio, 163
acidophilus, 163
acupuncture treatments, 214
acute renal failure, 199
acute stress conditions, 27
Adams, Rod, 84
adaptive response, 33, 91, 129-132, 250, 252, 253, 259-262, 265, 268-270, 274, 275, 284
adenocarcinoma colorectal cancer, 214
adenoids, 169
adrenal cancer, 115
adrenal fatigue, 21
adrenaline, 21
aerobic exercise, 168, 170
aflatoxin, 114, 152
Africa, 46, 155, 248, 253, 255
aggravation period, 116, 144
aging, 21, 23, 27, 29, 71, 80, 94, 97, 104, 111, 112, 116, 123, 143, 160, 170, 176, 195, 199, 216, 249
agriculture, and radiation hormesis, 15
AIDS, 101, 117
Air Force, 16, 88, 239, 244
air-born microorganisms, 175
alcohol, 20, 90, 93
alcoholics, 93
Aleve, 218
algae, 52, 89
alkaline, 163, 164, 272
alkaline foods, 164
alkaline reserve, 163
alkalizing colonic, 237
allopathic medicine, 79
aloe leaf, 165
aloe skin, 165
aloe smoothie, 165
alpha particles, 47, 57
alternative treatments, 193
Alzheimer's, 117
America, 4, 20, 28, 40, 43, 49, 53, 59, 75, 83, 95, 147-149, 152-154, 193, 229, 232, 245, 247, 251, 255
American doctors, 154
American Nuclear Society, 43
Americans, 28, 83, 147, 153, 229
amoebas, 110
amygdala, 175
anaerobic, 167
ancient cultures, 155
ancient peoples, 71, 153
ancient yogic tradition, 156
anemias, 77
anesthesiology, 202
angioma, 115
animal fat, 153
animal fats, 162
animals, 52, 79, 80, 98, 113, 127, 128, 152, 154, 164, 176, 177
Antarctica, 84
anti-aging effects, 94
anti-fungal dietary-cleansing plan, 162
anti-nuclear activity, 65
anti-wrinkle therapy, 104
antibiotics, 32, 52, 78, 79, 114, 251
antioxidant defense, 21
anxiety, 117
apoptosis, 98-100, 104, 253, 259-261, 263, 265, 268-270, 273-275, 277, 280, 281, 283, 284
appendix, 5, 169, 176, 183, 223, 229, 231, 233
apple cider vinegar, 163
appliances, 174
Arkansas Hot Springs, 72
Armenia, 83
Army and Navy General Hospital, 72
Arndt, Rudolf, 91
Arndt-Schultz Law, 91, 92, 142
arsenic, 92, 140, 224
arterial cells, 34
arterial plaque, 34
arterial walls, 169

arteries, 34, 111, 171, 177
arthritis, 45, 76, 104, 113, 117, 118, 198, 247, 251
ascites, 205
Asia, 63, 249
aspergillus, 108, 110
assimilation, 127, 167
asthma, 117, 162
astronauts, 22
atherosclerosis, 114, 117, 153, 162
atomic bomb, 55, 58-60, 62-64, 79, 229, 232
atomic bomb blasts, 60
atomic chain reaction, 82
atomic energy, 56, 83-85, 119, 120, 232, 247, 250
Atomic Energy Commission, 83, 120, 232
atomic radiation, 47, 59, 255
atoms, 47, 56, 101, 158
atonement, 153
ATP, 103, 142
Australia, 131, 251
Austria, 72, 83, 122, 233, 247
autoimmune disease, 117
Avastin, 205
axons, 128
Ayurvedic tradition, 153
babies, 64, 134, 154
back injury, 211
back pain, 176, 217-219
background radiation, 47, 61, 64, 86, 95, 119, 122, 123, 136, 250, 252, 255
bacteria, 78, 79, 101, 103, 110, 112, 140, 158, 163, 164, 173, 254
Bad Gastein Spa, Austria, 122
Bad Gastein, Austria, 72
baked goods, 174
Baltimore, MD, 64
Bangkok, Thailand, 66
barium enema, 136
baseball, 22
bath, 46, 72, 155, 162, 237
Bath, England, 72
bathtub, 162
Battle Creek Sanitarium, Battle Creek, MI, 154
beans, 164
beauty, 10, 39, 44, 75, 101, 137, 179
Because People Are Dying (Goldberg), 12
Becquerel, Henri, 74
beer, 162
bees, 15
Behounek's Sanatorium, 234
Belarus, 64
bentonite, 165, 208
benzene, 128
Berkeley, CA, 11
beta particles, 47
beta rays, 57
Bettelheim, Bruno, 28, 29
Big Fast, 153
Bikini Atoll, 122
bioenergetic communication network, 158
bioenergetic principles, 159
biological toxins, 153
biology, 2, 16, 19, 97, 119, 147, 159, 232, 247, 248, 251-253, 255
bioplasma, 129
biopsies, 199
biopsy, 14, 187, 188, 190, 199, 214, 216
birds, 154, 191
Black Plague, 172
black salve, 111, 216
black sand, 87
bladder, 115, 117, 155, 178, 191, 280
bladder disease, 117
bladder disorder, 191
blood, 14, 34, 40, 88, 103, 111, 113, 150-152, 156, 162, 168, 169, 171-175, 177, 178, 190, 200, 203, 204, 212, 256, 268, 278
blood cells, 103, 111, 150, 171
blood plasma, 171
blood sugar, 200
blood supply, 34, 156, 168
blood vessels, 34
blood work, 203, 212
bloodroot, 111
bloodstream, 113, 115, 162, 168, 170
blue-green stone, 45, 50
boils on neck, 117
Boltwood, Bertram, 101
bomb factories, 90

bone, 21-23, 77, 93, 111, 112, 130, 159, 197, 211, 256, 263, 264, 267
bone and joint fractures, 159
bone cells, 111
bone grafts, 211
bone marrow cells, 130, 256, 264, 267
bones, 22, 23, 57, 58, 90, 93, 157, 158
boost fat burning, 20
Boulder, Montana, 76
bowel cleansing, 163, 165
bowel movements, 154, 155
brain, 24, 25, 32, 34, 104, 107, 109, 115, 117, 120, 129, 136, 151, 168, 172, 175, 177-179, 188, 189, 191, 235, 256, 274
brain anemia, 177
brain cancer, 188
brain cells, 25
brain chatter, 179
brain disorders, 24, 117
brain fog, 117
brain tumor, 115
brainstem gliomas, 109, 188
Brazil, 87, 123, 136, 164, 234
Brazil nuts, 136
bread, 162, 174, 175
breast cancer, 111, 114, 115, 145, 155, 185, 187, 193, 215-217, 248, 250
breast milk, 151, 152
breasts, 155
breast-fed babies, 154
breathing, 68, 76, 134, 167, 168, 171, 175
breathing oxygen, 171
Broad Stroke theory, 105
broccoli, 138
bronchial conditions, 162
Brucer, Marshall, 120
Bufferin, 148
bursitis, 75, 76, 104, 232
butter, 162, 164, 251
Byers, Eben, 78
CA 125, 204-206
CA 125 level, 205
CA 125 test, 204
caffeine, 92, 93
California, 19, 30, 75, 84, 231, 247
calmness, 157
calorie restriction, 21, 24, 97
Camby, Bruno, 43
cancer, 2, 4, 5, 12, 14, 15, 26, 27, 31, 33, 34, 42, 45, 48, 50, 51, 59-61, 64, 65, 68, 69, 71, 78, 80-82, 87-89, 94, 95, 98-100, 102, 104, 107-115, 117, 120, 122-127, 131, 138-140, 145, 147, 150, 151, 155, 158, 162, 167, 179, 184-188, 190, 193, 195-197, 199, 200, 203-207, 210, 212-217, 221, 225, 231, 235, 239, 241, 247-250, 252-254, 266, 272, 273, 276-278, 280-283
cancer cells, 99, 100, 102, 104, 167, 190, 205, 277, 278, 280
cancer deaths, 60, 95, 98, 124, 252
cancer free, 213, 215
Cancer is a Fungus (Simoncini), 114
cancer level, 190
cancer of the large intestine, 155
cancer patients, 2, 12, 26, 31, 33, 50, 51, 100, 108, 110, 112, 131, 196, 235
cancer rates, U.S., 147
cancer suppression, 94, 250
Cancer Treatment Center of America, 193
cancer tumor cell, 140
cancer tumors, 45, 111
cancer, as a radiologic-induced disease, 94
cancers, 21, 24, 33, 40, 51, 55-57, 59, 60, 64, 65, 68, 69, 77, 93, 95, 103, 106, 107, 114, 115, 120-122, 124, 129, 134, 137, 150, 152, 153, 204, 214, 283
candida, 21, 117, 158, 214, 241
Canon City, Colorado, 72
Capitol, Washington, D.C., 86, 87
capryillic acid, 163
carbohydrates, 162
carboplatinum resistant, 205
cardiac pacemakers, 136
cardiomyopathy, 199
Carrel, Alexis, 100

cascara sagrada, 166
cashews, 152, 164
catarrh, 179
Catholicism, 153
CATSCAN, 189
cattle, 15, 51, 52, 79, 120
cattle ranching, 51
cat's eyes, 66
cell death, 99, 283
cell membranes, 104, 140, 169, 174
cells, 25, 32-34, 57, 93, 94, 97-104, 111-113, 115, 116, 126, 128-132, 140, 142, 150, 155, 158, 160, 167, 169-174, 187, 188, 190, 197, 205, 247, 250, 254, 256-280, 282-284
cellular metabolism, 160
cellular protection, 21
cellular systems, 159
Center for Disease Control and Prevention, 128
Central Research Institute of Electric Power Industry, 88
chart of radiation exposures, 136
cheese, 162, 164
chemical agents, 19
chemicals, 22, 24, 25, 71, 150, 151, 156, 157, 163, 174, 248
chemistry, 40, 46, 114, 115, 159, 251, 257, 258, 262-264, 266, 271, 279, 282
chemo, 184, 185, 188, 189, 193, 195, 205, 206, 214, 215
chemo advocates, 206
chemotherapy, 32, 99, 100, 131, 150, 207, 214, 216, 266
Chernobyl Forum, 64, 250
Chernobyl nuclear accident, 131
Chernobyl nuclear power plant, 63
Chernobyl radiation, 65, 85, 254
Cheshire, Molly, 35
chick-peas, 164
chicken pox, 27
Chief Cloudpiler, 53
childhood diseases, 27
childhood febrile diseases, 33
children, 28, 29, 64, 67, 93, 102, 134, 152, 195, 248
China, 87, 123, 247, 250, 255
Choctaw, 53
cholera, 45, 259
cholesterol, 34, 114, 162
chromium, 92, 224
chromosome aberrations, 130, 260
chronic Brights disease, 72
chronic degenerative disease, 167
chronic diarrhea, 72
chronic fatigue, 117, 177, 191, 200
chronic fatigue syndrome, 191, 200
chronic headaches, 191
chronic inflammation, 15
chronic skin lesions, 73
chronic stress, 21
chrysoberyl gems, 66
chrysocolla, 45, 46
cigarette, 92
cinnamon-laced wax paper, 175
circulation, 167, 177
cities, 57, 59, 141, 166, 167, 229
citrus fruits, 164
clay water, 165
cleansing, 153, 155, 157, 162-165, 169, 237
coal, 136, 223, 225-227
Cobalt-60, 121, 125
coffee, 90, 93, 158, 165
coffee drinkers, 93
coffee enemas, 165
Cohen, Bernard, 35, 68, 69, 81, 104, 122, 136
colema board, 165
collagen, 142
collagen producing cells, 142
Colombia, South America, 49, 135
Colombian hot stones, 49
colon, 107, 115, 153-155, 164, 165, 176, 178, 214, 237
colon cancer, 107, 115
colon cleansing, 153, 164, 237
colon therapists, 155
colon tract, 155
colon walls, 154, 165
colonic irrigation, 237
colony collapse disorder, and bees, 15
Colorado, 7, 16, 17, 21, 39, 51, 72, 83, 84, 87, 106, 124, 138, 208, 214, 216, 243, 244
colostomy, 214, 215

colostrum, 200
combustible fuels, 136
Concordia Foundation, 12, 237
congenital malformations, 48
consciousness, 154, 179
Consumer Reports magazine, 66
contraceptives, 75
copaxone, 202
COPD, 191
corn, 152
corn byproducts, 152
corn oil, 152
Cornwall, England, 123
cortisol, 21, 27
cosmic rays, 56, 86, 87
Costantini, A. V., 114
cotton, 143
countertops, 66, 67
cows, 52, 62, 73, 120
Cox, Faye, 221
Crick, Francis, 102
CRIEPI, 88
Crohn's Disease, 117, 152
crops, and radiation hormesis, 15
CT exams, 59
CT scan, 199, 203, 212
CT-guided brush biopsies, 199
cures, 9, 71, 76, 101, 191
Curie Sanatorium, 233
Curie, Marie, 74, 231
Cushing's Disease, 117
Cuttler, Jerry, 62
cycle of renewal, 112
cycling, 23
cycloheximide, 101
cysts, 32
Czech Republic, 72, 83, 161, 233, 234
daphnia magna, 121
Day, Tanya, 131
degenerative diseases, 15
dehydration, 175
Delpha, M., 62
dental x-ray, 136
dentists, 77
Denver, Colorado, 87
Department of Energy, 88, 124, 252
depression, 117, 118, 191, 225, 279
depressive disorder, 199
desire, 153, 154
detoxification, 21, 100, 101, 103, 116, 144, 151-155, 164, 178, 237
Devon, England, 123
diabetes, 24, 104, 117, 152, 199, 212, 241
diabetes mellitus type 2, 199
diaphragm, 168
diaphragmatic breathing, 168
diarrhea, 72, 211, 218
dietary fiber, 164
Diflucan, 163
digestion, 24, 73, 164, 167, 277
digestive disorders, 117
digital radiation detector, 140
diluted toxicants, may be beneficial, 92
diphtheria, 74
disautonomia, 200
disease, 24, 26, 31, 33, 34, 72, 82, 94, 95, 103, 113, 117, 118, 128, 145, 148, 152, 158, 160, 167, 168, 172, 173, 176, 177, 191, 196, 200, 201, 203, 225, 249
disease mongering, 148
distilled water, 155
diverticulitis, 155
dizziness, 144
DNA, 21, 97, 101-104, 130, 131, 150, 249, 250, 253, 257, 259-261, 263-266, 268-270, 272-277, 280, 284
DNA damage, 21, 104, 130, 131, 250, 253, 284
DNA synthesis, 103, 257, 260
DNA-Repair theory, 101
DOE, 88, 125, 253
dried foods, 152
dried prunes, 164
drug companies, 78
drugs, 20, 100, 106, 148-150, 158, 163, 203
dry-brush, 179
Dupuyytren's contracture, 14
dust particles, 110
d'Angelo, Raphael, 16, 17, 195-197, 244
earth, 22, 34, 39, 46, 47, 67, 68, 72, 81, 84, 87, 110, 147, 166, 174, 204, 223, 226, 237, 245

earth's magnetic field, 160
eating, 20, 21, 24, 87, 88, 136, 138, 153, 163, 174, 193, 198, 217
eating lightly, 153
economic systems, 30
eczema, 117
Edison, Thomas, 75
eggs, 121, 164
Egypt, 45, 218
Egyptian tombs, 110
Egyptians, ancient, 45
Eilat stone, 46
Eilat stones, 50
Eilat, Israel, 46
Einstein, Albert, 157, 246
Einstein's quantum model, 159
EKG, 194
electricity, 46, 61, 141, 142, 167
electromagnetic field, 140
electromagnetic waves, 58
electrons, 104, 158, 167
elimination, 27, 85, 101, 142, 164, 167
elimination of waste products, 142
endorphins, 104
enemas, 164, 165
energy, 17, 28, 40-43, 47, 55-58, 61, 65, 73, 81, 83-85, 88, 93, 98, 101, 103, 117, 119, 120, 124, 128, 138, 141-145, 150, 157-162, 166, 168, 176, 178, 183, 184, 188, 194, 198, 200, 201, 203, 212, 213, 225, 232, 237, 247-250, 252, 253, 255
energy fields, 159
England, 72, 123, 250
enkephalins, 104
environmental problems, 61, 147
Environmental Protection Agency, 67
enzymatic systems, 170
enzymes, 104, 127, 130, 169, 253, 277, 285
EPA, 67, 68, 78, 88, 249
Epstein-Barr, 158
Erlich, J., 91
escharotics, 111, 185
esophogeal cancer, 115
ESP, 10
essential oil application, 237
essential oils, 173-175
essential trace elements, 98
Europe, 63, 72, 85, 159, 172, 179, 189, 226, 227, 247, 249, 256
European Bank, 85
eustress, 29
EWOT, 170-172, 237
exercise, 20-25, 31, 53, 90, 91, 97, 150, 164, 165, 168-170, 172, 203, 235, 237
Exercise with Oxygen Therapy, 170, 237
exposure, 19, 20, 28, 33-35, 56, 57, 59, 60, 63, 65, 67, 71, 78, 80, 83, 84, 86, 90, 94, 95, 97, 98, 100-105, 119-121, 125, 126, 129-131, 133, 134, 136, 137, 142, 143, 152, 203, 231, 232, 247-251, 254-257, 260-263, 265-268, 270, 271, 274, 275, 278, 279, 283
eye blisters, 220
eyelids, 221
eyes, 14, 66, 106, 172, 187, 221
face mask, 144
facials, 237
fairy tales, 28-30, 247
fatalities, 148, 227
fatigue, 21, 33, 117, 167, 177, 191, 200, 202, 203
fats, 162
FDA, 80, 127, 159
feathers, 53
Federal Drug Administration, 80
fermented foods, 152, 162
Fermi Laboratory, 82
fertility problems, 117
fertility rate, 123
fever, 32, 144
fevers, 27
fiber, 162, 164
fibro-cystic masses, 187
fibromyalgia, 117, 191, 200
filberts, 164
fish, 162, 163
fish oils, 162
flaxseed, 165
flaxseed cereal, 165
flaxseed tea enemas, 165

Flinders University, 131
floatation, 237
flu, 128, 158, 211
fluid, 155, 169, 205, 259, 260
fluoroscopes, 75
fluoroscopy, 75
food chain, 152
Food Irradiation, 127
food supplements, 175
foot baths, 212, 237
foot detoxification, 237
formaldehyde, 128
Foundation for Advancement of Cancer Therapies, 26
Free Enterprise Radon Health Mine, 76
free radical scavenger, 163
free radicals, 97, 104, 128
Freiburg, Germany, 115, 248
French Academy of Medicine, 107
frequencies, 2, 15, 157, 158, 174
Freud, Sigmund, 99
fructose, 152, 162
fruit, 88, 162
Fukushima, Japan, 35
full-body scan, 56, 59
fumonisin, 152
fungal growth, 162
fungal infestation, 152
fungal infestations, 113
fungal overgrowth, 53, 117
fungal spores, 117
fungi, 91, 110, 112-115, 152, 153, 162, 164, 254
fungi growth, 91
fungi-mycotoxins, 115
fungus, 101, 108, 110-114, 116-118, 150, 152, 162, 163, 185, 186, 210, 220, 254
fungus colonies, 114
fungus infection, 114
Furstenzeche Bergwerk, 233
G-force, 169
galaxy, 67
gallbladder cancer, 115
gallbladder diseases, 155
gamma rays, 47, 58, 121, 138
gangrene, 74, 251
garlic, 162, 163
Gasteiner Heilstollen, 233
gastric dyspepsia, 72
Gatorade, 137
Geiger counter, 47, 51, 140, 230
gel electrophoresis, 101, 284
Genentechs, 205
genes, 22, 119, 257, 259, 265, 273, 274, 276-278, 282
genetic aberrations, 130
Geritol, 148
Germany, 83, 115, 123, 233, 234, 248
Gerson, Max, 112
glands, 156, 175, 210
glandular system, 156
goat yogurt, 165
God, 17, 93, 195-197, 207, 208, 210, 212, 213, 215, 221
gold, 2-5, 9, 12, 13, 16, 17, 35, 42, 75, 92, 173, 235, 237, 238, 245, 251
Goldberg, Jane G., 3, 9-11, 13, 16, 35, 42, 237, 245
Goldman, Marvin, 151
golf elbow, 210
gout, 72, 114, 117
grain-fed animal products, 162
grains, 162, 164
Gramercy Park, 11, 12
Grand Central Station, 87
Grand Central Station, NYC, 136
grand mal seizure, 108, 192
granite, 66, 86, 136
grape seed extract, 163
graphite, 82
gravitational pressure, 170, 176
gravity, 22, 168, 169, 176-178
gray stone, 141, 145
gray stones, 139
gray water stones, 140
grays, 135, 266
green eliat stone, 202
Green Peace, 82
green stone, 45, 48, 50, 140-143, 146, 161, 187, 201, 202, 209, 210, 218, 219, 239
Green Stone treatments, 201
green stones, 140, 141, 221
green tea, 190
green-blue stones, 43
Guarapari, Brazil, 234

guilt, 28, 153
guinea pigs, 74, 120, 248
Gutierrez, Jay, 3, 10, 12-16, 21, 31, 35, 39, 42, 43, 45, 46, 48-51, 53, 71, 105-108, 110, 111, 115-117, 129, 131, 133-135, 137, 139-141, 143-145, 150, 190, 195, 200, 204, 207, 215, 219, 221, 239, 244, 245
gynecologist, 214
hair loss, 117
Halpern, David, 30
hamsters, 120
headache, 116
headaches, 144, 191, 192, 211
healers, 46, 115, 116, 157, 158, 237, 239
healing, 2-4, 10, 13-16, 22, 23, 31, 33, 37, 41, 43, 45, 46, 49, 56, 71, 72, 80, 96, 116, 128, 132, 139, 142, 144, 154, 156, 157, 159, 161, 173, 175, 177, 183, 185-190, 198, 205, 211, 212, 217, 219, 237, 239, 241
healing crisis, 116, 139
healing powers, 10, 45, 188
healing properties, 46, 71, 173
healing stones, 56, 183, 217
health, 8-10, 12, 13, 19, 20, 22-25, 30, 31, 39-43, 49, 58-62, 64, 69, 72-76, 78-85, 91, 93, 95, 98, 99, 101, 102, 104, 105, 113, 114, 117, 118, 121, 124, 126, 127, 134, 137, 147-157, 159, 160, 163, 167, 176, 178, 188, 191, 192, 197, 200, 214, 216, 218, 221, 226, 232, 235, 239, 241, 247-255, 266, 271, 305
health benefits, from low-level radiation, 93
health care, 9, 40, 76, 147-149, 159
health crisis, 41, 149, 191
Health Effects of Low-Level Radiation (Kondo), 121
Health Physics Society, 43
health professionals, 134
health revolution, 40-42
health springs, 72
heart, 10, 12, 23, 31, 32, 34, 95, 100, 117, 155, 156, 168, 169, 172, 177, 189, 194, 200, 206, 207, 217, 221, 241
heart disease, 31, 34, 95, 117, 168
heart fibers, 169
heart muscle, 32
heart rate, 156, 169, 194
heat, 57, 73, 153, 161, 162, 249
heavy metals, 97, 125
Henry, Hugh, F., 133
hepatic metastases, 199
herbs, 96, 162, 166, 174, 175, 220
Herxheimer, Carl, 115
Hevesy, Georg de, 74
hiatal hernia, 155
high blood pressure, 200
high fiber foods, 162
high intensity exercise, 23
high-background radiation areas, 119
high-dosage radiation, 61
high-dose radiation, 59, 63, 74, 80, 259, 266
high-level radiation, 59, 71, 79, 80, 93, 96, 100, 125, 126, 128, 129, 131
Hiroshima, Japan, 57-61, 63, 79, 82, 121, 230
Hiserodt, Ed, 119
Hispanics, 152
holistic centers, 155
holistic health, 12, 20, 41, 151, 200, 235
holistic health movement, 151
holistic practitioners, 116, 151
homeopathic treatment, 91
homeopaths, 79
homeopathy, 20, 79, 92, 159
homeostasis, 26, 27, 29, 142
honey, 41, 164, 165
hope, 12, 114, 195-197, 204, 207, 210, 248
hormesis, 1-5, 7, 12-16, 19-21, 23-26, 29-31, 33-35, 37, 41, 48, 52, 62, 79, 80, 90-92, 94-98, 100, 101, 103, 105, 107-112, 116, 118-120, 125, 129, 132, 134, 139, 159, 173, 180,

183, 187, 196, 197, 203, 206, 207, 217, 219, 221, 232, 237, 239, 241, 245, 247-254, 259, 260, 266, 270, 285, 305
hormesis effect, 1, 2, 4, 7, 12-14, 16, 20, 21, 23, 29, 33, 37, 79, 90-92, 97, 125, 241, 305
hormesis stones, 109, 118, 129, 241, 245
hormesis water, 41, 52, 96, 139, 219
hormetic effect, 25, 27, 29, 34, 79, 92, 101, 260
hormetic model, 94
hormetic principle, 94
hormetic principle, defined, 94
hormology, 94
hormone problems, 117
hormones, 27, 28, 104, 169, 173
hospice care, 199
hospitals, 42, 83
hot springs, 35, 72, 83, 155
Hot Springs, Arkansas, 72
hot stones, 52
hot water, 72, 141, 156, 165, 201
human body frequency, 158
hydrogen bomb test, 122
hydrotherapy, 156
hyperactivity, 117
hyperaldosteronism, 117
hyperlipidemia, 114, 117
hypertension, 104, 113, 117, 162, 199
hyperthyroidism, 95
hyponatremia, 199
Illinois, 50
illness, 35, 40, 98, 117, 159, 160, 225
immortal apple, 51, 53
immune deficiency, 191
immune stimulation, 120
immune system, 27, 49, 97, 98, 103, 104, 108, 113, 114, 116, 118, 132, 150, 170, 203, 214, 218, 251, 259, 265, 266, 273, 276, 279, 281
immune systems, 69
immunizations, 20, 32
immunology, 91, 262, 276
IMS Health, 148
India, 87, 122, 123, 245, 252, 253
indigenous peoples, 154
indigestion, 194
industrial chemicals, 151
industrial radiography, 86
infant health, 64
infant mortality, 149
infants, 102, 168
infections, 74, 95, 110, 113, 173
inflammation, 15, 31, 32, 110, 113, 142, 165, 211, 249
inflammatory bowel disease, 117
inflammatory disease, 113
inflammatory diseases, 74
inflammatory process, 32
injured tissue, 32
inorganic toxins, 92
insects, 89
insulin, 104, 193, 200
insulin potentiated therapy, 193
integrative family medicine, 15
integrative/holistic medicine, 244
intensive colonic, 237
interferon, 202, 273, 276, 281-283
interferon treatment, 202
intermittent fasting, 24
internal bleeding, 189
internal organs, 55, 153, 178
intestinal bacteria, 164
intestinal cancer, 115
intestinal disorders, 117
intestinal stream, 153
invertebrates, 89
Inyushin, Victor, 129
iodine, 64, 66, 92, 95
ion exchange, 142
ion foot baths, 237
ionizing radiation, 47, 66, 76, 80, 85, 89, 93, 95, 98, 101, 103, 134, 203, 247-262, 264, 266-275, 277-280, 282-284
Iran, 87, 123
Irons, V. E., 165
irradiated cells, 103
irradiated food, 127, 128, 227
irradiating food, 126
irradiation, 89, 90, 94, 95, 98, 103, 120, 127, 128, 131, 134, 249, 250, 253-285
irradiation supplementation, 98

Ishnaan, 155
isolation, 31, 32
isotopes, 47, 82, 87
Israel, 46
Israelites, 46
Jachymov, Czech Republic, 161
JAMA, 133, 249, 252
Japan, 35, 58, 61, 62, 72, 83, 88, 122, 160, 167, 229, 249, 251, 252, 255
Japanese, 57, 59, 61, 62, 64, 122, 183, 229, 251, 252
Japanese fishermen, 122, 251
jaundice, 199
Jaworowski, Zbigniew, 64
Jensen, Bernard, 115, 116, 150, 176, 178, 179
Jesus, 254, 305
jewelry, 10, 44, 45, 48, 66, 172, 239
jewelry making, 48
Jewish tradition, 153
Jews, 153
Joachimstal, Czech Republic, 72
Johnson and Johnson, 148
Joint Committee on Atomic Energy, 85
joint pain, 117, 201
Journal of Nutrition, 127
jumping, 168
junk food, 158
Kazakhstan University, 129
Kellogg, John Harvey, 154
Kerala, India, 123, 252
kidnapping, 28, 30
kidney cancer, 115
kidney stones, 117
kidneys, 172
Kiev, Ukraine, 85
King Solomon, 46
King Solomon Stone, 46
King Solomon's mines, 48
Klein, Dale, 88
Kondo, Sohei, 60, 100, 121
kriyas, 153
Kurbad Schlema, 234
Kurmittelhaus Sibyllenbad, 234
La Casa Day Spa, 5, 10, 21, 39, 42, 83, 84, 155, 156, 161, 166, 233, 235-238, 245
lactic acid, 164
lactobacillus acidophilus, 163
Lalley, Greg, 10
Lalley, Gregg, 238
lambs, 73
Lamisil, 163
Lane, Arbuthnut, 154
larger organs, 169
laryngeal cancer, 115
Law of Mass Action, 171
laxatives, 165, 166
lead, 14, 21, 42, 74, 75, 110, 137, 153, 224, 263
lead mine, 75
legumes, 164
lemon, 31, 165, 175
Lent, 27, 153, 168, 223, 232
lesions, 73, 141
leukemia, 55, 60, 64, 95, 115, 123, 252
Levine, Stephen, 167
Lewis, Wade V., 75
life, 2, 5, 13, 17, 19-21, 23, 27-31, 33, 34, 40-43, 45, 46, 49, 62, 66, 69, 73, 76, 80, 88-90, 92, 95, 96, 98, 99, 105, 110, 117, 121, 127, 128, 131, 134, 138, 140, 145, 149-151, 156, 157, 166, 167, 170-173, 175, 183, 184, 189, 191, 193-198, 206, 207, 209, 215, 218, 219, 221, 223, 225, 231, 237, 239, 246, 252
life expectancy, 149
Life magazine, 76
life-threatening disease, 167
Lilly, 35, 40-42, 238
Limu, 200
linear no-threshold assumption, 107
Lipetz, Philip, 102
lipid peroxide, 104, 256
lipid peroxides, 128
lipids, 104, 114, 174
Lipitor, 149
liquefied petroleum, 137
liquid sunshine, 75
liver, 21, 57, 111, 115, 165, 203, 204, 274
liver cancer, 115
Llope, W. J., 67
longevity, 21, 97, 120, 133, 248

Los Alamos National Laboratory, 121, 124, 125
loss of memory, 168
loss of proprioception, 202
Lovelock, James, 43
low blood pressure, 113
low carbohydrate dietary program, 162
low energy, 168, 198
low stamina, 202
low thyroid, 200
low-dose radium-infused products, 75
low-dose x-rays, 73, 259
low-level nuclear power, 62
low-level radiation products, 89, 137
low-level radioactivity, 62
lower frequencies, 158
low-dose irradiation, 90, 94, 95, 134
low-dose radiation, 61, 74, 97, 98, 119, 132, 186, 250, 252, 253
low-level radiation, 34, 247, 250-252, 254, 255
Luan, Y. C., 124
Luckey, T. D., 79, 89, 94, 103, 124, 232
lump, 186-188, 193, 214, 216
lung cancer, 68, 69, 81, 82, 95, 115, 122, 123, 145, 162, 207, 212, 247, 250, 277, 278
lung cancers, 68, 122
lungs, 57, 68, 110, 111, 162, 168, 195, 207, 209
Lyme's disease, 200
lymph fluid, 169
lymph nodes, 118, 169, 187, 188, 193, 214
lymph system, 169
lymphocytes, 103, 170, 254, 256, 259, 260, 262, 266, 268, 271, 273, 275, 276, 283
lymphocytic lymphoma, 123
lymphoma, 115, 123, 247, 256, 266, 268, 278, 280, 283
m-enkephalins, 104
magic, 46, 48, 156
magical stone, 48
magnesium, 132
magnetic fields, 157, 160
magnetic massage magnetic pulse therapy, 237
Magnetic Pulse Therapy, 159, 237
magnetics, 158
malachite, 45, 46, 140
malic acid, 163
mammary cancer, 120
man-made radiation, 93
Manhattan Project, 60, 121, 255
Manhattan, NY, 11
mass retention, 20
massage, 173, 183, 193, 194, 218, 237
massage therapist, 193, 194
Mattson, Mark, 25
Mayo Clinic, 55, 74
McKinley, Wes, 138
McMurdo Sound, Antarctica, 84
measles, 27
meat, 73, 152, 162
meats, 162, 163
medical error rates, 149
medical X rays, 138
medication, 28, 114, 201
medicine, 15, 19, 20, 32, 33, 52, 53, 55, 56, 59, 65, 69, 71, 74, 78, 79, 82, 86, 91, 107, 113-115, 119, 134, 136, 149, 157, 159, 195, 202, 232, 244, 245, 247-249, 251, 252, 255, 256, 273, 277, 279, 281, 285
Medicine Men, 53
meditation, 179, 180
melanoma, 21, 261, 268, 272, 273, 276, 278, 281-283
membrane permeability, 104
memory loss, 117, 191, 201
men, 44, 53, 80, 99, 150, 156, 208, 229, 249
menstrual cramps, 198
mental dysfunction, 117
mental problems, 168
Merck, 148
Mercola, Joseph, 149
mercury, 92, 152, 224
Merkel Cell, 184
metabolic acid wastes, 179
metabolic function, 167
metabolic waste products, 157
metallic poisoning, 72
metastasis, 131, 266, 281

metastatic presacral lymph node, 215
mice, 103, 119, 120, 130, 131, 134, 247-249, 251, 252, 256-265, 267-279, 281-284
microbes, 128, 175
microorganisms, 115, 126, 127, 175
mid-brain, 175
milk, 63-66, 84, 151, 152, 162
Mineral Palace, 7, 39, 51, 83, 138, 155, 161, 221, 242, 245
minerals, 5, 7, 14, 21, 24, 41, 96, 132, 173, 215, 221, 239-241, 244
miners, 80, 226
mines, 13, 46, 48, 76, 80, 81, 83, 104, 106, 134, 137, 140, 252
mini-trampoline, 168
Misasa Radon Springs, Japan, 122
Misasa, Japan, 72
modern diseases, 154
modern medicine, 32, 33, 78
modern radiation therapy techniques, 102
modern technology, 159
mold, 53, 110, 162, 174, 175
mold spores, 110
molding, 175
molds, 78, 110, 113
molecules, 102, 150, 158, 174, 251, 257-260, 263, 264, 266, 276
Mollaret's Meningitis, 117
monazite, 234
Montana, 75, 76, 83, 104, 137, 252
morphine, 108, 191
Mother Nature, 138
Mound Laboratory, 121
mouth, 100, 164
MPT, 159, 160
MS symptoms, 202
mud mask, 144
mud pack, 48, 143, 173, 184, 187, 188, 200-202, 211, 219, 221
mud packs, 139, 140, 142, 143, 184, 212
Muller, Herman J., 93
multiple sclerosis, 117, 202, 203
mumps, 27
muscle layers, 169
muscle stiffness, 118
muscles, 23, 24, 90, 157, 165, 169, 172, 202, 203, 213, 214
muscular dystrophy, 117
muscular pain, 202
mutagens, 127
mutant cells, 197
mutations, 93, 105, 130
mycotoxicoses, 152
mycotoxin, 114, 153
mycotoxin cyclosporine, 114
mycotoxin medications, 114
mycotoxins, 113-116, 152, 153, 163
myelin, 128
myth, 28, 223, 224
NAFERA, 53
Nagasaki, Japan, 57-60, 63, 79, 82, 121, 230
nail fungus, 118
Nakagawa, Kyochi, 160
NASA, 115, 170, 232
nasal cancer, 115
nasal canula, 170
National Academy of Sciences, 128, 161
National Academy of Sciences Center for Theoretical Physics, 161
National Cancer Research Institute, 88
National Council on Radiation Protection, 119, 125, 232
National Institute of Radiological Science, 88
Native American Free Exercise of Religion Act, 53
Native Americans, 153
natural antibiotic, 46
natural foods, 113
natural gas, 136
natural radiation, 69, 86, 106, 239, 249
natural remedies, 163
naturally occurring radiation, beneficial, 93
nausea, 116, 144, 198, 201, 211
NCRP, 119, 232
necklace, 74, 134, 145, 173, 187, 198, 209, 212
necklace stone, 187, 198, 209
necklaces, 212
negative thinking, 153
nematodes, 110
Nemenhah Band and Native American Traditional Organization, 53,

245
nerve cancer, 115
nerve cells, 32
nerves, 157
nervous system, 33, 151, 167
neuralgia, 72, 122
neurotrophic factors, 25
neutrons, 47, 58
New Jersey, 67, 76
New Mexico, 84, 120
New Orleans, LA, 11
New Realities, 10, 237
New York City, NY, 64, 136
Newtonian-Cartesian worldview, 157
nicotine, 92, 93
Night Hawk Minerals, 5, 7, 14, 21, 132, 215, 221, 239-241, 244
Nizoral, 163
norepinephrine, 27
Nrf2, 21
nuclear bombs, 56-58, 138
nuclear energy, 17, 42, 43, 55, 65, 225, 248
nuclear energy plants, 65
nuclear fission, 58
nuclear medicine, 56, 65, 74, 82, 86, 136, 248, 256
nuclear power, 5, 34, 56, 61-65, 67, 81, 82, 86, 87, 90, 119, 124, 137, 161, 223, 224, 226, 249, 255
nuclear power plant workers, 67, 124
nuclear power plants, 34, 56, 65, 81, 90, 119, 124, 137, 161, 226
nuclear radiation, 56
nuclear reactors, 56, 82
Nuclear Regulatory Commission, 88, 125, 248, 251, 253, 255
Nuclear Shipyard Workers Study, 124
nuclear transformation, 56
nuclear weapons, 81, 250
nutrients, 95, 100, 101, 127, 142, 154, 160, 169, 173-175
nuts, 136, 152, 162, 164
Nystatin, 163
oak bark, 91
obese, 57, 189
obesity, 118
ochratoxin, 152
oils, 102, 117, 162, 164, 172-175
olfactory bulb, 175
olive leaf extract, 163
oncology, 26
onion, 162
oral cancer, 115
oregano oil, 163
Oregon Institute of Science and Medicine, 69
organ transplantation, 114
Organic Consumers Association, 127
organic corn, 152
organs, 21, 31, 33, 55, 58, 101, 153, 154, 156, 158, 169, 178, 256, 257, 259, 282
osteoarthritis, 113
osteogenic cancer, 115
outer space, 56
ovarian cancer, 115, 120, 204
oxidation, 167
oxidative damage, 163
oxidative stress, 23, 97, 283
oxygen, 97, 108, 117, 142, 157, 160, 166-174, 178, 192, 237, 283, 284
oxygen booths, 167
oxygen concentrator, 170
oxygen deprivation, 170
oxygen ions, 97
oxygen-rich air, 168
oxygen-rich environment, 167
oxygenation, 142, 172
ozone detoxification baths, 237
p53 protein, 103, 258, 261, 262, 268, 269, 275, 283, 284
pain, 13, 32, 45, 104, 108, 109, 111, 117, 118, 132, 141, 142, 157, 176, 183, 186, 188-192, 194, 195, 198-203, 205, 208-210, 217-219, 241, 249
paint, 77
pain-reliever, 141
Panchakarma cleansing, 153
pancreas, 115, 190, 200, 203, 204
pancreas cancer, 115
pancreatic cancer, 199, 203
pancreatic mass, 199
pap smear, 214
Paracelsus, 91

parasite testing, 16
parasites, 118, 127, 158
parasitic diseases, 15
parasitic infection, 15
parathyroid cancer, 115
ParaWellness Research Program, 16, 244
pascalite/bentonite clay, 208
pathogenic cells, 33, 140, 150
pathogenic microorganisms, 126
pathogens, 27, 31, 33, 98, 100, 101, 112, 116, 118, 126, 164, 227
pau d'arco, 163
peanuts, 152
pecans, 164
pendant, 48, 74, 145, 146, 173
pendants, 140
penicillin, 79, 92
Pennsylvania, 67, 111, 185
peristaltic cramping, 166
peristaltic movement, 176
peroxides, 97, 128
perspiration, 157
PetScan, 214, 215
Pfizer, 149
pharmaceutical industry, 80, 148
pharmaceuticals, 32
pharmacological literature, 92
pharmacological substances, 159
pharmacology, 20, 114, 202
pharmacology industry, 114
Philadelphia, PA, 64
phosphate fertilizer, 136
photons, 57
photosynthesis, 73
photovoltaic solar plant, 65
physical activity, 193
physicists, 5, 159, 231
physics, 43, 157, 159, 161, 231, 247-252, 255
physiologic biliary drainage, 199
physiology, 159
picoCurie, 135
piezoelectric, 141
pigs, 74, 79, 120, 248
pilots, 86, 95
pineal glands, 175
Pittsburgh University, 68
pituitary cancer, 115
pituitary gland, 127
plants, 24, 34, 39, 53, 56, 65, 73, 77, 81, 90, 110, 119, 124, 137, 161, 173, 175, 180, 223-227, 230, 250
plasma, 171, 282
platinum, 75
pleasure, 35, 154, 190
plutonium, 121, 122, 124, 125, 232, 255
poison, 61, 67, 91, 164
poisons, as cures and stimulants, 92
Poland, 83
politicians, 85, 134
pollution, 166, 226
Pollycove, Myron, 58, 125
pornography, 30
Port Hueneme, California, 84
post-bomb radiation, 121
post-traumatic growth syndrome, 29, 31
postpartum depression, 118
potassium, 47, 87, 88, 136
potatoes, 164
prayer, 84, 180, 193, 213
predators, 24
pregnant females, 134
pregnant women, 64, 67
premature aging, 170
premature deaths, 95, 148
prescription drug business, 148
prescriptions, 148, 149
primordial soup, 156
Princess Diana, 192
Pritchett, Colorado, 7, 17, 21, 39, 72, 83, 136, 243
pro-oxidants, 97
prolapsed bowel, 178
prolapsus of the internal organs, 178
prostate, 14, 115, 178, 189, 190, 204
prostate cancer, 14, 115
prostate cancers, 204
protein, 21, 101, 103, 142, 203, 257-265, 267-269, 271, 272, 274, 275, 277-280, 282-284
protein synthesis, 101, 142, 259, 268, 274
protoplasm, 101
protozoa, 31, 110
prunes, 164, 165

PSA, 14, 190, 210
PSA blood test, 14
PSA score, 190
PSA test, 14, 190
psoriasis, 118
psychoanalysis, 179, 180, 237
public health officials, 134
pulsed magnetic energy, 40, 160
pulsed magnetic therapy, 40
putrefied material, 165
Pycnogenol, 163
pyramids, 218
pyroelectric, 141
quack cures, 76
quantum physics, 157
quarries, 66
quartz, 142, 218
quartz crystals, 218
Qvick, Lars I., 115
Radiant Float, 237
radiation, 5, 12-15, 20, 21, 34, 35, 41-43, 46-50, 55-67, 69, 71-74, 76, 78-90, 93-112, 116, 117, 119-141, 143-145, 147, 150, 155, 159, 160, 162, 173, 180, 183, 185-188, 193, 195-197, 200, 203, 206-208, 214-217, 219, 221, 223, 225, 227, 231, 232, 237, 239, 241, 245, 247-264, 266-285
radiation deficiency, 95
radiation emission, 86, 134, 139
radiation hormesis, 5, 12, 13, 15, 48, 62, 95, 98, 100, 101, 103, 105, 107-112, 116, 119, 120, 129, 132, 134, 159, 173, 180, 183, 187, 196, 197, 203, 206, 207, 217, 219, 221, 232, 237, 239, 241, 248, 249, 252, 260, 266, 285
Radiation Hormesis (Luckey), 95
radiation leakage, 34, 65
radiation protection standards, 88
radiation sickness, 126
radiation therapy, 71, 80, 83, 98, 102, 137, 273, 276, 283
radioactive air, 76
radioactive cancer treatments, 42
radioactive isotopes, 47, 82
radioactive material, 63
radioactive mines, 76
radioactive particles, 61, 63
radioactive potassium, 87, 136
radioactive products, 76
radioactive rays, 58
radioactive stones, 2-4, 13, 16, 37, 49, 139, 241
radioactive trash, 84
radioactive water, 72, 122, 144
radioactivity, 5, 19, 42, 43, 46-48, 55-57, 62, 65, 67, 72, 74-76, 88, 89, 93, 101, 105, 106, 136, 142, 223, 224, 226, 227, 229, 251, 253
radioisotopes, 87, 226, 255
radiologic burns, 58
radiologic exposure, 60
radiologic rays, 57
Radiological Society of North America, 59
radiologically-induced cancers, 59
radiologist, 200
Radiology magazine, 59
radiophobia, 80, 83
radium, 42, 47, 72, 74-78, 80, 87, 121, 136, 137, 234, 250, 252
radium 226, 87
radium dial painters, 121
radium painters, 76
Radium Palace, 234
radium poisoning, 78
radium roulette, 75
radium workers, 80
radium-induced deaths, 78
radium-laced toothpastes, 137
radon, 5, 35, 42, 47, 57, 67-69, 72, 75, 76, 80-84, 95, 104, 122, 123, 134, 135, 161, 162, 183, 226, 233, 237, 247-253
radon bath, 162, 237
radon eliminator, 35
radon exposure, 83, 247
radon gas, 57, 68, 81, 83
radon health mines, 76
radon mines, 80, 104
radon spas, 72, 83, 161, 226
radon steam baths, 83

radon-abatement industry, 68
rads, 121, 135
Raindrop Therapy, 237
rainwater, 63
Ramsar, Iran, 123
rape, 30
rapid heart beat, 200
rats, 120, 127, 131, 164, 250
raw vegetables, 164
Raynaud's Syndrome/Disease, 118
rays, 42, 47, 56-58, 73-75, 85-87, 89, 93, 98, 121, 134, 138, 150, 211, 231, 249, 250, 253-255, 257-265, 267-272, 274-285
Reading Prong, Pennsylvania, 67
rebounding, 168-171
rectal cancer, 115
rectum, 164, 214
red blood cells, 171
Red Sea, 46
refined foods, 178
reflexology, 237
regeneration, 31, 33, 154, 173
rehab, 22, 191
rejuvenation, 153
relaxation, 157
rems, 135, 139
residential radon, 67, 68
respiration, 156, 167
respiratory disease, 168
respiratory disorders, 118
rest, 14, 32, 40, 57, 62, 63, 81, 83, 102, 124, 153, 154, 165, 177, 178, 184, 189, 195, 197, 198, 209, 217
resting, 153
restorative systems, 159
resveratrol, 20
Revigator, 75
revitalized blood, 156
rheumatism, 72, 122
rheumatoid arthritis, 118
rings, 16, 86, 156, 197
road construction materials, 136
Robinson, Arthur, 69
rocket fuel, 151
rocks, 47, 49, 52, 66, 188, 212, 213
Rockwell, Ted, 60, 96, 101, 223, 225, 232
Rocky Flats, 121, 124, 125, 250
rodents, 131
Rodgers, Brenda, 130
Roentgen, Wilhelm C., 73
Romans, ancient, 72
rotator cuff, torn, 13
Royal English Archives, 172
rubidium, 47
running, 22, 31, 73, 90, 170, 191, 194, 205, 219
Russia, 22, 63-66, 83-85, 250
Russian space program, 22
Russians, 66
Sackman, Ruth, 26, 33
Sacramento, CA, 65
Sagan, Leonard, 19
salamanders, 31
salivary cancer, 115
salt sauna, 237
sarcoid arthritis, 118
sarcoidosis, 118
sarcoma; skeletal, 115
Saxon Giant, the, 178
schizophrenic paranoia, 66
Schmeidler, Gertrude, 10
Schultz, Hugo, 91
science, 10, 48, 55, 58, 63, 69, 71, 88, 90, 91, 97, 151, 156, 157, 177, 247, 250-255
Science magazine, 151
scientists, 19, 55, 56, 59, 60, 62, 64, 74, 79, 95, 103, 104, 111, 128, 150, 155, 157, 166, 239, 253
Sea Raven Press, 2-4, 7, 239, 254, 305
Seaborg, Glen, 232
Seabrook, Lochlainn, 3
sebum, 179
secretions, 22, 156
seeds, 162, 188
seizure, 108, 192
seizures, 191
selenium, 96, 224
Selye, Hans, 29, 98
senility, 168
senna, 166
sensory loss, 191
servs, 135
sexual assault, 30

sexual violence, 30
Shrader, William, 74
sick building syndrome, 118
sickness care, 148
silica, 142
silver, 45, 46, 75, 220
Simoncini, Tulio, 114
sinus trouble, 113
sinusitis, 113, 118
Sivinanda Yoga, 153
skeletal system, 157
skeleton, 22
skin, 13, 14, 21, 32, 55, 57, 58, 73, 111, 112, 115, 118, 143, 144, 165, 171, 173, 175, 178, 179, 184, 186, 190, 191, 202, 205, 212, 213, 231, 249, 283
skin brushing, 178, 179
skin cancer, 115, 184
skin cancers, 21
skin cells, 32, 283
skin disease, 118
skin disorders, 191
skin irritation, 205
slant board, 177, 178
sluggishness, 160, 168
smokers, 93, 95
smoking, 20, 113
sodium chloride, 179
soil bacteria, 78
soil, and radiation hormesis, 15
Southam, C., 91
soy powder, 216
spas, 72, 83, 106, 155, 161, 226
spermatocytes, 130, 265, 269, 270, 275, 280
spices, 162
spider bite, 207
spinal meningitis, 191
spine pain, 191
spiritual life, 193
spiritual traditions, 153
spleen, 33, 169, 257, 259, 274, 282
split peas, 164
Sporanax, 163
spores, 110, 117
Stage III Invasive Ductal Carcinoma Breast Cancer, 216
stage-4 cancers, 106
starfish, 31
Steinfeld, Alan, 10
sterility, 95
stillbirths, 123
stimulatory radiation, 104
Stockholm, Sweden, 115
stomach cancer, 115
stomach lining, 111
stones, 2-4, 10, 13-16, 35, 37, 43-53, 56, 62, 66, 71, 87, 100, 107-109, 116-118, 126, 129-134, 138-142, 145, 150, 162, 173, 183, 184, 187-190, 196, 198, 200, 207-212, 215, 217, 220, 221, 239, 241, 245
stored foods, 152
stress, 21-25, 27, 29, 35, 90, 97, 98, 116, 129, 150, 170, 176, 194, 213, 283
stress, good, 98
stressors, 21, 26, 27, 31, 97, 98
submarines, 90
sugar, 112, 117, 162, 164, 200
sun, 11, 21, 73, 86, 178, 223, 251, 258, 261, 262, 268, 273, 274, 279, 281, 283, 285
sunburn, 21
sunlight, 105
super-oxide dismutase, 103
supernova, 67
supplemental radiation, 96
supplementation, 95, 96, 98, 138, 283
supplements, 175, 186, 193, 200, 202, 214
suppositories, 75
suppurating wounds, 74
surgery, 154, 183, 185, 187, 188, 193, 204, 207, 211, 214-216
sweat lodges, 153
Swedish Radiobiology Society, 97, 147
swimming, 23
swollen lymph nodes, 118
systemic sclerosis, 118
T cells, 99, 103, 271
Taiwan, 123, 124
Taleb, Nassim Nicholas, 25, 26, 29, 32
Tamagawa, Japan, 72
Tarceva, 205

Taylor, Lauriston, 119, 232
technology, 30, 41, 59, 82, 139, 147, 159, 224, 232, 250-252
teens, 134
temperature shock, 97
temporary toxicity, 116
tenderness, 32
tendons, 157
tennis, 22, 90, 210
tennis elbow, 210
testicular cancer, 115
Texas Tech University, 130, 254
The Collected Works of Jane G. Goldberg, Ph.D. (Goldberg), 12
The Dark Side of Love (Goldberg), 12
therapeutic use of water, 155, 156
Thompson, J. J., 72
thorium, 46, 47, 87, 93, 202
thorium 232, 87
thorium stone, 202
thrombocytopenic purpura, 118
thyroid cancer, 64, 65, 95, 115, 225
thyroid problems, 145
Time magazine, 78, 120
tissues, 21, 33, 58, 99, 102, 113, 116, 140, 154, 158, 167, 169, 171, 172, 257, 259, 274
tobacco, 113
Tobias, Cornelius A., 231
Tomey, George H., 72
tomography, 136
tonsils, 169
Townsend Report, 61
toxic chemicals, 151
toxic gas, 173
toxic poisons, 116
toxic wastes, 116, 224
toxicogenic fungi, 152, 153
toxicological studies, 19
tracheal cancer, 115
traditional western diet, 178
trampoline, 168-170
trees, 39, 91
Trinity A-Bomb test, 120
Tsakona, Paula Gloria, 12, 238
tumor, 14, 26, 102, 111, 114, 115, 127, 131, 140, 145, 184, 188, 200, 214-216, 220, 250, 256, 258, 261, 266, 268-270, 272, 273, 276-284
tumors, 32, 45, 104, 107, 109, 111, 131, 141, 178, 188, 189, 204, 207, 212, 219, 220, 261, 263, 268, 271, 273, 276, 278, 281-283
turquoise, 44-46
Turski, Fukasz, 161
U.S., 4, 42, 59, 60, 65, 66, 68, 69, 72, 74, 76, 78, 81, 83-89, 93, 122, 124, 136, 137, 148, 149, 151, 159, 219, 223, 224, 229, 239, 247, 255
U.S. consumers, 148
U.S. government, 61, 89
UK, 124, 225, 266
Ukraine, 64
ultra sound, 188
umbilical-cord blood, 151
Under-Exposed (Hiserodt), 119
United States, 16, 65, 149, 176, 179, 249
United States Air Force, 16
University of California, 30
University of Missouri School of Medicine, 79
University of Oklahoma College of Medicine, 244
University of Wisconsin-Madison, 128
UNSCEAR, 59, 64, 65, 254, 255
uranium, 47, 51, 61, 67, 74, 82, 84, 86, 87, 93, 120, 123, 136, 223, 226, 247
uranium dust, 120
uranium fuel, 61
uranium mine, 51
uranium mining, 84, 86, 123
uranium ore, 51, 67
urea, 82, 179, 232, 252
uric acid, 162
urinary cancer, 115
urogenital cancer, 115
urologist, 189, 190
Utah, 49, 140
uterine cancer, 115, 120
uterine fibroid tumors, 178
uterus, 178
vaccinations, 20, 27, 33, 52

vaccines, 91, 148
vaginal cancer, 115
Valenti, Jessica, 30
varicose veins, 155
vegetable oils, 164
vegetables, 24, 73, 162, 164
vibration, 21, 22, 92, 157, 159, 237
vibrational frequency, 92
vibrational re-balancing, 237
vibrational therapies, 237
vibrational-energy medicine, 157, 159
Vietnam, 16, 244
viruses, 112, 158, 164
visual difficulties, 202
vitamin A, 96
vitamin C, 163, 205, 283
vitamin D, 21, 105
vitamin E, 98, 138, 283
vitamins, 24, 96, 127, 138, 158, 173, 283
Walinder, Gunnar, 97, 147
Walker, David, 149
walking, 23, 41, 51, 57, 84, 86, 172, 189, 191, 200, 201, 218
walnuts, 164
Warburg, Otto, 117, 167
Warren, Stafford, 229
Warsaw, Poland, 161
Washington, D.C., 4, 64, 66, 247, 249, 253, 255
waste material, 157
water, 2, 15, 35, 41, 46-49, 52, 62, 72, 75, 77, 78, 96, 106, 122, 128, 129, 136, 139-141, 144, 155, 156, 159, 161, 162, 165, 166, 175, 180, 183, 187, 200-204, 207, 211, 213, 219, 220, 223, 224, 227, 237, 245, 247, 250, 252, 256
water spas, 106
water stone, 35, 48, 144, 161, 187, 200, 201, 204, 220
water stones, 52, 140
water therapy, 156
Watson, James, 102
weight, 21, 23, 52, 114, 118, 178, 179, 197, 199, 203, 212, 281
weight gain, 52
weight loss, 21, 199
weightlessness, 169
well water, 72
Western Europe, 85
whey, 164
whiskey, 92
white blood cells, 103, 150
whole body vibration, 21
Wieland, Heinrich, 115
wildlife, 65
Windham, Christopher, 59
windmills, 65
wine, 162
Wolff's Law, 22
women, 64, 67, 76, 77, 108, 123, 151, 155
World Health Organization (WHO), 114
World War II, 76-78, 92
Wyoming, 43, 140
x-rays, 42, 57, 73, 89, 93, 98, 138, 231, 257-265, 267-272, 274-285
Yalow, Roslyn, 82, 95
yams, 164
yeast cultures, 92
yeast-related health problems, 118
yeasts, 113
yoga, 153, 177, 202, 203
Yogic science, 177
yogic tradition, 153, 155, 156
yogis, 153, 157
Yom Kippur, 153
young adults, 134
Young, Robert, 115
youthfulness, 156
Zeigfeld, Florenz, 179
zero gravity, 22
zinc chloride, 111

If you enjoyed *The Hormesis Effect* you will be interested in these spiritual, physical, and mental health related titles:

JESUS AND THE LAW OF ATTRACTION
CHRIST IS ALL AND IN ALL
THE BIBLE AND THE LAW OF ATTRACTION
JESUS AND THE GOSPEL OF Q

Available from Sea Raven Press and wherever fine books are sold.

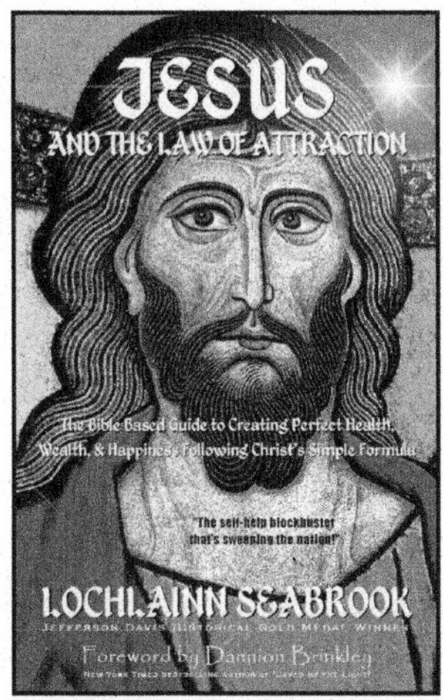

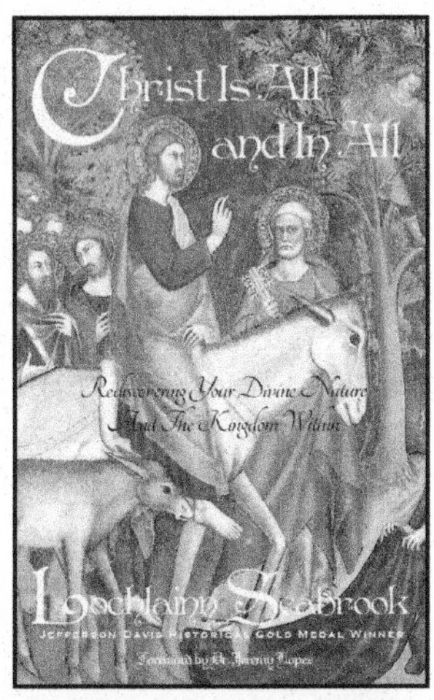

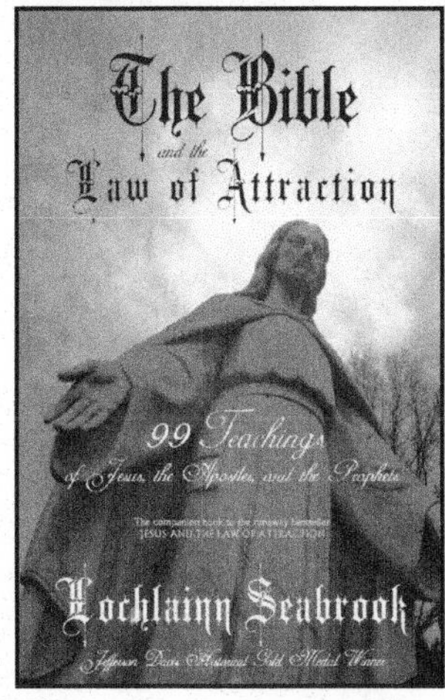

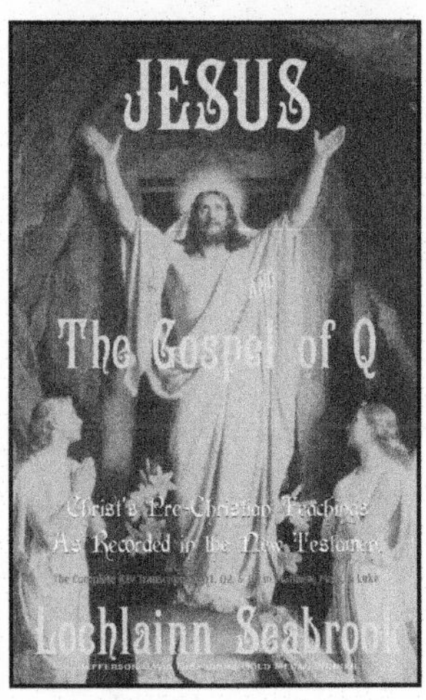

SeaRavenPress.com

CPSIA information can be obtained
at www.ICGtesting.com
Printed in the USA
FSOW03n1925070617
34815FS

9 780991 377923